TISSUE CULTURE OF THE NERVOUS SYSTEM

CURRENT TOPICS IN NEUROBIOLOGY

Series Editors:

Floyd Bloom

Chief, Laboratory of Neuropharmacology
National Institute of Mental Health
Division of Special Mental Health Research, IR
Saint Elizabeth's Hospital — WAW Building
Washington, D.C.

and

Samuel H. Barondes

Professor of Psychiatry
School of Medicine
University of California, San Diego
La Jolla, California

Volume 1 — Tissue Culture of the Nervous System • 1973
Edited by Gordon Sato

TISSUE CULTURE OF THE NERVOUS SYSTEM

Edited by
GORDON SATO
Department of Biology
University of California, San Diego
La Jolla, California

PLENUM PRESS • NEW YORK-LONDON

Library of Congress Cataloging in Publication Data

Sato, Gordon.
  Tissue culture of the nervous system.

  (Current topics in neurobiology, v. 1)
  Includes bibliographies.
  1. Nerve tissue—Cultures and culture media. 2. Cell culture. I. Title. [DNLM:
1. Nervous system—Cytology. 2. Neurochemistry. 3. Tissue culture. W1Cu82P v. 1
1973/WL101 T616 1973]
QM575.S27   591.1'88   73-79426

ISBN-13: 978-1-4684-2906-0   e-ISBN-13: 978-1-4684-2904-6
DOI: 10.1007/978-1-4684-2904-6

© 1973 Plenum Press, New York
A Division of Plenum Publishing Corporation
227 West 17th Street, New York, N.Y. 10011

Softcover reprint of the hardcover 1st edition 1973

United Kingdom edition published by Plenum Press, London
A Division of Plenum Publishing Company, Ltd.
Davis House (4th Floor), 8 Scrubs Lane, Harlesden, London, NW10 6SE, England

CONTRIBUTORS

G. Augusti-Tocco
*Laboratorio di Embriologia Molecolare, C.N.R., Arco Felice
Naples, Italy*

Gary Brooker
*Department of Pharmacology
School of Medicine, University of Virginia
Charlottesville, Virginia*

L. Casola
*Istituto Internazionale di Genetica e Biofisica, C.N.R.
Naples, Italy*

Glyn Dawson
*Departments of Pediatrics and Biochemistry
LaRabida–University of Chicago Institute
and Joseph P. Kennedy, Jr. Mental Retardation Research Center
Pritzker School of Medicine, University of Chicago
Chicago, Illinois*

Jean de Vellis
*Laboratory of Nuclear Medicine and Radiation Biology
and Department of Anatomy, University of California
Los Angeles, California*

Albert Dorfman
*Departments of Pediatrics and Biochemistry
LaRabida–University of Chicago Institute
and Joseph P. Kennedy, Jr. Mental Retardation Research Center
Pritzker School of Medicine, University of Chicago
Chicago, Illinois*

Barbara P. Grauling
*The Departments of Biological Chemistry and Neurosciences
and Laboratory of Nuclear Medicine and Radiation Biology
    School of Medicine, University of California
Los Angeles, California*

A. John Harris
The Salk Institute, San Diego, California

Stephen Heinemann
The Salk Institute, San Diego, California

Harvey R. Herschman
*The Departments of Biological Chemistry and Neurosciences
and Laboratory of Nuclear Medicine and Radiation Biology
    School of Medicine, University of California
Los Angeles, California*

Y. Kidokoro
The Salk Institute, San Diego, California

Michael P. Lerner
*The Departments of Biological Chemistry and Neurosciences
and Laboratory of Nuclear Medicine and Radiation Biology
    School of Medicine, University of California
Los Angeles, California*

R. Levi-Montalcini
*Laboratorio di Biologia Cellulare, C.N.R.
Rome, Italy*

John D. Minna
Laboratory of Biochemical Genetics
National Heart and Lung Institute
National Institutes of Health
Bethesda, Maryland

P. G. Nelson
Behavioral Biology Branch,
National Institute of Child Health and Human Development
National Institutes of Health
Bethesda, Maryland

E. Parisi
Laboratorio di Embriologia Molecolare, C.N.R., Arco Felice
Naples, Italy

James Patrick
The Salk Institute, San Diego, California

S. E. Pfeiffer
Department of Microbiology
University of Connecticut Health Center
Farmington, Connecticut

M. Romano
Istituto Internazionale di Genetica e Biofisica, C.N.R.
Naples, Italy

Roger N. Rosenberg
Department of Neurosciences and Pediatrics
and University Hospital, University of California at San Diego
*   School of Medicine*
La Jolla, California

David Schubert
The Salk Institute, San Diego, California

Nicholas W. Seeds
Department of Biophysics and Genetics
and Department of Psychiatry
University of Colorado Medical Center
Denver, Colorado

K. R. Seshan
Department of Biology, Washington University
St. Louis, Missouri

Joseph Henry Steinbach
The Salk Institute, San Diego, California

Allen C. Stoolmiller
Departments of Pediatrics and Biochemistry
LaRabida–University of Chicago Institute
and Joseph P. Kennedy, Jr. Mental Retardation Research Center
Pritzker School of Medicine, University of Chicago
Chicago, Illinois

F. Zucco
Laboratorio di Embriologia Molecolare, C.N.R., Arco Felice
Naples, Italy

Preface

The impetus for compiling this book was the recent development of culture strains of neuroblastoma and glial cells and the immediate and enthusiastic way they have been taken up as model systems. After the first sudden rush of activity, it seems appropriate to pause, to assess progress, and to contemplate the future contributions that may be possible using these culture techniques.

Long before the advent of established strains, cultures of nervous tissue had already contributed to neurobiology. Ross Harrison, in 1906, in a single experimental series, established tissue culture as a promising new technique in cell biology and settled the Golgi–Cajal controversy as to whether axonic processes originated as outgrowths from the cell body or were formed first in the intercellular spaces and were later connected to the cell body. Harrison observed process growth from nerve cells in cultures, thus settling the matter in favor of Cajal. Of great importance to neurobiology is the discovery by Rita Levi-Montalcini of nerve growth factor. Cultures of spinal ganglia played a major role in the discovery, isolation, and characterization of the factor (Levi-Montalcini *et al.*, 1954). In my opinion, this discovery, although very well known, has not yet been adequately recognized for its germinal influence on neurobiology and embryology.

Progress since the advent of clonal cultures has been more modest. I would like to cite two pieces of work which emphasize the technical advantages of these cultures. The culture techniques have separated the neural and glial elements of nervous tissue, have freed the cells from restrictions found *in vivo*, and have enormously increased the ease with which these cells can be manipulated. To illustrate the first point, Jean de Vellis and coworkers demonstrated the stimulation of glycerol phosphate dehydrogenase in rat brain by adrenocortical steroids. It was not known whether this reaction was taking place in neurons or glia or both. Culture experiments have shown that glia respond and neurons or neuroblastoma cells do not (de Vellis and Inglish, 1969). The second point is illustrated with work on vitamin B_{12}

deficiency. Nervous tissue along with hemopoetic tissue is adversely affected by vitamin B_{12} deficiency, and the biochemical nature of the lesion has escaped elucidation. If neuroblastoma or glioma cultures are made vitamin B_{12} deficient, they can accumulate large quantities of odd chain fatty acids in their plasma membranes. Cultures of nervous tissue origin are more prone to accumulate odd chain fatty acids than cultures from other tissues. This phenomenon was more readily discovered in culture than in the whole animal because the whole animal probably cannot tolerate this substitution to any great extent and would be dead before levels of odd chain fatty acids became easily detectable. Cells in culture, freed from the responsibility of performing sensitive functions vital to life, can tolerate substitution to a much greater extent (Barley *et al.*, 1972). This example illustrates to an extreme degree the ease of manipulation in culture. Here membrane constituents can be varied at will and correlated with physiological function.

Given the technical advantages of these cultures, what can we expect in the future? Are problems such as the regulation of synapse formation, the mechanism of neurotransmitter substances, the biochemistry of action-potential generation, and the function of glia amenable to culture experimentation? What about higher cognitive processes? Are these even in the realm of biochemistry and cell biology? These questions are the ultimate concern of our contributors. Although all share in common the *in vitro* culture methods, their individual approaches and concerns are, appropriately for this stage, diverse.

GORDON SATO, Professor
Department of Biology
University of California/San Diego
La Jolla, California

REFERENCES

Harrison, R. G. 1906. Observations on the living developing nerve fiber. *Anat. Rec.* **1**: 116–124.

Levi-Montalcini, R., Meyer, H., and Hamberger, V. 1954. *In vitro* experiments on the effects of mouse sarcoma 180 and 37 on the spinal and sympathetic ganglia of the chick embryo. *Cancer Res.* **14**:49–57.

de Vellis, J., and Inglish, D. 1969. Glycerolphosphate dehydrogenase induction in a cloned glial cell culture by glucocorticoids, pp. 151–152. Second Intern at. Meet. Soc. Neurochem., Milan, Italy.

Barley, F. W., Sato, G., and Abeles, R. H. 1972. Effect of vitamin B_{12} deficiency in tissue culture. *J. Biol. Chem.* **247**:4270.

Contents

Chapter 3

Differentiation and Interaction of Clonal Cell Lines of Nerve and Muscle

David Schubert, A. John Harris, Stephen Heinemann, Y. Kidokoro,
James Patrick, and Joseph Henry Steinbach

Chapter 4

Biochemical Characterization of a Clonal Line of Neuroblastoma

G. Augusti-Tocco, E. Parisi, F. Zucco, L. Casola, and M. Romano

Chapter 5

Regulation of Neuronal Enzymes in Cell Culture

Roger N. Rosenberg

Chapter 6

Electrophysiological Studies of Normal and Neoplastic Cells in Tissue Culture

P. G. Nelson

Chapter 7

Genetic Analysis of the Mammalian Nervous System Using Somatic Cell Culture Techniques

John D. Minna

Chapter 8

Nervous System–Specific Proteins in Cultured Neural Cells

Harvey R. Herschman, Barbara P. Grauling, and Michael P. Lerner

Chapter 9

Clonal Lines of Glial Cells

S. E. Pfeiffer

Chapter 1

Long-Term Cultures of Embryonic and Mature Insect Nervous and Neuroendocrine Systems

R. Levi-Montalcini
Laboratorio di Biologia Cellulare
C.N.R. Rome, Italy

and

K. R. Seshan
Department of Biology, Washington University
St. Louis, Missouri, U. S. A.

I. INTRODUCTION

More than a half century of extensive work on the vertebrate nervous system cultured *in vitro* under different experimental conditions has brought to light the merits and the limitations of these techniques. While a considerable amount of information has been gathered on growth and differentiation of nerve cells, on axonal growth, on the relationship between glial and nerve cells, and, recently, also on bioelectrical properties of neuronal circuits *in vitro* (Crain and Peterson, 1964, 1967; Crain *et al.*, 1970), little has been learned concerning the organization of nerve cells at the supracellular level and no attempts have been made to explore, with the aid of these techniques, the problem of neuronal specificity and the building of wiring circuits between nerve cell populations and between nerve cells and their end organs. The reasons which suggested restriction of the study to only a few neurobiological

This work was supported in part by grants from the National Institutes of Health (NS-03777) and the National Science Foundation (GB-16330X).

problems are numerous. To mention only some of the limiting factors, we remind the reader that this system in vertebrates is from its very inception a highly organized system and cannot operate when submitted to dissociation into small fragments, with each one cultured alone or in proximity to other parts of the same system or of nonnervous structures. Disruption of the continuity of the neuraxis and destruction of the blood capillary network, which permeates the entire system and provides the nutrition and blood supply of individual nerve units, are most damaging factors which cannot possibly be mitigated by any technical skill or ingenious device. In order to permit survival if not proper function of the nerve cell populations, which must rely on diffusion rather than on blood vascular channels, the explants must be reduced to what has been defined as "the critical cubic millimeter" (Lumsden, 1968). The fragments of the nervous system undergo, as a rule, flattening and thinning in long-term cultures. This condition favors exchanges with the medium, and nerve cells located at the periphery of the explants survive reasonably well, but cell-to-cell interconnections through nerve circuits are grossly altered and nothing can be learned about their normal function, leaving aside the more complex problem of the operation of neuronal circuits between distant nuclei and between these and their end organs.

In the hope of finding a more suitable object for the *in vitro* study of the organization and functional properties of the nervous system, we started 4 years ago a research project on the insect nervous system. For reasons to be mentioned in the following section, the object of choice was the cockroach, *Periplaneta americana*. A synthetic medium devised in our laboratories proved to support not only long-term survival of explants of brain, ganglia, and the neuroendocrine system of this insect but also nerve cell migration and vigorous axonal growth from nerve cells located in intact explants or migrated out into the medium. Ganglia dissected out from cockroach embryos became interconnected by cable-like fiber bundles similar to the connectives which form in ontogenesis between these ganglia; nerve fibers emerging from thoracic ganglia assembled in nerves and innervated limb primordia positioned at some distance from them.

The results to be reported below should be considered as preliminary excursions in a field which is opening for the first time to exploration. Although cells and organs from a variety of insects are now routinely cultured in many laboratories with a success which stands comparison with that scored long before with vertebrate cells and organs (Silvana, 1971; Echalier and Ohanessian, 1970), *in vitro* studies on the insect nervous and neuroendocrine systems have not until now been the object of specific investigations. While in fact Marks and coworkers have since 1965 presented evidence for nerve fiber outgrowth from regenerating leg tissues dissected out from cockroach nymphs and cultured *in vitro* under different experimental conditions, this and subsequent papers by the same authors focused mainly on the effects of hormones and of humoral substances released by explants on nerve fiber outgrowth from the cut stump of the leg regenerates (Marks and Reinecke, 1965; Marks *et al.*, 1968).

In contrast to these and other investigations whose main object was the *in vitro* study of hormonal action on various insect tissues (Marks, 1970; Schneider, 1967; Williams and Kambysellis, 1969) inclusive of nerve tissue, our research program has centered entirely on problems which are unique to the nervous system and apply to that of insects as well as of lower and higher vertebrates. Among the advantages presented by the insect nervous system is the fact that it consists of fairly small ganglionic masses the whole of which can be explanted *in vitro*, thus avoiding disruption of nerve tissue and injury to cell populations and neuronal circuits. Lack of a closed circulatory system in arthropods has, according to Treherne (1968), favored the evolution of rapid diffusion processes of ions and molecules within the solid nerve structures. Metabolites and gas exchanges in brain and ganglia explanted *in vitro* from insect embryos or nymphal forms do not therefore differ from those in the living organisms to the extent that they differ in vertebrate nerve tissues. An additional reason which may account for the long-term survival *in vitro* of intact insect brain and ganglionic nerve cells is their location in a cortical rind: thus nerve cells are far more accessible to metabolites and oxygen than the vertebrate nerve cells embedded in the dense matrix of the neural tube.

In this chapter, we shall consider the results of some of the investigations performed on embryonic and mature insect nervous and neuroendocrine systems. Authors of these studies, partly in association with the writers, are J. S. Chen, R. S. Chen, and P. Amaldi.

II. THE OBJECT OF CHOICE: *Periplaneta americana*

Practical considerations as well as the availability of an extensive literature on *Periplanata americana* suggested its selection as the test object of these studies.

This insect is widespread throughout the world in temperate and tropical climates, it survives and breeds remarkably well under laboratory conditions, and large colonies can be maintained with no specially trained technical help. The insect, which is 30–35 mm long, has a life span of 12–14 months and does not face the cataclysm of metamorphosis but goes through a slow and continuous developmental process which transforms the embryo into the adult without substantial changes in the structural organization of its nerve structures. The nervous system of the embryo (which spends 29–45 days in the ootheca depending on the outside temperature: at 29°C the embryos hatch at the end of the first month, whereas it takes $1\frac{1}{2}$ months to complete the development at 15°C) is a miniature but otherwise faithful copy of the nervous system of the mature insect. Molting, which occurs first in embryonic life and then repeatedly during the 12 subsequent months in the nymph, makes possible the stepwise size increase of the immature insect, which emerges from the last molt with a well-developed, although rather inefficient flight apparatus but is similar in other respects to the tiny embryo.

Another advantage, which became apparent as we learned more about this insect from early embryonic life up to maturity, is its remarkable resistance to environmental changes and to infectious and other noxious agents. The embryos can be extracted from the oothecae, where they are aligned in two tightly packed parallel rows, and can be reared from the second week to hatching in a CO_2-conditioned humidified incubator at 29°C. Throughout this time, they can be manipulated, submitted to surgical intervention and microinjections of various drugs, and examined for hours under the stereomicroscope without, in most instances, lethal consequences. Mortality is in fact very low, even when limbs or antennae are amputated or additional organs implanted at the beginning of the third week of incubation. The fact that each ootheca contains 14–16 embryos, available for *in vivo* and *in vitro* experiments, gives this insect a remarkable advantage over other blattoids or orthopterans, which are either viviparous or hatch from individual eggs.

A considerable amount of work has been invested in the study of the nervous system of this cockroach, which is in fact better known at the structural, ultrastructural, biochemical, and electrophysiological levels than most other insects. Here are listed only some of the treatises and articles which are pertinent to the objects of our studies: Beattie (1971), Callec *et al.* (1971), Cornwell (1968), Farley and Milburn (1969), Frontali and Mancini (1970), Hyde (1972), Pearson (1972), Pearson and Iles (1970), Pichon and Callec (1970).

Closely related to the nervous system from a structural and functional viewpoint is the neuroendocrine or retrocerebral complex, which plays a key role in the life of insects, comparable in many respects to that of the vertebrate hypophyseal system. The similarity between the vertebrate and invertebrate neuroendocrine systems extends also to their relationship with brain structures and to the segregation in both phyla of this organ complex in a neural and a nonneural derivative. In insects, the paired corpora cardiaca have a neural origin and share some aspects in common with the neurohypophysis, while the corpora allata, small paired glands, possess important morphogenetic and nonmorphogenetic hormonal functions. "While the structural analogy between parts of the endocrine systems of insects and vertebrates is an interesting one," writes Smith, "it should not be pressed too far; for, unlike the corpus cardiacum, the neurohypophysis possesses no intrinsic secretory cell bodies and, of course, the hormones associated with the two complexes are entirely different in their effects" (Smith, 1968a, p. 96).

III. MATERIAL AND TECHNIQUES

Oothecae protruding from the ovipositor are detached from the insect body, cleaned, and stored in a humidified incubator at 29°C. At the moment of use, the oothecae are rinsed in iodine, alcohol, and distilled water; the seams of the dorsal cristae of the oothecae are carefully split with sterilized forceps and the embryos are collected in Schneider's insect solution For the present experimental studies on the nervous system and nonnervous tissues (alimentary canal and limb and antenna primordia), 16-day-old embryos were used, while the neuroendocrine complex was isolated from 12- and 20-day embryos.

Whole brains and subesophageal, thoracic, and abdominal ganglia are dissected out under the stereomicroscope. Together, in some instances, with the brain is explanted also the rostral part of the alimentary canal, the pharynx, which closely adheres to the posterior brain vesicle known as the tritocerebrum. Other segments of the alimentary canal, the esophagus, the gizzard, the midgut, and the posterior gut, are also dissected out and stored until the moment of use. All the embryonic explants are of a size not exceeding 1–1.5 mm. The neuroendocrine complex, consisting of corpora cardiaca and allata from nymphal and adult specimens, is dissected out under rigorously sterile conditions from nymphal and adult forms and cultured in the same medium used for embryonic tissues. This consists of 5 parts of Schneider's insect solution and 4 parts of Eagle's basal medium, mixed at the moment of use. Tissues dissected out from embryos or post-hatching forms are cultured in small cylindrical glass vessels 13 mm in diameter and 7 mm high, half filled with culture medium. The tissues are pressed on a coverslip laid on the bottom of the culture dish until they firmly adhere to its surface. Five to six culture vessels are then arranged in petri dishes 64 mm in diameter, and cotton soaked with sterile water is placed inside the dishes between each vessel to maintain a vapor-saturated atmosphere; the dishes are then stored in a desiccator filled with 95% air and 5% CO_2 and placed in an incubator at 29°C. The cultures are examined daily at the inverted microscope and then at higher magnification, still in living condition, with the Nomarski interference microscope. The same cultures are studied again upon fixation and staining with routine histological techniques or, more frequently, with the silver Cajal-DeCastro technique. Many cultures are also fixed and used for electron microscopic studies according to the technical procedures given in previous articles (Chen and Levi-Montalcini, 1969, 1970; Levi-Montalcini and Chen, 1969).

IV. SPECIFIC PROBLEMS

A. Cell Migration and Axonal Growth from Embryonic Brain and Ganglia

Cell migration and nerve fiber outgrowth do not substantially differ, at least in their essential features, whether they take place from brain, ganglia, or other organs such as the alimentary canal, where autonomic ganglia and sensory nerve cells are also present among nonnervous tissues. Since the purpose of this chapter is not to examine different explants in detail on a comparative basis but rather to outline the main features of axonal growth and cell migration, we will consider these processes without making reference to the nature of the explants, which were in most instances brain and ganglia, combined *in vitro* in numbers of six to ten for each culture; nerve fiber outgrowth and cell migration are in fact more vigorous when several embryonic tissues and organs are cultured together rather than in isolation.

1. The Nerve Cells

. On the basis of extensive studies on the vertebrate nervous system cultured *in vitro*, it has been stated that

> It cannot be overstressed at the outset that what characterizes neurons *in vitro*, except those of sympathetic ganglia, is the immobility of the soma or cell body. . . . The immobility of somatic nerve cell bodies is already evident at the neuroblast stage and applies also to tumor neuroblasts. It thus appears to be a fundamental property even of somatic cerebrospinal neurons in the formative stage . . . But this immobility *in vitro,* in conditions which are so ideal for migration and dispersion of other cell types, serves above all to emphasize the principle that, of all living cells, the somatic neuron is unique in having to establish its communications (to exchange information) with other cells in the body solely by means of projecting long processes which have to establish physical contact with their correspondent or target cells or tissue. The neuron soma cannot migrate to meet its confederate. (Lumsden, 1968, pp. 74–75)

The invertebrate embryonic neuron seems to provide a noticeable exception to this principle, so forcefully asserted in the above statement, and raises some doubts as to the validity of the arguments submitted by Lumsden in support of his contention.

Before reporting on the results of the present investigations, it may be of interest to see to what extent one is justified in extrapolating from results *in vitro* to the living organism, particularly when the conditions are vastly different as in the above experiments and negative findings could be accounted for by technical causes or drastic changes in the environmental conditions, rather than by intrinsic properties of the cells. While in fact Lumsden is correct in stating that there is no evidence for migratory activity of the embryonic neurons *in vitro*, few cells have provided more striking instances of migratory activity in the living organism than these. Immature neurons with unmistakable marks of their nature in the structural characteristics of the cell body, neurofilaments, and axonal process migrate by the thousands in orderly lines in the brain stem and in the cortical cerebellar layers of the avian and mammalian developing nervous system (Levi-Montalcini, 1963; Sidman, 1970). Migration is in fact the rule rather than the exception in vertebrate neurogenesis and accounts for the active displacement of entire cell populations from their site of origin to their final destination, where the still immature neurons undergo further differentiation and become stationary for the rest of their lives. The fact that nerve cell migration apparently does not take place in the conditions of culture suggests that certain environmental conditions, such as the proximity to other nerve cells or perhaps factors present in the ground substance, are needed for the realization of these oriented movements.

Our insect cultures differ greatly from those of the embryonic vertebrate nervous system. Between the end of the first and fourth weeks *in vitro*, the migratory areas around brain and ganglionic explants show an increasingly larger number of cells intermingled with elongated slender processes. Three distinct cell types have been identified: nerve, glial, and tracheolar cells. We shall first consider nerve cells. The criteria for their identification, listed in detail in previous publications (Chen and Levi-Montalcini, 1969, 1970; Levi-Montalcini and Chen, 1969), are based on observations in living cultures with the Nomarski microscope, on the study of fixed and silver-stained material, and on electron microscopic studies. These cells differ from others also present in large number in the migratory area around the explants in their round or ovoid shape, regular contour, dense texture, and large nuclei and nucleoli. The electron microscope revealed the presence of microtubules regularly spaced in the cytoplasm. A most unusual feature which sets them in a category apart from all other vertebrate and invertebrate cells in culture is the lack of "contact inhibition," at least toward another cell type. They stand in fact on a thin cytoplasmic layer which belongs to cells of very large size with distinct glial features (Fig. 2). In a previous article, we considered the possibility that the presence of a large number of nerve cells in the migratory area around brain and ganglia could be due to passive, rather than active, migration. The cells could have been dragged out from the explant by those to whose surface they closely adhere: their ancillary and omnipresent glial cells. The observation that toward the periphery they lose contact with the underlying cells could, in turn, be explained as consequent to the withdrawal of the glial cell cytoplasm or to the pulling of the distal, actively growing nerve

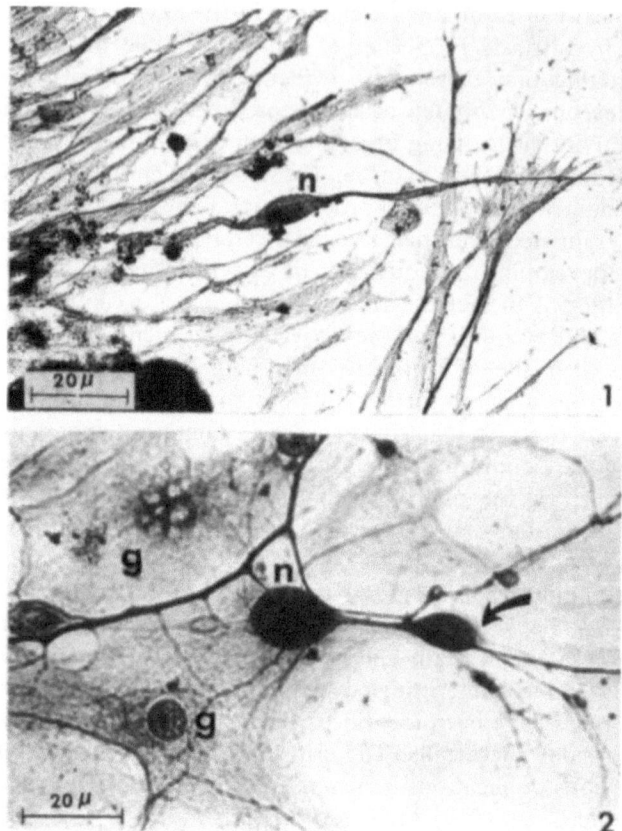

Figs. 1 and 2.   Details of migratory zone around foregut (Fig. 1) and brain explant (Fig. 2) from 16–day embryos cultured for 24 days *in vitro*. n, Nerve cells; g, glial cells. Arrow in Fig. 2 points to large ellipsoidal body along the course of axon emerging from the nerve cell. Further explanation is given in the text. Cultures stained with silver Cajal–DeCastro technique.

cell process. However, subsequent studies of hundreds of cultures showed nerve cells entirely free in the medium, at some distance from other cells, with the two oppositopolar processes well apparent in all their length; since in these instances the cells are not anchored to others, active rather than passive cell displacement seems to account for their position at a considerable distance from the explants. Figure 6 shows one of these cells. Also, the study of the alimentary tube and of limb and antenna primordia from the same donors showed that cells exhibiting features of nerve cells, presumably sensory neurons, are found in the migratory zone around these explants. In these instances, the cells do not show the relationship with other cell types as described above but are seen free in the medium from the moment they emerge from the explants (Fig. 1).

2. The Glial Cells

Of the three glial cell types described in a previous article (Levi-Montalcini and Chen, 1969), we shall consider here only those which are present in large number around brain and ganglionic explants and are also seen in the migratory areas of leg and antenna primordia, but not around segments of the alimentary canal. Four distinctive features mark these cells from others,

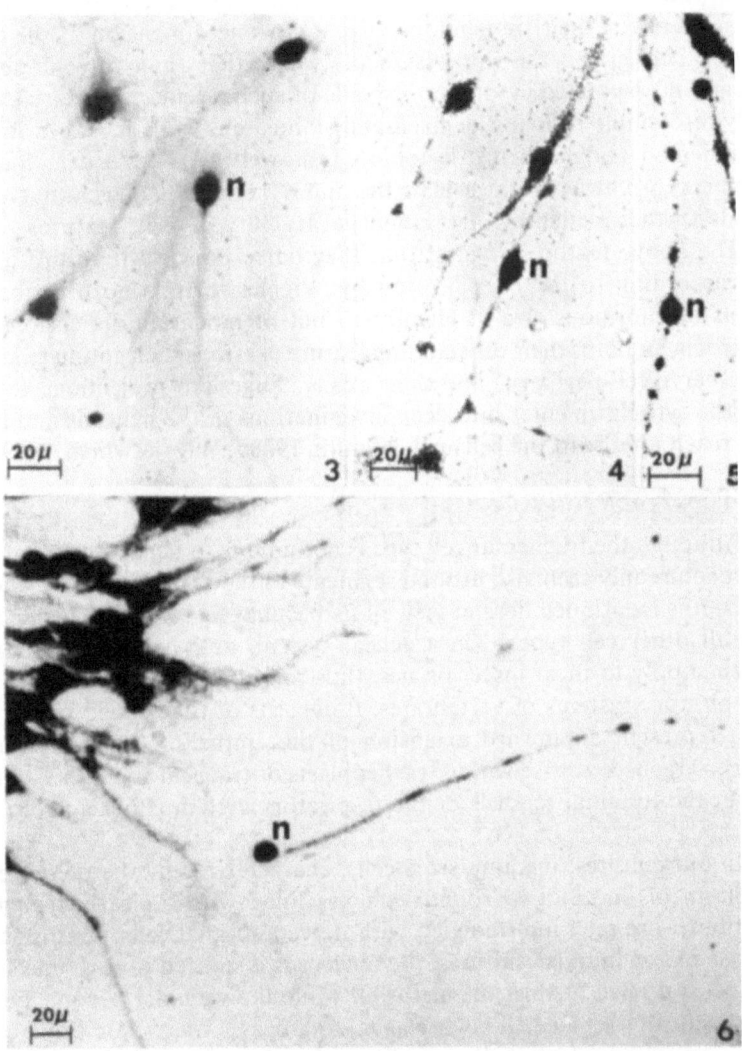

Figs. 3, 4, 5, and 6.   Uridine-H³ incorporation into neurons migrated from a brain explant from a 16-day embryo cultured *in vitro* for 8 days. Time of incubation with uridine-H³ was 30 min (Fig. 3), 4 hr (Fig. 4), 12 hr (Figs. 5 and 6). n, neurons. Further explanation is given in the text.

namely, their exceptionally large size, the flattened and thin cytoplasmic area, the indented and broken contours, and the fibrillar network sculptured on their surface by nerve fibers adhering to them to such an extent as to give the impression that they are part of the cell body. The adhesion of cells, identified as nerve cells, to their surface has already been mentioned. All the above features are perhaps the result of the unique property of these cells to adhere to other living or inert material which happens to be on their path. Thus their tendency to flatten as they leave the explant and move out on the glass surface may account for their tremendous increase in one dimension at the expense of the other, giving the impression of two- rather than three-dimensional objects. The expanded cytoplasm is made of such a tenuous material as to be barely discernible in living or fixed and stained cultures, as shown in Fig. 2. The indented and broken cell contours, as well as the frequent finding of fragments torn away from their bodies and adhering to adjacent nerve fibers, provide further evidence for the unusual fragility of their texture.

The above features suggest that they correspond to the third glial cell type, according to the classification by Wigglesworth, who describes these cells as of enormous size in Hemiptera but of moderate dimensions in the cockroach. In both, their outstanding feature *in vivo* is their intimate adhesion to the nerve cell perikarya and their axons: fingerlike projections extending from the cytoplasm enter into deep invaginations of the neurons and in some cases reach almost to the cell nuclei (Smith, 1968b; Wigglesworth, 1959, 1965).

3. The Tracheolar Cells

Although the tracheolar cell type is not unique to nervous explants and is in fact commonly seen also around segments of the alimentary tube and other tissues, it is mentioned here in view of its peculiar features which single it out from all other cell types. The tracheal system, as is well known, provides oxygen supply to most insect tissues, thus serving a role comparable to that of respiratory systems of vertebrates. It consists of tubes lined with a cuticle which represent an inward extension of the epithelium covering the body surface. Tracheoles arise within tracheoblasts or tracheal end cells from which fan out the terminal tendrils of the respiratory system (Locke, 1958; Smith, 1968a).

In our cultures, medium-sized cells, characterized by the presence in the cytoplasm of one or two round vacuoles lined with a clearly recognizable membrane, are seen intermingled with nerve and glial cells. As the vacuoles increase in size in older cultures, the nucleus is displaced toward one side and becomes flattened against the cell wall, while the vacuoles become confluent and practically replace the cytoplasm. Aggregates of two or three cells are often seen, although they do not line up in tubes. These features, as well as their presence in large number around all embryonic explants, suggest that they may represent tracheolar cells.

4. The Nerve Fibers

In explanting brain and ganglia *in vitro*, we expected to see nerve fibers emerging first and foremost from the connectives which in the living organism interconnect the brain with the subesophageal, thoracic, and abdominal ganglia and were cut at the moment of their dissection from the embryos. As a rule, however, the fibers did not branch out preferentially from the cut connectives but from the entire surface of the explants at random. At times, fibers grow out as single thin filaments which then aggregate in nerve bundles of different size, to split again at some distance; in other instances, they emerge from the explants as colossal fiber bundles, which then break into hundreds of thin filaments spreading, fanlike, on the glass surface. Nerve bundles of all sizes give origin to a large number of collaterals which bridge the distance between the stem fiber and neighboring fibers. Two main fiber types are seen in cultures of brain and ganglia: the first type closely resemble nerve fibers growing out from explants of embryonic vertebrate tissue in their strong affinity for silver salts, which gives them a dark, almost black, color in Cajal preparations. They differ, however, from vertebrate fibers in one respect: they seldom branch out freely into the medium; more frequently, they adhere to the surface of glial cells. The delicate and sometimes exceedingly tenuous fiber ramifications on the surface of these cells give the impression that they have lost their independence and are incorporated in the cell cytoplasm. They regain it, however, as they reach the cell edge, to reestablish similar connections with like cells. The other fiber type which is also frequently seen emerging from explants of the alimentary canal is characterized by a much larger caliber, lighter color, and round or ellipsoidal dilations of variable but often remarkably large size, unevenly spaced, along the path of the fibers. In living cultures examined with the Nomarski microscope, these round or ovoidal bodies show the presence of highly refringent small organelles, while in silver preparations they take an even dark brown color. One of these unusually large dilations located at a short distance from the cell of origin is shown in Fig. 1. Its size is in fact only slightly smaller than that of the cell of origin. The different natures of these two apparently similar structures were elucidated by destaining the slide; the larger ovoidal body showed the presence of a large nucleus which almost entirely filled the area and a distinct nucleolus, while the smaller body was of uniform texture. Other similar dilations are evident in Figs. 3–6 which will be considered again below.

With the electron microscope, neurotubules are seen in transverse sections of these fibers as circular profiles about 150 A in diameter enclosing an electron-transparent core. They are evenly spaced, as in nerve fibers dissected out from living specimens. Well-preserved mitochondria are present in the axoplasm among the neurotubules. Axon-to-axon junction sites, which occur in large number in these cultures, exhibit typical synaptic features:

clusters of electron-transparent vesicles are seen in one of the two axons, associated with a thickening of the "presynaptic" fiber, which is separated by a narrow cleft from the postsynaptic fiber.

The histological and electron microscopic studies briefly summarized here were supplemented with autoradiographic studies. The main aim of this investigation, reported in detail in an article by Amaldi (1970), was to explore the nature of the ellipsoidal bodies along the course of the fibers and the site of protein and ribonucleic acid synthesis. Only the results of this second group of experiments will be considered here.

Seven-day-old cultures of embryonic brain and ganglia with a large number of nerve cells and axonal processes in the migratory area around the explants were selected for these experiments. Uridine-H^3 at the concentration of 10 μc/ml was added to the culture medium, and the cultures were incubated for times varying from 30 min to 24 hr. The cultures were then discontinued, fixed, and processed according to the usual autoradiographic technique.

Silver grains were concentrated on the nucleolar region in the first 30 min (Fig. 3) and over all the nuclear region after 2 hr of labeling. At 4 hr, the label also appeared on the cytoplasm and on the nerve fiber (Fig. 4). After 12 hr of incorporation, the blackening of cells and fibers increased progressively (Fig. 5), and after 24 hr intense labeling was seen on the cell body and entire fiber (Fig. 6). Addition of actinomycin D to the culture medium shortly before the radioactive precursor or ribonuclease treatment of the labeled culture after fixation and before it was dipped into the autoradiographic emulsion resulted in a marked reduction of silver grains on cells and fibers.

These results raise the question of the significance of this high ribonucleic acid concentration in the ellipsoidal bodies along the fibers and at the same time raise the possibility of exploring this problem and others related to protein and ribonucleic acid synthesis and axonal transport in conditions far more favorable than those provided by vertebrate nerve fibers. The insect fibers are in fact of considerably larger diameter than avian or mammalian fibers. Since some of their cells of origin are found free in the medium, at a distance from the explants, it is possible to analyze the time sequence of the incorporation of labeled precursors in intact neurons and to examine whether incorporation occurs also in axons severed from their cell perikarya.

Fibers growing out from isolated explants of brain and ganglia increase in number and length between the end of the first and fourth weeks of culture but do not further elongate in subsequent weeks; on the contrary, they undergo partial regression. An entirely different situation obtains when the same explants are combined *in vitro* with like or different embryonic organs or tissues. The building of large fiber bundles between some paired explants and the oriented growth of axons toward some but not other tissues will be considered below.

B. Selective Outgrowth of Nerve Fibers and Interconnections *In Vitro* Between Thoracic Ganglia and Limb Bud Primordia

While the experiments considered above were directed mainly to analysis of the structural characteristics of cells and axonal processes in the migratory zone around brain and ganglionic explants, the aim of these sets of experiments was to examine whether chance or oriented growth is responsible for the formation of fiber interconnections between paired explants. Attempts to investigate this problem by *in vitro* techniques with the vertebrate nervous system have so far failed: no preferential distribution was seen in fibers growing out from segments of the mouse fetal spinal cord toward some but not other muscular tissues (Crain and Peterson, 1967; Crain *et al.*, 1968; Peterson and Crain, 1970). This may be due to the fact that explantation *in vitro* of clumps of nerve tissues destroys the final specificity involved in the functional hookups between nerve fibers and their target organs. A more advantageous situation is presented by insect ganglia in view of their simpler construction plan and characteristic segregation of motor and internuncial neurons in the outside cellular rind, where the two cell types are segregated from each other: motor neurons are located in the anterior half of the ganglia and interneurons in the posterior half of the same ganglia. Thoracic and abdominal ganglia differ from each other in volume, size of the motor nerve cell population, cell number, and peripheral distribution of their fibers. Thoracic ganglia provide for the innervation of the three pairs of legs by means of large nerves which originate from motor neurons. Thin motor nerve bundles branch out instead from the lateral surface of the abdominal ganglia and end in the axial musculature; some of these fibers also make connection in the muscular layer of the intestinal tract. Interneurons present in large number in both types of ganglia give origin to fibers of small and large caliber which form interconnections between ganglia, send collaterals into the synaptic field of adjacent and distant ganglia, and may extend to the subesophageal and brain regions.

In order to test whether fibers growing out from thoracic and abdominal ganglia branch out at random and make casual connections with neighboring explants or whether connections are established preferentially with some organs or tissues, like and unlike ganglia, leg bud primordia, brain, foregut, and posterior segments of the alimentary canal were combined *in vitro*. The ganglia in numbers of 10 or 12 and others organs dissected out from 16-day embryos were explanted according to different designs and at distances of 0.8–1 mm from each other. The combined cultures were examined daily, while living, with the inverted microscope and with the Nomarski optics, and upon fixation in silver-stained preparations.

The study of hundreds of cultures between the second and eighth weeks showed that in the first 2–3 weeks, fibers grow out radially in all directions from the entire surface of both types of ganglia. At the end of the third week, fibers growing out from paired ganglia establish multiple axon-to-axon contact at their distal ends. Figure 7 shows one of these combined cultures: among fibers growing at random in all directions, some have assembled in

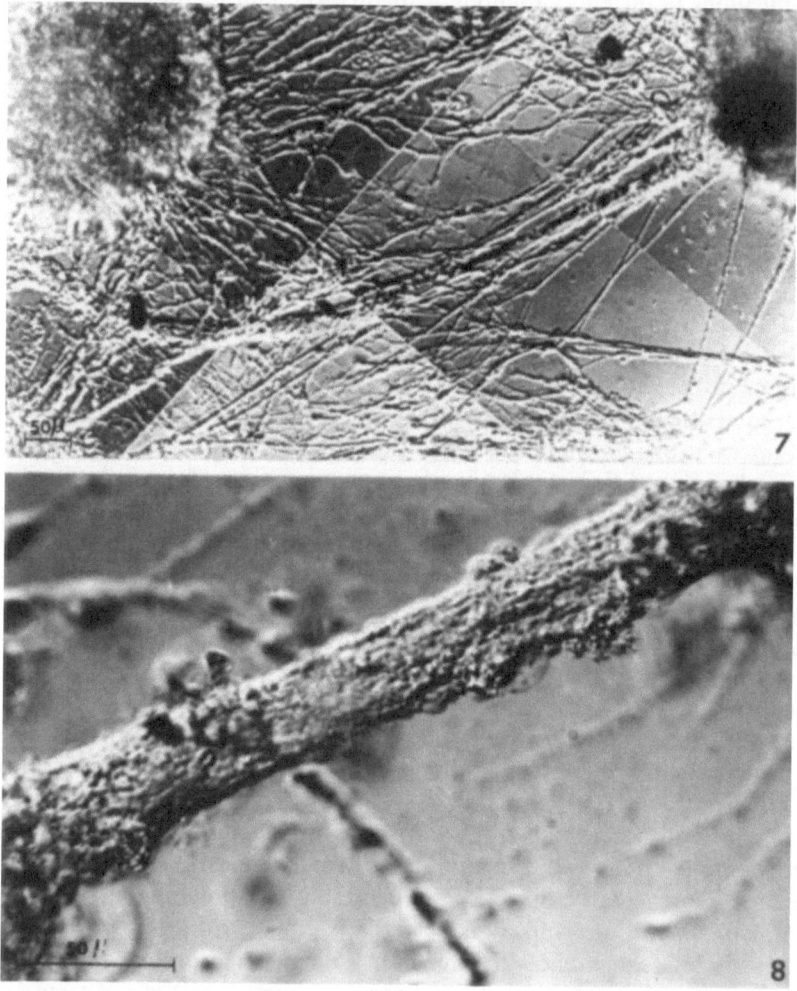

Figs. 7 and 8. Photomicrographs with Nomarski microscope of details of two living cultures of combined thoracic and abdominal ganglia from 16-day embryos cultured *in vitro* for 24 days (Fig. 7) and 45 days (Fig. 8). An early stage in the formation of fiber bundles interconnecting paired abdominal and thoracic ganglia is shown in Fig. 7. Figure 8 shows a large cable-like fiber bundle between two abdominal ganglia. Note small satellite cells adhering to the surface of the nerve bundle.

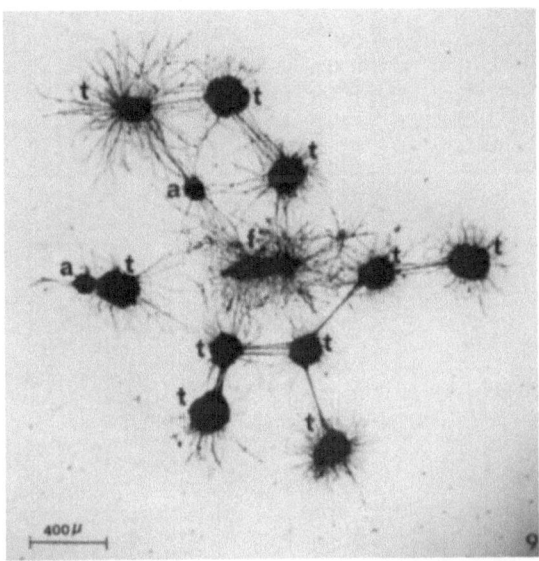

Fig. 9. Multiple thoracic (t) and abdominal (a) ganglia from 16–day embryos fixed after 28 days *in vitro* and stained with silver Cajal–DeCastro technique. All ganglia are interconnected by fiber bundles, while the centrally located foregut segment (f) receives only random fibers from adjacent ganglia.

small bundles which interconnect the paired explants. Figure 8 shows a 45-day-old culture which differs to a marked extent from that in Fig. 7. All fibers growing at random have disappeared from the scene, while fibers interconnecting paired ganglia have reached a remarkably large size. The similarity between this structure and the connectives connecting adjacent ganglia *in vivo* is too obvious to need comment; the organized and oriented growth of nerve fibers assembled in this voluminous fiber bundle is made more impressive by the alignment of small glial-type cells which line up on its surface and remain free from the glass surface. Figure 9 depicts a 28-day-old culture in which 12 mixed thoracic and abdominal ganglia were combined *in vitro* with a foregut segment. All ganglia are interconnected with each other, while only a few fibers branch into the foregut explant, in spite of the fact that it is positioned at a short distance from five ganglia. These results, which were obtained with only slight variations in all cases, indicate a preestablished connectivity pattern between thoracic and abdominal ganglia which materializes even under the unfavorable conditions of the experiments. Since in most instances only random fibers entered into adjacent foregut explants, the results are against the hypothesis that connections between like and unlike ganglia may be of an aspecific nature and that mechanical rather than biochemical factors may be responsible for their formation.

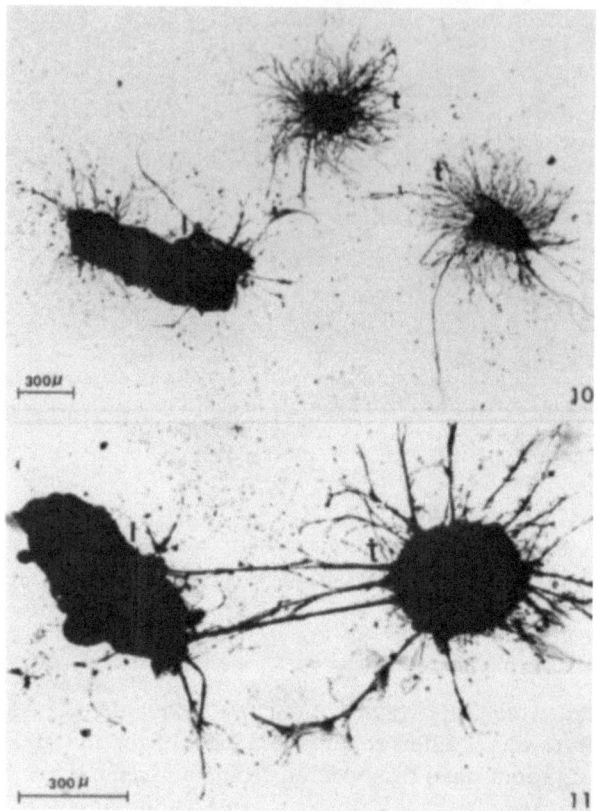

Figs. 10 and 11.   Combined cultures of thoracic ganglia (t) and limb primordia (l) from 16–day embryos cultured for 2 weeks (Fig. 10) and 6 weeks (Fig. 11) and stained with silver Cajal-DeCastro technique. Fibers growing out at random from the entire surface of the ganglia shown in Fig. 10 decrease in number in older cultures as that shown in Fig. 11 and make connection with the limb tissues.

When thoracic ganglia are facing explants of leg primordia, the results are at first sight similar to those depicted above in the temporal and spatial pattern of nerve fiber outgrowth from ganglia. During the first 2–3 weeks of culture, fibers emerge at random from the entire surface of the ganglia as shown in Fig. 10. Nerve fiber outgrowth and cell migration from the leg explant are rather poor and do not markedly increase in subsequent weeks. Figure 11 shows a 6-week-old culture. Three fiber bundles emerging from the ganglion connect with the leg tissues. The same results were obtained when the distance between the combined explants was considerably longer and the fibers growing out from the ganglion had to describe a curved path to enter in the leg proximal stump: a favorite, even if not exclusive, entrance site. Evidence for the strong affinity of thoracic fibers for leg tissues is more extensively documented in a previous publication (Levi-Montalcini and Chen, 1971).

When thoracic ganglia were positioned at the same distance from other ganglia and leg primordia, they produced in most cases two distinct and well-segregated fiber bundles which made connections with both explants. The most obvious hypothesis is that "leg" and "ganglion" fibers which stem out from different neuron pools make selective connections only with their matching end organs. This hypothesis finds support in the observation that abdominal ganglia, given the same choice, always produce large fiber bundles which connect with like or unlike ganglia but only seldom connect through thin bundles with leg tissues. Differences between thoracic and abdominal ganglia in this connection could result from quantitative rather than qualitative differences in the motor neurons; since the size of the motor pool is much smaller in abdominal ganglia, failure to make connections in most instances with leg tissues could be due to this cause rather than to intrinsic differences between thoracic and abdominal neurons.

A problem raised, but still not entirely settled, is whether matching organs or tissues exert an attractive effect "at distance" on ganglionic fibers, thus directing their course from their origin to their termination. Evidence for such an *in vivo* effect came from the experiments by Sperry and coworkers (Sperry, 1963; Attardi and Sperry, 1963) on optic nerve regeneration in fishes. It was in fact shown that the severed optic fibers not only establish appropriate connections with nerve cells in the optic tectum but also select "at distance" the central pathways which bring them to the correct terminal sites (Sperry, 1965). In our experiments, evidence for such a remote effect is indicated by the observation that fibers emerging from thoracic ganglia describe in many instances nonlinear devious courses to enter into the proximal stump of a leg primordium; in some other cases, the distance bridged by growing thoracic fibers to connect with the same tissues is longer than that covered by the same fibers not facing these explants.

C. *In Vitro* Studies on the Insect Neuroendocrine System

Among nerve tissues and glands endowed with neuroendocrine activities in all animal phyla, perhaps none is more favorable for experimental analysis than the insect cardiacum–allatum complex. Its easy accessibility, its large size, and the multiple and diversified roles played by these dual organs in controlling morphogenetic events and in releasing physiologically active factors apparently not related to morphogenesis made of it a favorite object of experimentation at different levels.

The development of a chemically defined medium, which proved to support survival of parts of the nervous system and of various organs of insect embryos and vigorous cell migration and nerve fiber outgrowth from these explants, suggested the use of the same techniques to explore this system. The first aim of these investigations, which are at present being actively pursued in our laboratory, was the study of the structural organization of this organ complex in isolation from the associated brain neurosecretory cells. It is all too well known that an additional complexity faced by those who engage in the study of this system at the structural, biochemical, and functional levels is to ascertain to what extent the biologically active products released by the cardiacum–allatum complex are manufactured *in situ* or exported from their site of origin in the protocerebral neurosecretory cells and stored as such or further elaborated and released by these glands. While in fact the last-mentioned possibility is the most plausible, the roles played, respectively, by the brain neurosecretory cells and the parenchymal or neuroglandular cells of corpora cardiaca in the production of these multiple factors remain to be defined.

The results of the experiments to be considered below showed that the cockroach nymphal and adult neuroendocrine complex, which consists of the paired corpora cardiaca and allata, adapts remarkably well to the conditions of culture, thus providing a baseline for future investigations at the biochemical and physiological levels. At the same time, they revealed some new features of the structural organization of the corpora cardiaca which may call for a revision of accepted schemes of their structure and function. Here we will consider in a condensed form the results of studies on corpora cardiaca of nymphal and adult specimens. Studies now in progress on the same embryonic glands will also be reported. First, we shall outline the structural organization of this gland on the basis of the extensive literature available on this topic. Only some of the recent contributions are listed here: Bern, (1966), Gabe (1966), Gilbert (1964), Highnam (1969), Meola and Lea (1972), Scharrer and Scharrer (1963), Scharrer and Weitzman (1970), Schneiderman and Gilbert (1964), Wigglesworth (1954, 1964), Williams (1969).

The corpora cardiaca are a neural derivative and consist of epithelioid elements and a medullary portion or neuropile, which in the cockroach is not clearly segregated topographically from the cells, belonging to two distinct types known as neuroglandular or parenchymal cells and interstitial or glial cells. A third cell type with features of true neurons is mentioned by some authors (Bern and Hagadorn, 1965; Gabe, 1966; Scharrer, 1962), but neither their structural characteristics nor the size and possible functional significance of this nerve cell population have been the object of investigation. Meola and Lea (1972) in a recent ultrastructural study of *Aedes sollicitans* consider the corpus cardiacum as a linearly arranged ganglion composed of either motor or internuncial neurons. However, detailed and highly accurate studies on the fine structure of neuroglandular cells are available (Aggarwal and King, 1971; Bowers and Johnson, 1966; Cassier and Fain-Maurel, 1970; Cazal et al., 1971; Normann, 1965; Scharrer, 1962, 1963; Smith, 1968a; Smith and Smith, 1966; Unnithan et al., 1971; Willey and Chapman, 1960). According to all authors, the neuroglandular cells differ from typical neurons in possessing stainable material synthesized within the cell bodies and passed out along the axon; as seen with the electron microscope, the material is contained in membrane-bound vesicles varying in size from 1000 to 3000 A. Not only the size but also the electron density of the vesicles' content differs in adjacent, apparently like neuroglandular cells and in the same cells and in their axons. While the problem of whether different neuroglandular cells manufacture and release substances endowed with different biological activity is not resolved by these studies, a possible answer is suggested by the identification in the gland homogenate of several physiologically active peptide factors displaying different and well-defined biological action on equally diversified target tissues (Brown, 1965; Highnam and Goldsworthy, 1972; Mordue and Goldsworthy, 1969; Natalizi and Frontali, 1966; Steele, 1961). Intermingled with the neuroglandular cells are a large number of axons; some of them originate from the above cells, while others have been traced to the neurosecretory cells located in the protocerebrum. It is generally assumed that the neurosecretory material which fills these extrinsic axons is in part released in the corpora cardiaca in close contact with blood vessels or hemocoels; however, since synaptic vesicles are also seen in some of the axon terminals in contact with the intrinsic cells of these glands, the question was raised whether this material is not also in part released in a conventional synaptic fashion at these sites (Bern and Hagadorn, 1965; Palay, 1957; Willey and Chapman, 1960).

A rather large contingent of the extrinsic axons does not end in the corpora cardiaca but passes through, and terminates in the adjacent corpora allata and also in other tissues and organs (Bern and Hagadorn, 1965; Johnson and Bowers, 1963; Thomsen, 1952). A most important and still unanswered question is whether axons of neuroglandular cells end entirely inside these glands or whether some of them leave the glands and reach peripheral end organs. According to Smith (1968a), the axon-like processes of the neuroglandular cells are short and bulbous and, unlike true axons, contain ribosomes and do not extend beyond the confines of the corpora cardiaca. The possibility, however, that some axons of the neuroglandular cells leave the glands and terminate in other organs is mentioned by some authors (e.g., Normann, 1965). Interstitial or glial cells are found scattered among neuroglandular cells in fairly large number. These cells do not substantially differ from satellite or glial cells of brain and ganglia; with the light microscope, they show a small

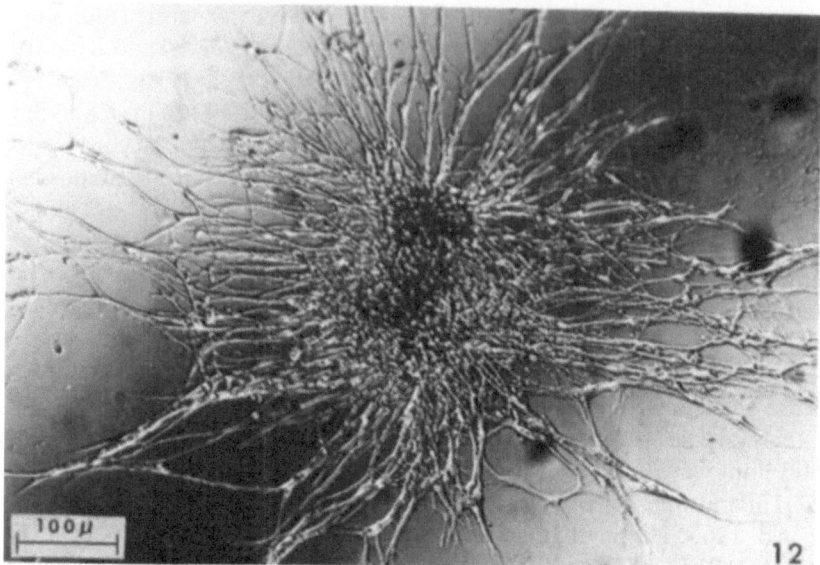

Fig. 12. Nomarski photomicrograph of a living culture of corpora cardiaca and allata dissected out from a fourth instar nymph and cultured 22 days *in vitro*. Note tubular profiles of fibers branching out in all directions from the explant.

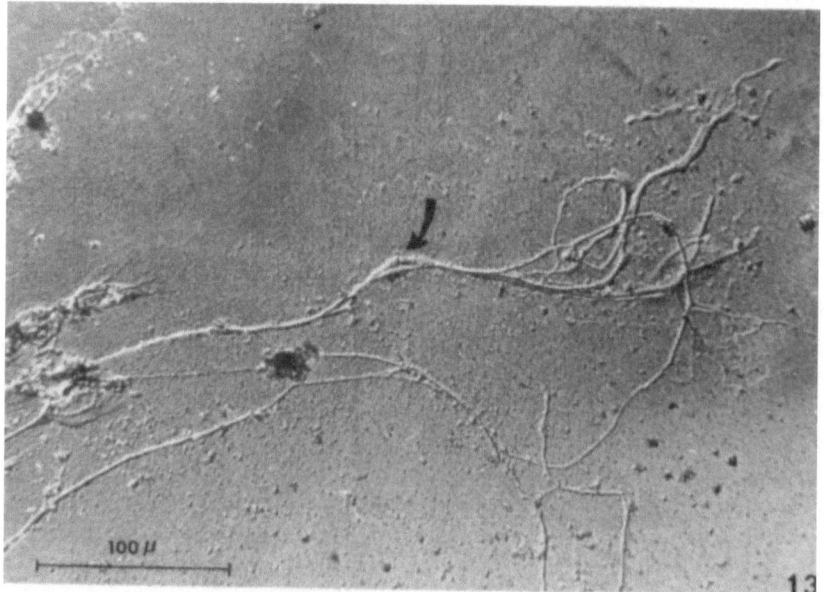

Fig. 13. Nomarski photomicrograph of distal part of migratory area around corpora cardiaca of fifth instar nymph cultured *in vitro* for 45 days. Arrow points to fusiform dilation along the course of a fiber which splits in two. Bulbous swellings on the tip of the branching ends of the same fiber are also apparent.

nucleus surrounded by a thin cytoplasmic ring which stains lightly with basic dyes.

In experiments reported in detail in a previous publication (Seshan and Levi-Montalcini, 1971), we combined *in vitro* corpora cardiaca and allata from nymphal and adult cockroaches together with embryonic organs from

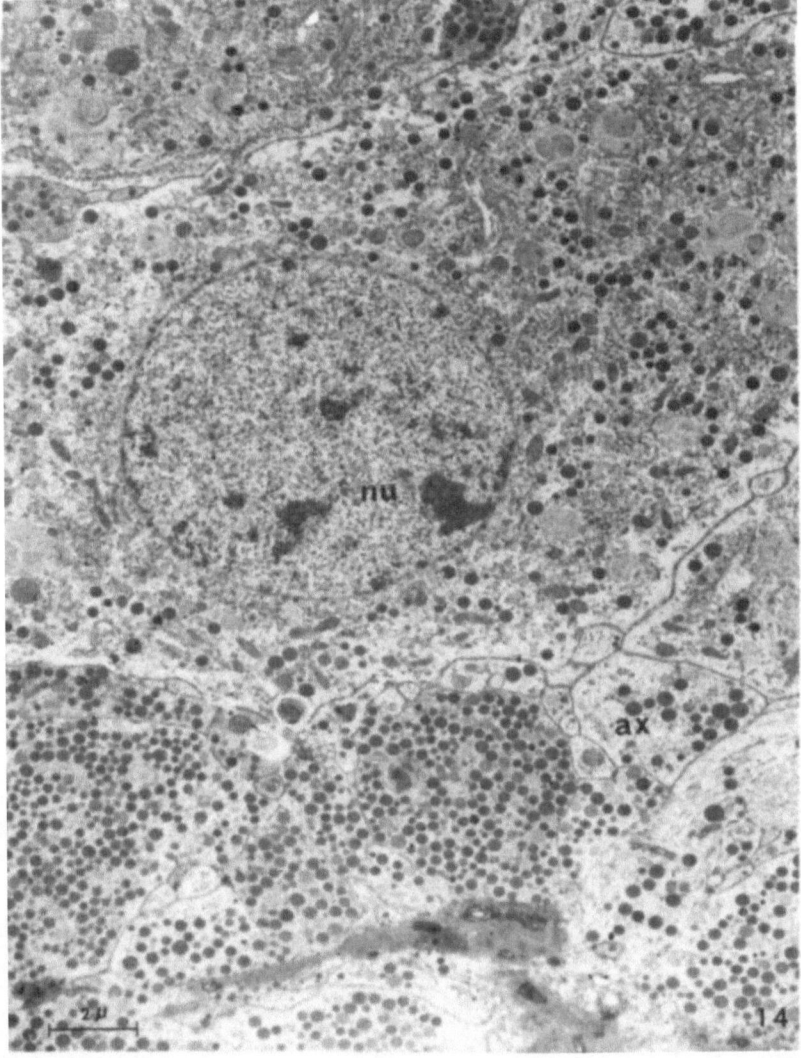

Fig. 14. Electron photomicrograph taken from culture of corpus cardiacum from a fifth instar nymph cultured *in vitro* for 34 days. nu, Nucleus of a neuroglandular cell with electron-dense bodies in the cell cytoplasm. Axon (ax) and membrane-bound areas tentatively identified as parts of other neuroglandular cells are also filled with large numbers of electron-dense granules suggestive of neurosecretory material.

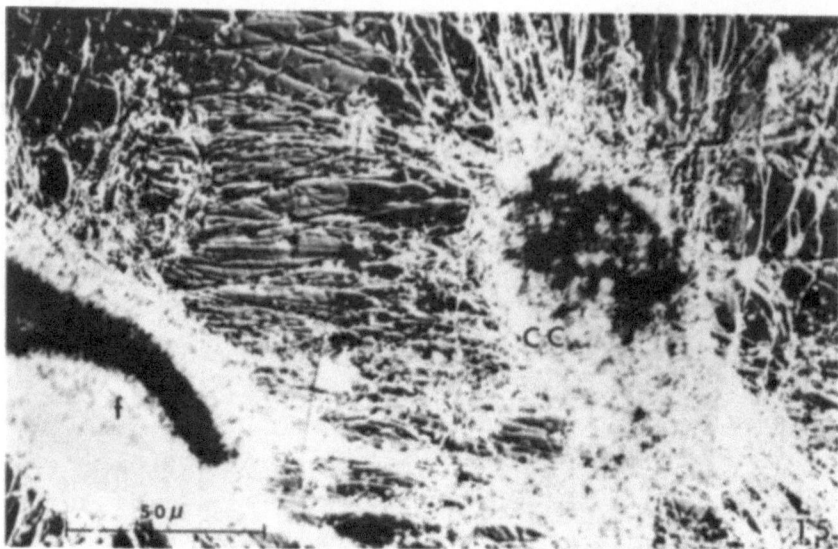

Fig. 15. Dark-field Nomarski photomicrograph of a living explant of corpora cardiaca (cc) from a fifth instar nymph cultured *in vitro* for 2 months, in combination with a foregut (f) and other explants from 16-day embryos. Fibers emerging from both explants bridge the distance between the combined organs.

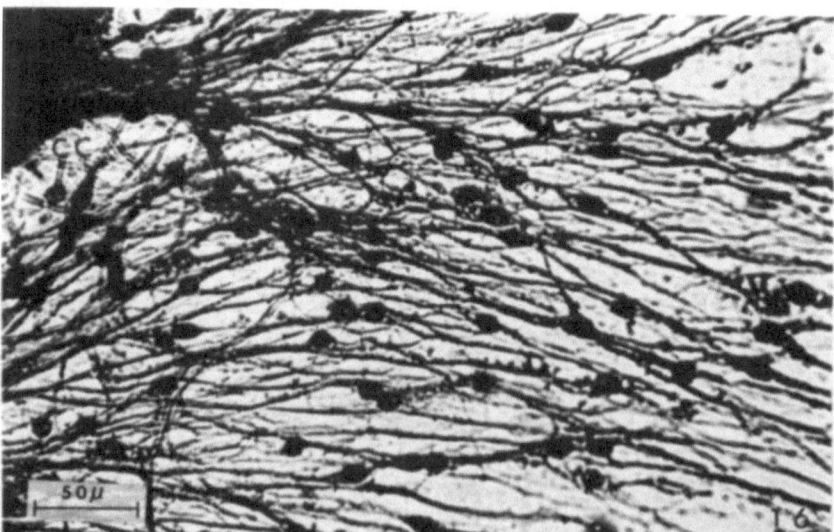

Fig. 16. Migratory area around explant of corpora cardiaca (cc) from an adult specimen. Culture fixed and stained with Cajal–DeCastro technique after 33 days of incubation *in vitro*. Small cells among fibers are identified as glial interstitial cells. Further explanation is given in the text.

donors of the same species. Brain, ganglia, foregut segments, and heart from 16-day embryos were positioned at distances of about 0.5–1 mm from the neuroendocrine complex. Toward the end of the first week of culture, slender processes emerged at random from the entire surface of the corpora cardiaca, but not of the allata, and underwent progressive elongation in the subsequent 7–8 weeks of culture. The identification of these processes as nerve fibers was strongly suggested by observations with the light microscope and was then definitely established by electron microscopic studies to be reported below.

Figure 12 shows a living culture of the cardiacum–allatum complex from a nymphal specimen, cultured *in vitro* for 22 days, and Figure 13 shows the peripheral branching of fibers from an explant of corpora cardiaca after 45 days of culture. The large size, the uneven fiber caliber, and the occurrence of fusiform dilations which taper down gradually at both ends give to these fibers a peculiar appearance markedly different from that of fibers growing out from embryonic brains and ganglia. A comparison of Figs. 2–6 and 13 illustrates these differences. It is of particular interest to note that while the brain fibers shown in Figs. 2–6 are thin and uniform in size in the short segments between the dilations, the fibers from corpora cardiaca show continuous variations in size from point to point even between the dilations. One gets the impression that accumulation of a viscous material flowing along the fibers in a proximodistal direction might be responsible for the fluctuation in size of these axons. An obvious hypothesis which suggests itself is that this material is the neurosecretory product, seen in large amount inside the cells and axons of corpora cardiaca explanted and cultured *in vitro* for several weeks, as in the case shown in Fig. 14 and in others kept for longer periods *in vitro*. Studies now in progress give evidence for the presence of vesicles filled with electron-dense and electron-transparent material also in axons in the migratory area at some distance from the explants. The vesicles, which present the same features as those seen in the cytoplasm of neuroglandular cells, are closely packed together or loosely arranged between microtubular structures. Not all fibers growing out from corpora cardiaca exhibit these features. Others, in fact more numerous, are much more similar to those emerging from brain and ganglionic explants, being smaller and uniform along the entire length of the axon. Fibers of this type extend at a distance from their site of origin and become lost to sight in the dense texture of adjacent embryonic explants: brain, foregut, and heart segments, as in the culture shown in Fig. 15. While in this case the distance between the pairing explants is very short, in others the space covered by the bridging fibers is considerably longer. Electron microscopic studies now in progress are directed to the analysis of the fine structure of these fibers and of their end terminals inside the embryonic organs. Are electron-dense bodies (suggestive of a neurosecretory function) present in these processes? Do these fibers establish conventional synapses with the embryonic tissues, or do they wander freely inside these explants?

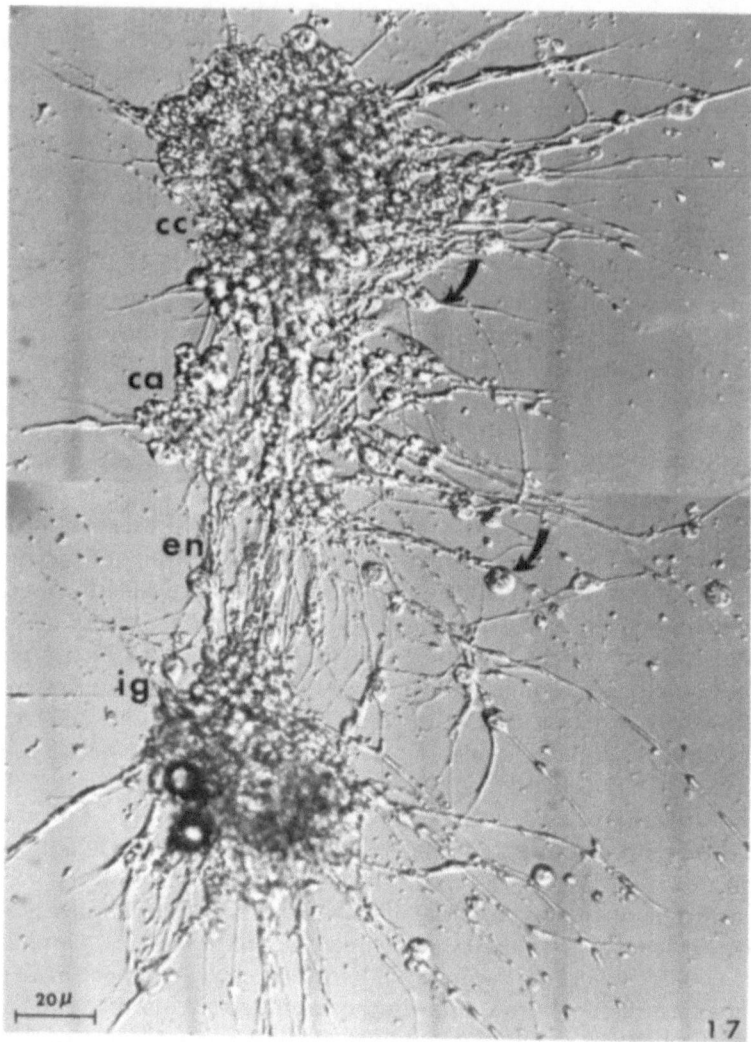

Fig. 17. Nomarski photomicrograph of a living culture of corpora cardiaca (cc), allata (ca), and the ingluvial ganglion (ig) of a 20-day embryo cultured *in vitro* for 12 days. The cardiacum–allatum complex is connected through the esophageal nerve (en) to the in-gluvial ganglion. Arrows point to nerve cells in the migratory zone around explants. Nerve and glial cells are also seen between fibers of the esophageal nerve.

Even if these questions are as yet unanswered, they bring to the fore the main contribution of these cultures, namely, to have shown that upon explantation *in vitro*, the corpora cardiaca, a neuroendocrine organ *par excellence*, behaves in a way similar to that of brain and ganglia dissected out from embryonic donors of the same species, in producing a large number of fibers and in establishing connections with adjacent explants. These findings at the same time raise other questions: What is the origin of these fibers? Do they all grow out from neuroglandular cells, or do the fibers which resemble conventional nerve fibers originate from "true neurons" which in the glands *in vivo* are overshadowed by the larger neuroglandular cell population? Are the glandular cells all of one type or of different types, each one manufacturing a different product? Before considering the results of some preliminary studies on the embryonic corpora cardiaca, a few words may be said on the characteristics of the cells which are found in large number in the migratory area around nymphal and adult corpora cardiaca, cutured *in vitro* for 2–8 weeks. Figure 16 shows a section of the migratory area around these glands, dissected out from an adult specimen and cultured *in vitro* for 33 days. The cells, all similar in appearance, are loosely scattered between the fibers and have no apparent close connection with them. In this respect, they differ markedly from glial cells migrating out from brain and ganglia of embryonic specimens. They were tentatively identified as interstitial or glial cells.

In close proximity to the explants, one also sees large round cells, similar in size and other features to cells identified as neurons, in the migratory areas around brain and ganglionic explants. These findings raise the question of whether these cells are neuroglandular cells or perhaps belong to the hypothetical small population of true neurons. The difficulty in recognizing cells of one or the other type in our cultures became more manifest from the study of the migratory areas around the neuroendocrine system of 12- and 20-day-old embryos. Figure 17 shows corpora cardiaca and allata, the esophageal nerve, and the ingluvial ganglion dissected out from a 20-day embryo and cultured for 12 days *in vitro*. Cells exhibiting typical features of nerve cells are present in rather large number around the neuroendocrine glands and the ingluvial ganglion. Long axon-like processes emerge from these cells and also from cells in the explants. The characteristics of cells and fibers around the neuroendocrine complex and the ingluvial ganglion are in fact so similar as to raise the question of whether these two organ primordia connected to each other by the esophageal nerve may not share a common origin. This possibility would, in turn, suggest that neuroglandular cells and "true neurons" are not, at least at this early stage of their differentiation, substantially different from each other. We will return to this point in the next and last section.

V. CONCLUDING REMARKS AND PERSPECTIVES

"A bacterium is a nondescript object," stated Williams. "The cells of a louse are, by comparison, of outstanding beauty" (Williams, 1963, p. 257).

The same compliment could be addressed to cockroach cells and, first of all, to nerve cells, which at this low phylogenetic level have already acquired all the essential and distinctive features which place them at the highest rank among other animal cells. The belief that these cells develop according to the same rules, whether they belong to an insect or to a mammal, and that neuronal circuits, although of an entirely different level of complexity, are under the same restraints and enjoy a comparable degree of freedom (the former dictated by the genetic code, the latter conferred by the operation of environmental factors which mitigate the rigor of genetic laws) suggested the selection of insects as test objects in a wide range of experimental conditions. Among insects, the despised cockroach, which has crawled, apparently unchanged, for at least 300 million years on earth, offered an ideal object for experimentation. Reasons for its selection were given in the Introduction and will not be repeated here, although it may be worthwhile to mention that the remarkable survival capacity of its cells and their adaptation to the synthetic medium of culture used in our experiments may well reflect the extraordinary resistance of this insect, which fares so comfortably under good as well as adverse conditions.

Comments added at the end of each section make unnecessary a critical reevaluation of the results obtained and of the merits and shortcomings of each one of the lines of investigations considered in this chapter. It may, however, be of interest, in forward reference to future work, to discuss briefly the perspectives opened in each of the three main lines of investigations presented above.

We reported first on cell migration and axonal growth from embryonic intact brain and ganglia in long-term cultures. Further analysis of these explants under the same experimental conditions will probably not add too much to what has already been learned, and, in view of these considerations, these experiments are at present discontinued. Autoradiographic studies of nerve cells migrating out from brain explants and cultured for short or longer times in the presence of labeled amino acids or uridine seem instead to present a most promising approach to the investigation of problems which until now have been explored mainly in the vertebrate phyla. We have mentioned the reasons why insect embryonic nerve cells cultured *in vitro* seem to offer a particularly favorable object for these investigations; we may add to that list that the slow growth rate of nerve fibers *in vitro* affords the opportunity of exploring the temporal and spatial patterns of these processes, whether we are dealing with ribonucleic acid and protein synthesis at the cellular level and their subsequent exportation along the fiber or whether evidence is obtained for synthesis *in situ* in the same axons. Also, we may hope to gain information on the reverse axonal flow from end organs to the nerve cells in charge of their innervation.

The results of experiments reported in the second section, dealing with the pattern of nerve fiber outgrowth and *in vitro* connectivity between all ganglia and between thoracic ganglia and limb primordia, gave evidence for the remarkable ability of nerve fibers to reestablish the same connections which they build during embryonic life in the developing organism. We may, however, ask whether further experimentation along this line will bring information on one of the most challenging and yet unsolved problems of neurobiology, namely, the mechanism of action and the nature of factors which are responsible for the building of wiring circuits among nerve cell populations and among these and their end organs. While insect systems present a distinct advantage over the vertebrate nervous system cultured *in vitro,* still they may be too complex for such a problem. A much higher level of sophistication is required to gain information on the geometry of synaptic circuits and on neural connections at the cellular level; for these reasons also, this line of investigation will not be pursued further unless— as is often the case with experimental work—a new approach to the problem with these *in vitro* systems suggests itself.

The *in vitro* analysis of the insect neuroendocrine sytem dissected out from embryonic, nymphal, and adult specimens seems to hold good promise of future development at different levels. It may in fact be worth recalling that neither the structural nor the functional organization of the organs which play a key role in this system, the paired corpora cardiaca, is at present satisfactorily known. Since elucidation of the structure and anatomical connection of these glands is a prerequisite to the study of their function, our future efforts will at first be aimed in the same direction as in the studies reported above. We expect in this way to gain additional information on these glands from their early inception to the nymphal and mature stages, and on cells and axons as they move out from the explants and, in so doing, reveal features hitherto unknown, or perhaps not even manifest, when cells and axons are packed in the dense fabric of these glands and the same are connected through multiple nerves with neurosecretory brain cells and with a constellation of other organs and tissues.

According to the description given by most authors, neuroglandular cells of corpora cardiaca are provided with short and bulbous axons which differ from normal axons in containing ribosomes and not extending beyond the confines of these glands; neurosecretory axons trespassing these limits and reaching the adjacent corpora allata and other more distant organs and tissues would belong to brain neurosecretory cells. The results of our *in vitro* analysis of these glands do not fit in this accepted scheme, in several ways.

The migratory area around nymphal and mature corpora cardiaca cultured *in vitro* for 1–2 months consists of a large number of fibers, identified using the optic and electron microscope as nerve fibers of numerous small glial-type cells and of a few cells in close proximity to the explants, tentatively identified as neurons. The migratory area around explants of the same embryonic glands shows instead a large number of round or ellipsoidal cells with features of true neurons in their shape and in the long processes which grow out from the cells' opposite ends and extend for a long distance into the medium. The questions raised by our findings are as follows:

What is the nature and the origin of fibers seen in such large number in the migratory area around nymphal and mature corpora cardiaca? Preliminary studies gave evidence for electron-dense granules in some of these fibers, thus suggesting a neurosecretory function. Axons branching out from these explants exhibit, however, different size and growth patterns; some show large dilations along the course of the fibers and bulbous endings, while others, as a rule of smaller caliber, become lost to sight as they enter adjacent embryonic or nymphal organs. Do these fibers stem out from different cell types—some true neurons and others neuroglandular cells? Or do the same fibers display alternatively a neurosecretory and a pure nerve function which can be switched on and off, or can they even display both functions simultaneously? Do the fibers which enter into adjacent explants exhibit at the junction sites the characteristics of true synapses, or do they end blindly in these tissues?

Another question of considerable interest and related to the more general and yet unsolved problem of the ontogenetic origin of the neurosecretory cells and of their relationship to true neurons is brought into focus by the observation that a large number of cells with distinct neuronal features are seen in the migratory area around embryonic but not nymphal and mature explants of corpora cardiaca. Are these cells conventional neurons which subsequently acquire the morphological characteristics of neuroglandular cells, maintaining or losing the capacity of carrying action potentials? Although evidence has been presented that neurosecretory cells can also convey nerve impulses (Hagadorn, 1967), little is known about this property in neuroglandular cells, also in view of the fact that their stout axons end at a short distance within the same glands. If evidence is obtained that nerve cells migrating out from the embryonic corpora cardiaca are indeed immature neuroglandular cells, an additional question is raised of the extent to which their differentiation is triggered by the axons of the brain neurosecretory cells, which establish connections with them and control their function. Would an early separation of the brain from this gland primordium reflect on the fate of these cells? Is there any evidence of an incipient neurosecretory function in cells migrating out from the embryonic neuroendocrine glands?

At the functional level, other problems can profitably be explored in this *in vitro* system.

The neuroglandular cell population is described as homogeneous on the basis of structural and ultrastructural criteria. And yet a variety of peptides endowed with different biological activities have been characterized in the gland extract (Gersch *et al.*, 1970; Kater, 1968; Keeley and Friedman, 1967; Mordue and Goldsworthy, 1969; Muller and Engelmann, 1968; Natalizi *et al.*, 1970; Normann and Duve, 1969). Evidence for the release of the cardioaccelerator factor *in vitro* was earlier obtained in some preliminary experiments with our long-term cultures of nymphal corpora cardiaca. The possibility that other factors may likewise be released and characterized is now the object of study. The same cultures will be used to explore synthetic processes and axonal transport in these unusually large axons branching and ending blindly in the medium.

The list of problems which lend themselves to investigation could be much longer. We prefer to end here and leave to future work to tell whether the *in vitro* nervous and neuroendocrine systems of this humble insect can provide the answers to or perhaps a lead to the elucidation of problems related to growth and differentiation of these insect systems, as well as of their homologues in higher living organisms.

VI. REFERENCES

Aggarwal, S. K., and King, R. C. 1971. An electron microscopic study of the corpus cardiacum of adult *Drosophila melanogaster* and its afferent nerves. *J. Morphol.* **134:** 437–446.

Amaldi, P. 1970. Incorporation of RNA and protein precursors into embryonic nerve cells of *Periplaneta americana* cultured *in vitro*. *Brain Res.* **21:**305–308.

Attardi, D. G., and Sperry, R. W. 1963. Preferential selection of central pathways by regenerating optic fibers. *Exptl. Neurol.* **7:**46–64.

Beattie, T. M. 1971. Histology, histochemistry, and ultrastructure of neurosecretory cells in the optic lobe of the cockroach, *Periplaneta americana*. *J. Insect Physiol.* **17 (10):** 1843–1855.

Bern, H. A. 1966. On the production of hormones by neurons and the role of neurosecretion in neuroendocrine mechanisms. *Symp. Soc. Exptl. Biol.* **20:**325–344.

Bern, H. A., and Hagadorn, I. R. 1965. Neurosecretion, pp. 353–429. *In* T. H. Bullock and G. A. Horridge (eds.). Structure and Function in the Nervous Systems of Invertebrates. W. H. Freeman & Co., San Francisco and London.

Bowers, B., and Johnson, B. 1966. An electron microscopic study of the corpora cardiaca and secretory neurons in the aphid, *Myzus persicae* Sulz. *Gen. Comp. Endocrinol.* **6:** 213–230.

Brown, B. E. 1965. Pharmacologically active constituents of the cockroach corpus cardiacum: Resolution and some characteristics. *Gen. Comp. Endocrinol.* **5:**387–401.

Bullock, T. H., and Horridge, G. A. 1965. Structure and Function in the Nervous Systems of Invertebrates, Vols. I and II. W. H. Freeman & Co., San Francisco. 1719 pp.

Callec, J. J., Guillet, J. C., Pichon, Y., and Boistel, J. 1971. Further studies on synaptic transmission in insects. II. Relations between sensory information and its synaptic integration at the level of a single giant axon in the cockroach. *J. Exptl. Biol.* **55:**123–149.

Cassier, P., and Fain-Maurel, M. A. 1970. Contribution à l'étude infrastructurale du système neurosécréteur rétrocérébral chez *Locusta migratoria migratoriodes* (R. et F.) 1. Les corpora cardiaca. *Z. Zellforsch.* **111:**471–482.

Cazal, M., Joly, L., and Porte, A. 1971. Étude ultrastructurale des corpora cardiaca et de quelques formations annexés chez *Locusta migratoria* L. *Z. Zellforsch.* **114:**61–72.

Chen, J. S., and Levi-Montalcini, R. 1969. Axonal outgrowth and cell migration *in vitro* from nervous system of cockroach embryos. *Science* **166**:631–632.

Chen, J. S., and Levi-Montalcini, R. 1970. Long term cultures of dissociated nerve cells from the embryonic nervous system of the cockroach *Periplaneta americana*. *Arch. Ital. Biol.* **108**:503–537.

Cohen, J. J. 1967. Correlations between structure, function and RNA metabolism in central neurons of insects, pp. 65–78. *In* C. A. G. Wiersma (ed.). Invertebrate Nervous Systems. University of Chicago Press, Chicago.

Cornwell, P. B. 1968. The Cockroach, Vol. 1. Hutchinson, London.

Crain, S. M., and Peterson, E. R. 1964. Complex bioelectric activity in organized tissue cultures of spinal cord (human, rat and chick). *J. Cell. Comp. Physiol.* **64**:1–13.

Crain, S. M., and Peterson, E. R. 1967. Onset and development of functional interneuronal connections in explants of rat spinal cord–ganglia during maturation in culture. *Brain Res.* **6**:750–762.

Crain, S. M., Peterson, E. R., and Bornstein, M. B. 1968. Formation of functional interneuronal connections between explants of various mammalian central nervous tissues during development *in vitro*, pp. 13–31. *In* G. E. W. Wolstenholme and M. O'Connor (eds.). Ciba Foundation Symposium on Growth of the Nervous System. J. & A. Churchill Ltd., London.

Crain, S. M., Alfei, L., and Peterson, E. R. 1970. Neuromuscular transmission in cultures of adult human and rodent skeletal muscle after innervation *in vitro* by fetal rodent spinal cord. *J. Neurobiol.* **1**:471–489.

Echalier, G., and Ohanessian, A. 1970. *In vitro* culture of *Drosophila melanogaster* embryonic cells. *In vitro* **6**:162–172.

Farley, R. D., and Milburn, N. S. 1969. Structure and function of the giant fiber system in the cockroach, *Periplaneta americana*. *J. Insect Physiol.* **15**:457–476.

Frontali, N., and Mancini, G. 1970. Studies on the neuronal organization of cockroach corpora pedunculata. *J. Insect Physiol.* **16**:2293–2301.

Gabe, M. 1966. Neurosecretion. Pergamon Press, Oxford, London, New York. 872 pp.

Gersch, M., Richter, K., Böhm, G.-A., and Stürzebecher, J. 1970. Selektive Ausschuttung von Neurohormonen nach elektrischer Reizung der Corpora Cardiaca von *Periplaneta americana in vitro*. *J. Insect Physiol.* **16**:1991–2013.

Gilbert, L. I. 1964. Physiology of growth and development: Endocrine aspects, pp. 149–225. *In* M. Rockstein (ed.). Physiology of Insecta. Academic Press, New York.

Hagadorn, I. R. 1967. Neurosecretory mechanisms, pp. 115–124. *In* C. A. G. Wiersma (ed.). Invertebrate Nervous Systems: Their Significance for Mammalian Neurophysiology. University of Chicago Press, Chicago.

Highnam, K. C. 1969. Neurosecretion in insects. *Progr. Endocrinol., Excerpta Med. Internat. Congr. Ser.,* No. 184, pp. 351–355.

Highnam, K. C., and Goldsworthy, G. J. 1972. Regenerated corpora cardiaca and hyperglycemic factor in *Locusta migratoria*. *Gen. Comp. Endocrinol.* **18**:83–88.

Hyde, A. C. Ta. 1972. Regeneration, post-embryonic induction and cellular interaction in the eye of *Periplaneta americana*. *J. Embryol. Exptl. Morphol.* **27**:367–379.

Johnson, B., and Bowers, B. 1963. Transport of neurohormones from the corpora cardiaca in insects. *Science* **141**:264–266.

Kater, S. B. 1968. Cardioaccelerator release in *Periplaneta americana* (L). *Science* **160**:765–767.

Keeley, L. L., and Friedman, S. 1967. Corpus cardiacum as a metabolic regulator in *Blaberus discoidalis* Serville (Blattidae). *Gen. Comp. Endocrinol.* **8**:129–134.

Landureau, J. C. 1966. Cultures *in vitro* de cellules embryonnaires de Blattes. *Exptl. Cell Res.* **41**:545–556.

Landureau, J. C. 1968. Cultures *in vitro* de cellules embryonnaires de Blattes (Insectes Dictyoptères). II. Obtention de lingnées cellulaires à multiplication continue. *Exptl. Cell Res.* **50**:323–337.

Levi-Montalcini, R. 1963. Growth and differentiation in the nervous system, pp. 261–295. *In* J. M. Allen (ed.). The Nature of Biological Diversity. McGraw-Hill, New York.

Levi-Montalcini, R., and Chen, J. S. 1969. *In vitro* studies of the insect embryonic nervous system, pp. 277–298. *In* S. H. Barondes (ed.). Cellular Dynamics of the Neuron. Academic Press, New York.

Levi-Montalcini, R., and Chen, R. S. 1971. Selective outgrowth of nerve fibers *in vitro* from embryonic ganglia of *Periplaneta americana*. *Arch. Ital. Biol.* **109**:307–337.

Locke, M. 1958. The formation of tracheae and tracheoles in *Rhodnius prolixus*. *Quart. J. Microscop. Sci.* **99**:29–46.

Lumsden, C. E. 1968. Nervous tissue in culture, pp. 67–140. *In* G. H. Bourne (ed.). The Structure and Function of Nervous Tissue, Vol. 1. Academic Press, New York.

Marks, E. P. 1968. Regenerating tissues from the cockroach *Leucophaea maderae*: Effects of humoral stimulation *in vitro*. *Gen. Comp. Endocrinol.* **11**:31–42.

Marks, E. P. 1970. The action of hormones in insect cell and organ cultures. *Gen. Comp. Endocrinol.* **15**:289–302.

Marks, E. P., and Reinecke, J. P. 1965. Regenerating tissues from the cockroach *Leucophaea maderae*: Effects of endocrine glands *in vitro*. *Gen. Comp. Endocrinol.* **5**:241–247.

Marks, E. P., Reinecke, J. P., and Leopold, R. A. 1968. Regenerating tissues from the cockroach *Leucophaea maderae*: nerve regeneration *in vitro*. *Biol. Bull.* **135**:520–529.

Meola, S. M., and Lea, A. O. 1972. The ultrastructure of the corpus cardiacum of *Aedes sollicitans* and the histology of the cerebral neurosecretory system of mosquitoes. *Gen. Comp. Endocrinol.* **18**:210–234.

Mordue, W., and Goldsworthy, G. J. 1969. The physiological effects of corpus cardiacum extracts in locusts. *Gen. Comp. Endocrinol.* **12**:360–369.

Muller, H. P., and Engelmann, F. 1968. Studies on the endocrine control of metabolism in *Leucophaea maderae* (Blattaria). II. Effect of the corpora cardiaca on fat-body respiration. *Gen. Comp. Endocrinol.* **11**:43–50.

Natalizi, G. M., and Frontali, N. 1966. Purification of insect hyperglycaemic and heart accelerating hormones. *J. Insect Physiol.* **12**:1279–1287.

Natalizi, G. M., Pansa, M. C., D'Ajello, V., Casaglia, O., Bettini, S., and Frontali, N. 1970. Physiologically active factors from corpora cardiaca of *Periplaneta americana*. *J. Insect Physiol.* **16**:1827–1836.

Normann, T. C. 1965. The neurosecretory system of the adult *Calliphora erythrocephala*. I. The fine structure of the corpus cardiacum with some observations on adjacent organs. *Z. Zellforsch.* **67**:461–501.

Normann, T. C., and Duve, H. 1969. Experimentally induced release of a neurohormone influencing hemolymph trehalose level in *Calliphora erythrocephala* (Diptera). *Gen. Comp. Endocrinol.* **12**:449–459.

Palay, S. L. 1957. The fine structure of the neurohypophysis, pp. 31–49. *In* H. Waelsch (ed.). Ultrastructure and Cellular Chemistry of Neural Tissue, Vol. II of Progress in Neurobiology. Paul B. Hoeber, New York.

Pearson, K. G. 1972. Central programming and reflex control of walking in the cockroach. *J. Exptl. Biol.* **56**:173–193.

Pearson, K. G., and Iles, J. F. 1970. Discharge patterns of coxal levator and depressor motoneurones of the cockroach, *Periplaneta americana*. *J. Exptl. Biol.* **52**:139–165.

Penzlin, H., and Stölzner, W. 1971. Frontal ganglion and water balance in *Periplaneta americana* L. *Experientia* **3**:390–391.

Peterson, E. R., and Crain, S. M. 1970. Innervation in cultures of fetal rodent skeletal muscle by organotypic explants of spinal cord from different animals. *Z. Zellforsch.* **106**:1–21.

Pichon, Y., and Callec, J. J. 1970. Further studies on synaptic transmission in insects. I. External recording of synaptic potentials in a single giant axon of the cockroach, *Periplaneta americana* L. *J. Exptl. Biol.* **52**:257–265.

Pipa, R. L., and Cook, E. F. 1959. Studies on the hexapod nervous system. I. The peripheral distribution of the thoracic nerves of the adult cockroach, *Periplaneta americana*. *Ann. Entomol. Soc. Am.* **52(6)**:695–710.

Scharrer, B. 1962. Neurosecretion. The fine structure of the neurosecretory system of the insect *Leucophaea maderae*. *Mem. Soc. Endocrinol.*, No. 12, pp. 89–97.

Scharrer, B. 1963. Neurosecretion. XIII. The ultrastructure of the corpus cardiacum of the insect *Leucophaea maderae*. *Z. Zellforsch.* **60**:761–796.

Scharrer, B., and Weitzman, M. 1970. Current problems in invertebrate neurosecretion, pp. 1–23. *In* W. Bargmann and B. Scharrer (eds.). Aspects of Neuroendocrinology. Springer-Verlag, Berlin, Heidelberg, New York.

Scharrer, E., and Scharrer, B. 1963. Neuroendocrinology. Columbia University Press, New York and London. 289 pp.

Schneider, I. 1967. Insect tissue culture, pp. 543–554. *In* N. Wilt and N. K. Wessells (eds.). Methods in Developmental Biology. Crowell, New York.

Schneiderman, H. A., and Gilbert, L. I. 1964. Control of growth and development in insects. *Science* **143**:325–333,

Seshan, K. R., and Levi-Montalcini, R. 1971. *In vitro* analysis of corpora cardiaca and corpora allata from nymphal and adult specimens of *Periplaneta americana*. *Arch. Ital. Biol.* **109**:81–109.

Sidman, R. L. 1970. Cell proliferation, migration and interaction in the developing mammalian central nervous system, pp. 100–107. *In* F. O. Schmitt, G. C. Quarton, T. Melnechuk, and G. Adelman (eds.). The Neurosciences—Second Study Program. Rockefeller University Press, New York.

Silvana, D. 1971. Cell culture of Diptera, pp. 247–265. *In* invertebrate Tissue Culture, Vol. 1. Academic Press, New York.

Smith, D. S. 1968*a*. Insect Cells: Their Structure and Function. Oliver and Boyd, Edinburgh.

Smith, D. S. 1968*b*. The trophic role of glial cells in insect ganglia, pp. 189–198. *In* J. W. L. Beament and J. E. Treherne (eds.). Insects and Physiology. American Elsevier, New York.

Smith, U., and Smith, D. S. 1966. Observations on the secretory processes in the corpus cardiacum of the stick insect, *Carausius morosus*. *J. Cell. Sci.* **1**:59–66.

Sperry, R. W. 1963. Chemoaffinity in the orderly growth of nerve fiber patterns and connections. *Proc. Natl. Acad. Sci.* **50**:703–710.

Sperry, R. W. 1965. Embryogenesis of behavioural nerve nets, pp. 161–186.*In* R.L.DeHaan and H. Ursprung (eds.). Organogenesis. Holt, Rinehart & Winston, New York.

Steele, J. E. 1961. Occurrence of a hyperglycaemic factor in the corpus cardiacum of an insect. *Nature* **192**:680–681.

Thomsen, E. 1952. Functional significance of the neurosecretory brain cells and the corpus cardiacum in the female blow-fly, *Calliphora erythrocephala* Meig. *J. Exptl. Biol.* **29**: 137–172.

Treherne, J. E. 1968. Axonal function and ionic regulation in insect central nervous tissue, pp. 175–188. *In* J. W. L. Beament and J. E. Treherne (eds.). Insects and Physiology. American Elsevier, New York.

Unnithan, G. C., Bern, H. A., and Nayar, K. K. 1971. Ultrastructural analysis of the neuroendocrine apparatus of *Oncopeltus fasciatus* (Heteroptera). *Acta Zool.* **52**:117–143.

Wigglesworth, V. B. 1954. The Physiology of Insect Metamorphosis. Cambridge University Press, London. 152 pp.

Wigglesworth, V. B. 1959. The histology of the nervous system of an insect, *Rhodnius prolixus* (Hemiptera). II. The central ganglia. *Quart. J. Microscop. Sci.* **100**:299–313.

Wigglesworth, V. B. 1964. The hormonal regulation of growth and reproduction in insects. pp. 247–335. *In* J. W. L. Beament, J. E. Treherne, and V. B. Wigglesworth (eds.) Advances in Insect Physiology. Academic Press, London and New York.

Wigglesworth, V. B. 1965. Cell associations and organogenesis in the nervous system of insects, pp. 199–217. *In* R. L. DeHaan and H. Ursprung (eds.). Organogenesis. Holt, Rinehart & Winston, New York.

Willey, R. B., and Chapman, G. B. 1960. The ultrastructure of certain components of the corpora cardiaca in orthopteroid insects. *J. Ultrastruct.* **4**:1–14.

Williams, C. M. 1963. Differentiation and morphogenesis in insects, pp. 243–260. *In* J. M. Allen (ed.). The Nature of Biological Diversity. McGraw-Hill, New York.

Williams, C. M. 1969. Nervous and hormonal communication in insect development, pp. 133–150. *In* A. Land (ed.). Developmental Biology. Suppl. 3, Communication in Development. Academic Press, New York and London.

Williams, C. L., and Kambysellis, M. P. 1969. *In vitro* action of ecdysone. *Proc. Natl. Acad. Sci.* **63**:231.

Young, D. 1969. The motor neurons of the mesothoracic ganglion of *Periplaneta americana. J. Insect Physiol.* **15**:1175–1179.

Chapter 2

Differentiation of Aggregating Brain Cell Cultures

Nicholas W. Seeds

Department of Biophysics and Genetics and Department of Psychiatry
University of Colorado Medical Center
Denver, Colorado

I. INTRODUCTION

Although nerve was the first tissue used for *in vitro* culture (Harrison, 1907), only recently have the techniques for the maintenance, growth, and development of nerve tissue *in vitro* advanced. Most studies of brain differentiation *in vitro* use small explants. These explants from various regions of fetal and newborn mouse brain can undergo structural and bioelectrical development during culture (Bornstein, 1964; Crain, 1966; Wolf, 1970). In addition, functional connections are formed between separated spinal cord, brain stem, and neocortex fragments (Crain *et al.,* 1968). However, the absence of sensitive biochemical procedures for detecting picomoles of product formation, in addition to the small size of the explants, has primarily limited the study of biochemical differentiation in explants to histochemical observations (Hosli and Hosli, 1970).

In an attempt to obtain larger amounts of nerve tissue for biochemical study and to assess the activity of specific cell types, several investigators

The author is a Career Development Awardee of the U.S.P.H.S. (1K04-GM40170), and his investigations are supported in part by a grant from the National Institutes of Health (NS-09818). This publication is from the Eleanor Roosevelt Institute of Cancer Research and the Department of Biophysics and Genetics (No. 516), University of Colorado Medical Center, Denver, Colorado.

35

(Wilson *et al.,* 1972; Werner *et al.,* 1971; Varon and Raiborn, 1969) have physically and enzymatically dissociated fetal brain tissue and cultured the cells as monolayers on the surface of glass or plastic petri dishes. Although monolayer cultures often show increases in specific activities of some enzymes related to neurotransmission during culture, these increases rarely surpass the specific activity of the undissociated fetal tissue (Rosenberg, this volume).

The limited biochemical development in monolayer cultures of brain cells suggests that three-dimensional cellular interactions destroyed by tissue dissociation may be required for differentiation. Such a requirement for specific cell interaction prior to ultimate differentiation would not be unique. There are several developing epithelial tissues (salivary gland, thyroid, kidney, skin, pancreas, thymus) that must interact for a specific time with mesenchymal cells prior to the onset of differentiation (Grobstein, 1964; Fleischmajor and Billingham, 1968). Furthermore, certain biochemical properties of cells are lost in monolayer cultures. One example is the ability of hydrocortisone to induce glutamine synthetase in explants of neural retina, a property that is rapidly lost when dissociated retinal cells are cultured in monolayers (Morris and Moscona, 1970).

II. AGGREGATION

Fortunately, an alternative cell culture technique is available that permits dissociated cells to interact in three dimensions. This procedure is called "aggregation culture" and has been studied in depth by Moscona and coworkers (Moscona, 1965). The tendency to aggregate is a property of all embryonic cells. However, the degree of aggregation largely depends on the tissue of origin and the age or state of differentiation of the cells. In general, the more undifferentiated the tissue the better the aggregation. Furthermore, the *in vitro* conditions greatly influence the rate and extent of aggregation (Table I).

Aggregate formation is enhanced by gently rotating suspensions of trypsin-dissociated cells in Erlenmeyer flasks on a gyrotary shaker. A speed (about 70 rpm) is selected such that the cells are brought into a vortex, thereby

TABLE I

Factors Influencing Cellular Aggregation

Tissue of origin
State of differentiation of cells
Rotation speed
Temperature
Ca^{2+}
Serum protein
Cell-specific aggregation factors

greatly increasing the number of collisions between cells. At higher speeds, the shearing forces increase; therefore, aggregate size decreases, but the number of aggregates per flask increases. The volume and composition of the cell culture medium are also important variables. Aggregation requires the presence of Ca^{2+} and is greatly enhanced by serum protein. Furthermore, aggregation is directly dependent on the incubation temperature, with maximal aggregation occurring at 37–38°C. Lower temperatures reduce aggregate size, and temperatures below 15°C completely block aggregation, suggesting that cell adhesion does not depend solely on ionic interactions but requires some metabolic processes (Moscona, 1961). This metabolic requirement may be the replacement of cell-surface molecules lost on dissociation. New protein synthesis appears to be a requirement for reaggregation, since puromycin inhibits this phenomenon (Moscona and Moscona, 1963).

The aggregation of cells from a specific tissue decreases with increasing differentiation. Dissociated cells from adult mouse brain aggregate poorly and from small aggregates less than 200 μ in diameter; however, brain cells from 16-day fetuses readily form aggregates greater than 1000 μ in diameter. Furthermore, the mixing of adult cells with fetal cells leads to decreased aggregation of the fetal cells. Similar results are obtained with coaggregates of fetal brain and neuroblastoma or glioma cells. The differences in aggregatibility of cells during differentiation probably reflects change in the composition of their cell surface. This proposal is supported by the finding that binding sites for plant agglutinins on embryonic and neoplastic cells are readily exposed; however, on adult cells these sites are masked and only uncovered by trypsinization (Moscona, 1971). Thus the cell interactions taking place during aggregation probably reflect the exposure of certain sites on the cell surface that function during morphogenesis and become masked when differentiation is complete.

The chemical nature of groups on the cell surface responsible for aggregation is not known. Although silalic acid moieties represent a major component of the cell surface, they do not appear to be involved in neural retina aggregation (McQuiddy and Lilien, 1971). However, Roth and coworkers (Roth et al., 1971) have demonstrated that β-galactosyl residues on the surface of neural retina cells are partially responsible for specificity of cell adhesion. Aggregation also involves macromolecules that occupy intercellular space. The enhancement of aggregation by serum has been attributed to its content of one such intercellular macromolecule, the mucopolysaccharide hyaluronic acid (Pessac and Defendi, 1972). However, we have found hyaluronidase-treated sera to be completely active in mouse brain cell aggregation.

An additional feature of some aggregating cells is their ability to secrete specific aggregation factors. Such factors have been isolated from sponges (Humphreys, 1963), chick neural retina cells (Lilien, 1968), and embryonic

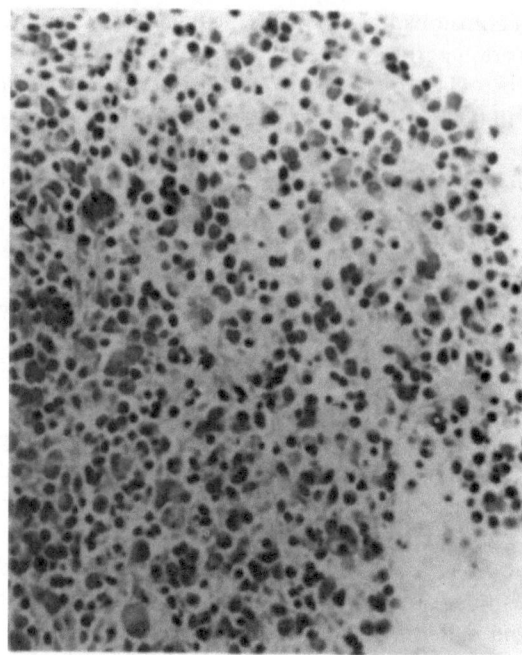

Fig. 1. Section through an aggregate after 1 day of culture. Stained with hematoxylin eosin Y, and azure II.

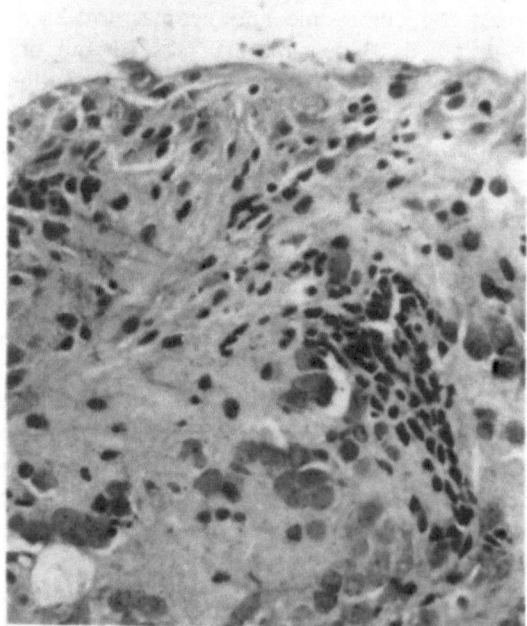

Fig. 2. Section through an aggregate after 12 days of culture.

mouse brain cells (Garber and Moscona, 1972b). These factors are produced only by cells in a certain developmental stage. Furthermore, they are specific and enhance aggregation of only homologous cell types of a specific age; that is, factor from retina promotes only aggregation of retinal cells. Although the aggregation factors obtained from sponge cells are species specific (Margoliash et al., 1965), these aggregation-enhancing factors from mouse cerebrum demonstrate tissue specificity but lack species specificity. Aggregation-factor preparations from 14-day embryonic mouse cerebrum cells enhance the aggregation of dissociated cells from mouse or chick cerebrum; however, the aggregation-enhancing material is without effect on mouse cerebellum, medulla, and liver as well as chick optic tectum, cerebellum, neural retina, liver, and kidney (Garber and Moscona, 1972b). The lack of species specificity suggests that the cell-surface properties related to histogenesis have been conserved during evolution.

The physicochemical characterization of these aggregation-enhancing factors has been limited. They appear to be glycoproteins that exist in complexes with molecular weights of several million. In the absence of calcium, the sponge factor completely dissociates into 4.2 and $2.3S_{20}$ components, the smallest being approximately 15,000 mol. wt. (Margoliash et al., 1965). The lipids detected represented less than 1 mole per mole of protein, and nucleic acid represented less than 5% of the material. However, at present it is not possible to attribute aggregation enhancement to a specific glycoprotein molecule.

III. MIGRATION

Aggregation is complete within 12–24 hr, and these initial aggregates are composed of loosely packed and randomly dispersed cells (Fig. 1). One notable feature at this early stage is the presence of small cellular extensions. After several days, there is an increase in cellular outgrowth, thus forming a more stable complex. During this time, the cells undergo extensive migration and segregate within the aggregate into clusters of similar cell types (Fig. 2). The ability of cells derived from different tissues to sort out in aggregates of mixed cell populations has been known for many years (Trinkaus and Groves, 1955; Moscona, 1956). Since there are many cell types in brain and the various brain regions develop at different rates, it is not surprising that cells of specific brain regions segregate themselves from cells of other regions (Garber and Moscona, 1972a). Due to the staining differences between chick and mouse cells (Moscona, 1957), this segregation is readily apparent in coaggregates of mouse cerebrum and chick optic tectum. In contrast, coaggregates of chick cerebrum and mouse cerebrum show no segregation, with both cell types dispersed throughout the aggregate.

More impressive is the ability of cells from a specific brain region to migrate and organize themselves into structures whose architecture closely resembles that of the brain area sampled. Such histotypic pattern formation has been most dramatically demonstrated in aggregates of hippocampal cells from 18.5-day fetal mice, where pyramidal neurons align in a configuration characteristic of Ammon's horn (DeLong, 1970). The formation of these histotypic structures is very age dependent and occurs only in aggregates derived from animals of a particular age. Furthermore, cerebral and cerebellar aggregates of cells from the "reeler" mutant mouse show the same lack of cellular alignment and orientation that characterizes the genetic defect *in vivo* (DeLong and Sidman, 1970).

The sorting out observed in coaggregates of different tissues or dissimilar areas of a given organ may be explained in terms of a differential adhesion hypothesis (Steinberg, 1970). This hypothesis implies that sorting out is a quantitative property where cells seek the most thermodynamically favorable situation. However, the formation of histotypic patterns appears to require specific cell–cell interactions for establishing the proper alignment of cells after they have sorted out. Thus alignment may be a qualitative selection process. Most notably, these studies suggest that the guiding force in histogenesis is a property of individual cells, not preexisting cellular matrices.

IV. BIOCHEMICAL DIFFERENTIATION

The ability of dissociated cells to reestablish specific cell–cell contacts and produce histotypic patterns characteristic of the original tissue suggested that aggregate cultures may show biochemical differentiation similar to that of the developing brain. Embryonic mouse brain was chosen as a source of cells for our biochemical studies for several reasons. Brain cells from fetal mice readily aggregate to form large (greater than 1000 μ), easily manageable aggregates. At present, the mouse is the only animal with complex neurological abilities suited for genetic studies; over 100 neurological mutants of the mouse have been characterized thus far (Sidman *et al.,* 1965). Furthermore, fetal mouse brain cells are relatively undifferentiated with respect to the biochemistry of neurotransmission. The greatest development of many biochemical activities related to neurotransmission occurs postnatally. This is seen in Fig. 3, where the activities of three neuronal enzymes–choline acetyltransferase, acetylcholinesterase, and glutamate decarboxylase increase ten- to twentyfold between the first and third weeks postnatally. This is the same time period during which most dendritic branching and synapse formation occurs (Aghajanian and Bloom, 1967).

Cholinesterase activity resistant to the acetylcholinesterase specific

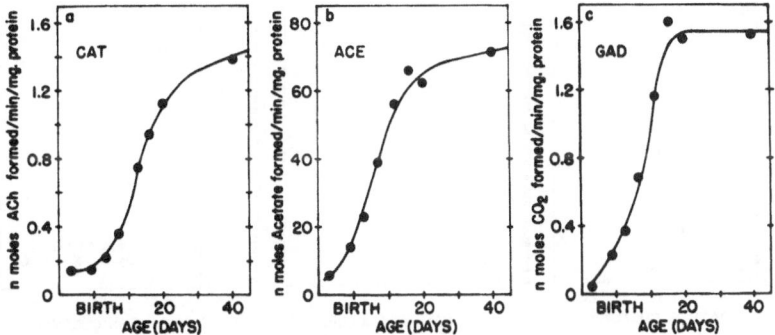

Fig. 3. *In vivo* development of choline acetyltransferase (a), acetylcholinesterase (b), and glutamate decarboxylase (c) in the whole brain of C57Bl/6J mice. (From Seeds, 1971.)

inhibitor BW-284-C51 has been subtracted from the values shown in Fig. 3b. The cholinesterase activity represents 5–8% of the total acetylcholine hydrolytic activity in fetal brain and 2–5% in adult mouse brain. Furthermore, brain tissue possesses two enzymatic activities capable of decarboxylating L-gluta-mate-1-C^{14}. One enzyme is glutamate decarboxylase (E.C. 4.1.1.15), which is inhibited by chloride and requires a pyridoxal phosphate cofactor. Glutamate decarboxylase is responsible for γ-aminobutyrate synthesis and appears to be a neuronal enzyme. The other activity which is stimulated by chloride and unaffected by the pyridoxal phosphate inhibitor amino-oxyacetic acid is thought to be of glial or mitochondrial origin (Haber *et al.*, 1970). The gluta-mate decarboxylase activity in Fig. 3c represents both activities. In 15-day-old fetal brain, 20% of the activity is of the glial form, whereas in the adult brain less than 5% of the activity is the glial enzyme.

Aggregate cultures derived from 17-day-old fetal mice show increases in choline acetyltransferase, acetylcholinesterase, and glutamate decarboxylase specific activities similar to those in developing mouse brain (Fig. 4). Choline acetyltransferase increases over twentyfold to an activity 70% that of adult mouse brain *in vivo*. Similarly, a tenfold increase in acetylcholinesterase activity is observed in the cultures. The maximum level is 40% of the adult brain. Furthermore, cholinesterase activity decreases from 9% of the total esterase activity in freshly dissociated fetal cells to less than 3% in 21-day-old aggregate cultures. Glutamate decarboxylase activity increases fivefold during aggregate culture and is one-third the specific activity of adult brain. In addition, the mitochondrial or glial activity decreases during cell culture. More recent culturing procedures give choline acetyltransferase and acetylcholines-terase specific activities that are 90% those of adult mouse brain. The radioactive products of the choline acetyltransferase and glutamate decarboxylase

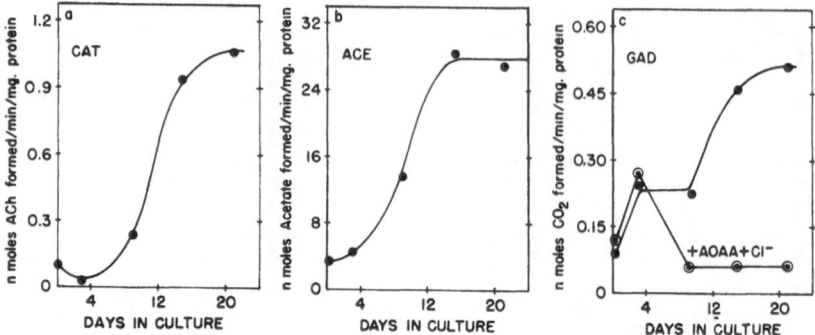

Fig. 4. *In vitro* development of choline acetyltransferase (a), acetylcholinesterase (b), and glutamate decarboxylase (c) in brain cell aggregates. The activities of the undissociated brain tissue are 0.18, 11, and 0.13, respectively. In (c), the filled circles represent neuronal decarboxylase activity as assayed in the presence of pyridoxal phosphate, and the open circles around dots represent the glial or mitochondrial decarboxylase activity, which is assayed in the presence of amino-oxyacetic acid and Cl^-. (From Seeds, 1971.)

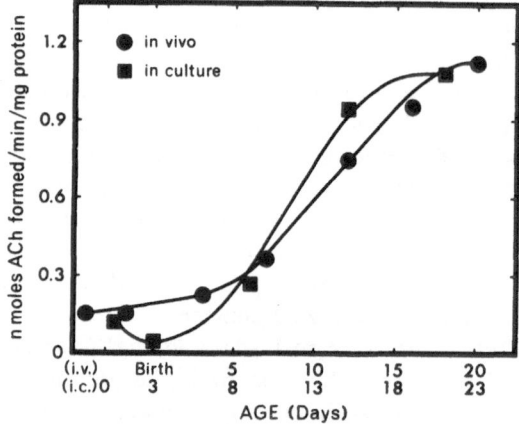

Fig. 5. The pattern of development of choline acetyltransferase activity in the aggregate culture and the living mouse brain. (From Seeds, 1972.)

reactions show cochromatography with acetylcholine and γ-aminobutyrate in several solvents. Absolute identification of the radio labeled products is necessary since in certain cell cultures the products are not always the expected material (Amano *et al.*, 1972; Wilson *et al.*, 1972).

Not only do the levels of enzyme activity approximate those *in vivo*, but the patterns of development are also remarkably similar to the *in vivo* situation (Fig. 5). These findings suggest that the cellular or intercellular mechanisms controlling the time course for expression of the differentiated state are retained in the *in vitro* environment. Furthermore, a 20-hr exposure to radio labeled thymidine shows that only 1–2% of the cells are labeled in 8- to 10-day-old aggregates. Thus there is very little cell division in the aggregate cultures during the time of increased enzyme specific activity.

If these aggregates are developing in a manner typical of neurons, the increased enzyme activity should be coupled with increased storage of the putative neurotransmitters. The accumulation of transmitters can be readily detected following tissue incubation with radiochemical precursors of suspected neurotransmitters (Hildebrand *et al.*, 1971). Using this procedure, acetylcholine-C^{14} has been extracted from the brain aggregates after incubation in basal Eagle's medium containing choline-C^{14}.

Since the three activities observed in Fig. 4 are relatively specific for neurons, the development of enzymes found in both neurons and glia is of interest. Of additional interest is the behavior of enzymes that either decrease or show no change in specific activity during development. Four enzymatic activities that fit these criteria have been observed in the aggregates. Monoamine oxidase is a mitochondrial enzyme that increases severalfold during brain maturation (Table II), with a pattern of development very similar to that of the three neuronal activities discussed above. The greatest increase in rat brain monoamine oxidase activity occurs between the first and third postnatal weeks (Bennett and Giarman, 1965). The enzyme is found in both neural and glial tumors; however, glial cells show severalfold-higher specific activities (Silberstein *et al.*, 1972; Seeds, 1973). In contrast, the activity of catechol-*O*-methyltransferase shows little change during brain development (Table II). This enzyme is also found in both neural and glial tumors (Blume *et al.*, 1970;

TABLE II

MAO, COMT, and PGP Development[a]

Tissue	MAO	COMT	PGP
In vivo			
Fetal brain	0.4	0.067	1.3
Adult	0.9	0.075	0.3
In vitro			
Dissociated			
cells	0.3	0.065	2.6
Aggregate	1.2	0.076	1.7

[a]The specific activities (nmoles product formed/min/mg protein) of monoamine oxidase, catechol-*O*-methyltransferase, and phosphogluconate pathway in 17-day fetal mouse brain, adult brain, freshly dissociated brain cells from 17-day-old fetus, and 20-day aggregate cultures are compared. (From Seeds, 1973.)

Silberstein *et al.*, 1972). Two enzymes, glucose-6-phosphate dehydrogenase and 6-phosphogluconate dehydrogenase, decrease during rat brain development (Kuhlman and Lowry, 1956; Bagdasarian and Hulanicka, 1965). The activity of these two enzymes can be followed using glucose-6-phosphate-1-C^{14} in a single assay designated the "phosphogluconate pathway." The phosphogluconate activity in mouse brain decreases greater than threefold after birth (Table II).

The behavior of these three non-neuron-specific enzymes in the aggregate cultures is also shown in Table II. Monoamine oxidase and catechol-*O*-methyltransferase show levels of activity and patterns of development that mimic the *in vivo* situation. The phosphogluconate activity decreases during *in vitro* culture; however, the specific activity of trypsin-dissociated cells is higher than in fetal brain (Table II). This increase upon dissociation may reflect a disproportionate loss of protein from cells during trypsinization. Alternatively, the increased activity may represent a demand for NADPH by lipid metabolism needed for membrane repairs. Thus brain aggregates continue to demonstrate a developmental behavior that is essentially identical to brain maturation.

Brain development is characterized by a shift in carbohydrate metabolism toward more oxidative metabolism. One enzyme related to this transition is lactate dehydrogenase, which increases two- to threefold during this period (Kuhlman and Lowry, 1956; Lehrer *et al.*, 1970). In addition, lactate dehydrogenase shows a change in isoenzyme patterns during development (Bonavita *et al.*, 1964). While the muscle type is predominant in neuroblastoma (N–18), glial tumor (C–6), and fetal brain, the heart-type subunit prevails in adult mouse brain. These two subunits are coded for by two different genes; therefore, this transition represents a specific change in mRNA synthesis or translation. For this reason, it is of interest to observe the behavior of the isoenzyme pattern of brain cell aggregates (Fig. 6). The brain cell aggregates have an isoenzyme pattern intermediate to that of fetal tissue and adult brain.

TABLE III

Development of Monolayer Cultures[a]

Cells	CAT	ACE	GAD	PGP	MAO	COMT
Dissociated cells	0.08	2.98	0.17	2.6	0.30	0.067
Monolayer	0.05	2.43	0.08	1.5	0.47	0.053

[a]Fetal brain tissue was dissociated into individual cells that were cultured for 11 days on the surface of plastic dishes. The specific activities (nmoles product formed/min/mg protein) of several enzymes were compared to the activities of freshly dissociated cells. (From Seeds, 1971, 1973.)

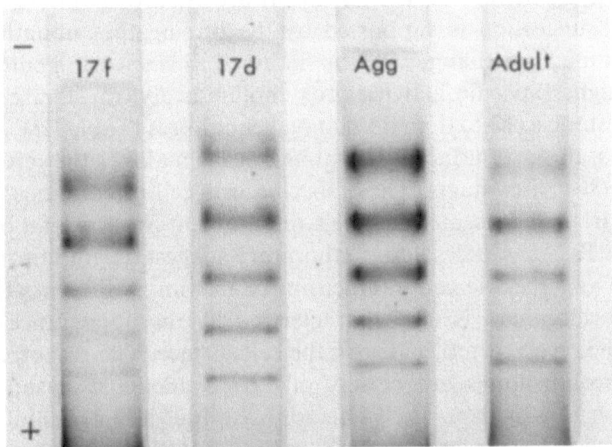

Fig. 6. Lactate dehydrogenase isoenzyme patterns of mouse brain and aggregate cultures. From left to right are 17-day fetal brain, 17-day postnatal brain, 24-day-old aggregate cultures, an adult mouse brain. Embryonic brain is characterized by the slower-moving muscle forms (M_4 and M_3H).

Further characterization of intermediate-age tissues shows that the aggregate pattern is similar to that of the 17-day-old whole brain. Similar isoenzyme changes have recently been demonstrated in explants of mouse cerebrum (Maker *et al.*, 1972).

As previously mentioned, monolayer cultures of normal brain tissue rarely acquire the characteristics of a differentiated state. Dissociated cells from 17-day fetal mice were cultured as monolayers on plastic dishes. The development of these cultures after 11 days *in vitro* is shown in Table III. Although the three neuron-specific enzymes increase in the aggregated cultures (Fig. 4), these same activities decrease during this time interval in monolayer cultures. Only the non-neuron-specific activities phosphogluconate pathway, monoamine oxidase, and catechol-*O*-methyltransferase resemble normal developmental trends.

The inability of monolayer cultures to demonstrate maximal biochemical development characteristic of neurons may be the result of several factors. Monolayer culturing favors cell division, whereas aggregation places cells in a contact-inhibited environment, thus restricting cellular division and possibly favoring differentiation. Therefore, the glial or epithelial cells may divide more readily and serve only to dilute the activity of the slowly dividing neuronal population. Another contributing factor is that neurons do not attach well to the plastic dishes; therefore, many neurons are discarded at the first medium change. This suggestion is supported by the finding that nonattached cells from the first medium change when maintained as suspension cultures for 11 days show higher specific activities for choline acetyltransferase (0.14) and acetylcholinesterase (12.5) than do monolayer cultures (Table III). A third and probably most important factor is that aggregation allows the reformation of preexisting cell–cell contacts. These specific cell–cell interactions, which are formed only in the aggregate, may be a requirement for maximal biochemical development. Recent studies in our laboratory suggest the importance of critical cell mass and specific cell interaction for maximal differentiation.

Brain development is also characterized by the appearance of specific neurohormone receptor molecules on the cell surface. The receptors for some of these neurohormones are closely linked to adenyl cyclase; thus these hormones presumably exert their effect by altering the intracellular levels of adenosine-cyclic-3',5'-monophosphate (cyclic AMP). Prostaglandins, histamine, norepinephrine, isoproterenol, and 5-hydroxytryptamine promote the rapid accumulation of cyclic AMP in brain slices (Rall and Sattin, 1970). Within minutes, norepinephrine produces a fivefold increase in the level of cyclic AMP in slices of cerebral cortex from both rat and mouse. This stimulation is not observed in brains of newborn rats and appears first in brain tissue 4 days of age, with maximal effect occurring at day 10 (Schmidt *et al.,* 1970). The acquisition of the cyclic AMP response is thought to reflect the formation of β-adrenergic receptors on the cell surface during postnatal days 4–10.

Since the increase of cyclic AMP levels in response to norepinephrine represents a developmental event occurring during brain maturation, the response of brain cell aggregates to norepinephrine or the β-adrenergic effector isoproterenol was examined (Seeds and Gilman, 1971). As expected, fetal mouse brain tissue does not respond to norepinephrine or isoproterenol (Table IV). Although aggregate formation is essentially complete, the catecholamines fail to elicit an increase of cyclic AMP levels in 15-hr cultures. However, after 9 days of culture the aggregates show a four- to sixfold increase in cyclic AMP levels following a 15-min incubation with either norepinephrine or isoproterenol, thus resembling adult mouse brain (Table IV). Neither increased culturing time nor the presence of theophylline alters the magnitude of the response.

Further studies by Gilman and coworkers (Gilman and Nirenberg, 1971; Gilman and Schrier, 1972) have demonstrated that clonal cell lines of rat glial tumors and fetal rat brain monolayer cultures, rich in glial cells, show large (50- to 200-fold) stimulating effects of catecholamines on intracellular levels of cyclic AMP. The isoproterenol response of these cells was inhibited by the β-adrenergic blockers sotatol and dichlorisoproterenol; however, the response

TABLE IV

Effect of Catecholamines on Cyclic AMP Levels[a]

| | Cyclic AMP (pmole/mg protein) | | |
| | | Cell culture | |
Additions	Fetal tissue	15 hr	9 days
None	11	12	8.5
Norepinephrine	11	10	38
Isoproterenol	14	14	45

[a]Brain cell aggregates and fetal tissue were preincubated for 30 min in Eagle's basal medium plus 10^{-3} M theophylline 30°C. Norepinephrine and isoproterenol were added at a concentration of 10^{-4} M each, and incubation was continued for 15 min. Tissues were then assayed for cyclic AMP content (Gilman, 1970) and protein. (From Seeds and Gilman, 1971.)

was unaffected by the α-adrenergic blocking agent phentotamine. Similar results have been found with a human glioma cell line (Clark and Perkins, 1971). These studies suggest that the cyclic AMP response in brain and in brain aggregates may be due primarily to glial elements. The more "normal" magnitude of the response seen in the aggregates probably reflects the more natural proportions of neurons and glial in these cultures.

A wide variety of biochemical events that characterize brain maturation have been examined in reaggregating mouse brain cell cultures. These events include biochemical activities that increase, decrease, and remain stationary during development; furthermore, many of these events occur in different types of brain cells. In all cases, the aggregate cultures were similar to the mouse brain in both magnitude and time course of development. Thus brain cell aggregates appear to be a faithful model system for studying the biochemical development of the brain.

V. MORPHOLOGICAL DIFFERENTIATION

The increased specific activities of choline acetyltransferase, acetylcholinesterase, and glutamate decarboxylase and the high degree of cellular organization in the aggregates suggest that brain cell aggregates may undergo morphological differentiation characteristic of brain maturation. The two most characteristic features of brain development are synaptogenesis and myelination. Both of these events occur rather late in brain differentiation.

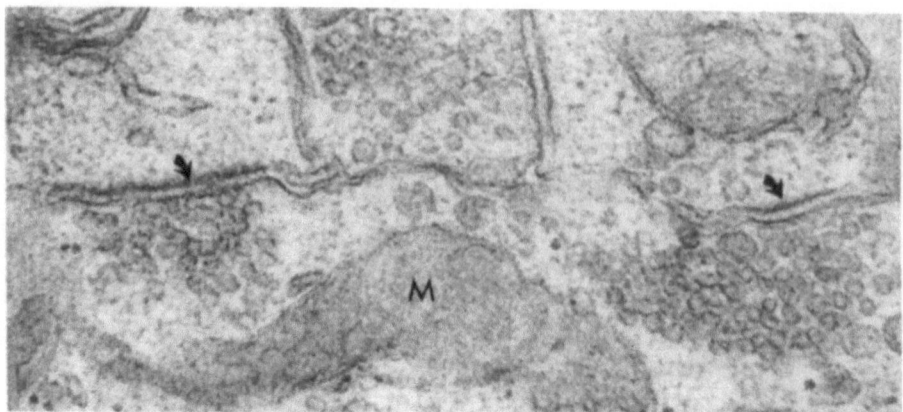

Fig. 7. Morphologically mature synaptic complexes in an aggregate after 35 days of culture. Note the mitochondrion (M), the numerous small vesicles, and the opposing dark membranes (arrow). (From Seeds and Vatter, 1971.)

Most synapse formation in mouse brain occurs between 10 and 20 days after birth (Aghajanian and Bloom, 1967; Woodward *et al.*, 1971). The time sequence for synaptic development correlates well with eye opening, maturation of the electroencephalograph recording, and development of adult behavioral patterns (Himwich, 1964). Myelinated axons are first observed in the mouse brain approximately 10 days after birth, and myelination continues for several weeks (Karlsson, 1967).

There are very few synapses in the 16-day-old fetal mouse brain, and these are generally restricted to the spinal cord (Crain *et al.*, 1968; Model *et al.*, 1971); however, trypsin-dissociated cells from 16-day-old fetal brain were examined by electron microscopy (Seeds and Vatter, 1971). Although a small number of cells occurred in clusters of two or more, the regions of contact did not show any specialization of cellular membranes suggestive of synaptic structures, thus ruling out the possibility that previously formed synapses were carried through the cell dissociation procedure.

After 12 days in culture, a few scattered asymmetrical junctional complexes are found in the aggregates. These synaptic structures are immature as judged by the scarcity of synaptic vesicles, waviness of cell membranes, and relative absence of opaque material associated with the opposing synaptic membranes. In contrast, 33-day-old aggregate cultures contain many morphologically mature synapses (Fig. 7). The number of synaptic vesicles is much greater, the synaptic cleft is wider (250 A), the presence of mitochondria in presynaptic terminals is more apparent, and much more opaque material is associated with the postsynaptic membrane. These structures are similar to the mature axodendritic synapses of adult mouse brain (Gray, 1959). Since the synapses are found in groups and not evenly distributed within the aggregate, a direct comparison of the number of synapses in aggregates of various ages is difficult; however, we estimate that there is about a fivefold increase from day 12 to day 33. The subcellular structure of aggregates at all ages resembles that in normal brain development and suggests that the aggregates are in good health.

An additional feature of the 33-day-old aggregate is the presence of myelin-like structures (Seeds and Vatter, 1971). These structures are not observed in the young tissue (day 12). The inner loops and the compactness and periodicity of the membranes as well as the presence of mitochondria are all identical to what is found in myelinated neurons in the adult brain. Thus aggregate culture derived from totally dissociated fetal mouse brain can perform two highly specialized morphological events requiring cell–cell interaction that are characteristic of mouse brain differentiation.

Recently, Bornstein and Model (1972) have demonstrated the presence of synapses and myelin in small aggregates of dissociated fetal spinal cord and brain stem. Both dendritic and axosomatic synapses are found. Furthermore, these aggregates show electrical activity, including rhythmic discharge patterns suggesting complex circuits of excitatory and inhibitory potentials (Crain and Bornstein, 1972).

VI. PROSPECTUS

The studies with aggregate cultures described in this chapter have merely shown that brain aggregate cultures behave in a manner very similar to developing brain, and for this reason the aggregates appear to be a reliable model system. As of now, the aggregates have done little to further our knowledge of brain development; therefore, their value rests solely with the future.

The biochemical and morphological development of aggregates makes them very suitable systems for observing the effects of various drugs and hormones on brain development in a relatively defined environment. Furthermore, the ability of cells to migrate and form histotypic patterns within the aggregates as well as the availability of neurological mutant mice that express their migratory defects *in vitro* should provide a much greater understanding of the genetic control of cell migration. In this regard, chemical characterization of cell membranes from normal and mutant cell types would appear to be a promising area.

Since the system can be dissociated and reconstituted, we are now in a position to ask questions about the role of specific cell types in the final product. Cell fractionation procedures by Barkley *et al.* (1972) and in our laboratory appear most promising. Then aggregates consisting of various permutations and combinations of cell types can be formed and the role of specific cell–cell interactions in development determined. The complexity of the system could be reduced and a simple system of a few cell types that form a predictable pattern of synapses achieved. Thus the aggregates' future in neurobiology appears bright.

VII. ACKNOWLEDGMENTS

I gratefully acknowledge the collaborative efforts of Drs. Albert Vatter and Alfred Gilman on portions of these studies. The technical assistance of Miss Susan Cotten is greatly appreciated.

VIII. REFERENCES

Aghajanian, G. K., and Bloom, F. E. 1967. The formation of synaptic junctions in developing rat brain: A quantitative electron microscopic study. *Brain Res.* **6**:716–727.

Amano, T., Richelson, E., and Nirenberg, M. 1972. Neurotransmitter synthesis by neuroblastoma clones. *Proc. Natl. Acad. Sci.* **69**:258–263.

Bagdasarian, G., and Hulanicka, D. 1965. Changes of mitochondrial glucose-6-phosphate dehydrogenase and 6-phosphogluconate dehydrogenase during brain development. *Biochim. Biophys. Acta* **99**:367–369.

Barkley, D. S., Rakin, L. L., Chaffee, J. K., and Wong, D. L. 1972. Cell separation of newborn mouse cerebellum by velocity sedimentation. *J. Cell Biol.* **55**:15a.

Bennett, D. S., and Giarman, N. J. 1965. Schedule of appearance of 5–hydroxytryptamine (serotonin) and associated enzymes in the developing rat brain. *J. Neurochem.* **12**: 911–918.

Blume, A., Gilbert, F., Wilson, S., Farber, J., Rosenberg, R., and Nirenberg, M. 1970. Regulation of acetylcholinesterase in neuroblastoma cells. *Proc. Natl. Acad. Sci.* **67**: 786–792.

Bonavita, V., Ponte, F., and Amore, G. 1964. Lactic dehydrogenase isoenzymes in nervous tissue IV. An ontogenetic study on the rat brain. *J. Neurochem.* **11**:39–47.

Bornstein, M. B. 1964. Morphological development of neonatal mouse cerebral cortex in tissue culture, pp. 1–11. *In* P. Kellaway and I. Petersen (eds.). Neurological and Electroencephalographic Correlative Studies in Infancy. Grune & Stratton, New York.

Bornstein, M. D., and Model, P. G. 1972. Development of synapses and myelin in cultures of dissociated embryonic mouse spinal cord, medulla and cerebrum. *Brain Res.* **37**: 287–293.

Clark, R. B., and Perkins, J. P. 1971. Regulation of adenosine 3':5'–cyclic monophosphate concentration in cultured human astrocytoma cells by catecholamines and histamine. *Proc. Natl. Acad. Sci.* **68**:2757–2760.

Crain, S. M. 1966. Development of "organotypic" bioelectric activities in central nervous tissues during maturation in culture. *Internat. Rev. Neurobiol.* **9**:1–43.

Crain, S. M., and Bornstein, M. B. 1972. Organotypic bioelectric activity in cultured reaggregates of dissociated rodent brain cells. *Science* **176**:182–184.

Crain, S. M., Peterson, E. R., and Bornstein, M. B. 1968. Formation of functional interneuronal connexions between explants of various mammalian central nervous tissues during development *in vitro*. pp. 13–40. *In* Growth of the Nervous System. Ciba Symposium; Little, Brown, Boston.

DeLong, G. R. 1970. Histogenesis of fetal mouse isocortex and hippocampus in reaggregating cell cultures. *Develop. Biol.* **22**:563–583.

DeLong, G. R., and Sidman, R. L. 1970. Alignment defect of reaggregating cells in cultures of developing brains of reeler mutant mice. *Develop. Biol.* **22**:584–600.

Fleischmajer, R., and Billingham, R. E. 1968. Epithelial–Mesenchymal Interactions. Williams & Wilkins, Baltimore. 326 pp.

Garber, B. B., and Moscona, A. A. 1972a. Reconstruction of brain tissue from cell suspensions I. Aggregation patterns of cells dissociated from different regions of the developing brain. *Develop. Biol.* **27**:217–234.

Garber, B. B., and Moscona, A. A. 1972b. Reconstruction of brain tissue from cell suspensions. II. Specific enhancement of aggregation of embryonic cerebral cells by supernatant from homologous cell cultures. *Develop. Biol.* **27**:235–243.

Gilman, A. G. 1970. A Protein binding assay for adenosine 3',5'-phosphate. *Proc. Nat. Acad. Sci.* **67**:305–311.

Gilman, A. G., and Nirenberg, M. 1971. Effect of catecholamines on the adenosine 3':5'-cyclic monophosphate concentrations of clonal satellite cells of neurons. *Proc. Natl. Acad. Sci.* **68**:2165–2168.

Gilman, A. G., and Schrier, B. K. 1972. Adenosine cyclic 3',5'–monophosphate in fetal rat brain cell cultures. I. Effect of catecholamines. *Molec. Pharmacol.* **8**:410–416.

Gray, E. G. 1959. Axo-somatic and axo-dendritic synapses of the cerebral cortex: An electron microscope study. *J. Anat.* **93**:420–439.

Grobstein, C. 1964. Cytodifferentiation and its controls. *Science* **143**:643–650.

Haber, B., Kuriyama, K., and Roberts, E. 1970. L-Glutamic acid decarboxylase: A new type in glial cells and human brain gliomas. *Science* **168**:598–599.

Harrison, R. G. 1907. Observations on the living developing nerve fiber. *Proc. Soc. Exp. Biol.* (N.Y.) **4**:140–150.

Hildebrand, J. G., Barker, D. L., Herbert, E., and Kravitz, E. A. 1971. Screening for neurotransmitters: A rapid radiochemical procedure. *J. Neurobiol.* **2**:231–246.

Himwich, W. H. 1964. Biochemical and neurophysiological development of the brain in the neonatal period. *Internat. Rev. Neurobiol.* **4**:117–158.

Hösli, E., and Hösli, L. 1970. The presence of acetylcholinesterase in cultures of cerebellum and brain stem. *Brain Res.* **19**:494–496.

Humphreys, T. 1963. Chemical dissolution and *in vitro* reconstruction of sponge cell adhension. I. Isolation and functional demonstration of the components involved. *Develop. Biol.* **8**:27–47.

Karlsson, U. 1967. Observations on the postnatal development of neuronal structures in the lateral geniculate nucleus of the rat by electron microscopy. *J. Ultrastruct. Res.* **17**:158–175.

Kuhlman, R. E., and Lowry, O. H. 1956. Quantitative histochemical changes during the development of the rat cerebral cortex. *J. Neurochem.* **1**:173–180.

Lehrer, G. M., Bornstein, M. B., Weiss, C., and Silides, D. J. 1970. Enzymatic maturation of mouse cerebral neocortex *in vitro* and *in situ*. *Exptl. Neurol.* **26**:595–606.

Lilien, J. E. 1968. Specific enhancement of cell aggregation *in vitro*. *Develop. Biol.* **17**:657–678.

Maker, H. S., Lehrer, G. M., Weissbarth, S., and Bornstein, M. B. 1972. Changes in LDH isoenzymes of brain developing *in situ* and *in vitro*. *Brain Res.* **44**:189–196.

Margoliash, E., Schenck, J. R., Hargie, M. P., Burokar, S., Richter, W. R., Barlow, G. H., and Moscona, A. A. 1965. Characterization of specific cell aggregating materials from sponge cells. *Biochem. Biophys. Res. Commun.* **20**:383–388.

McQuiddy, P., and Lilien, J. 1971. Sialic acid and cell aggregation. *J. Cell Sci.* **9**:823–833.

Model, P. G., Bornstein, M. B., Crain, S. M., and Pappas, G. D. 1971. An electron microscopic study of the development of synapses in cultured fetal mouse cerebrum continuously exposed to xylocaine. *J. Cell Biol.* **40**:362–371.

Morris, J. E., and Moscona, A. A. 1970. Induction of glutamine synthetase in embryonic retina: Its dependence on cell interactions. *Science* **167**:1736–1738.

Morris, J. E., and Moscona, A. A. 1971. The induction of glutamine synthetase in cell aggregates of embryonic neural retina: Correlations with differentiation and multicellular organization. *Develop. Biol.* **25**:420–444.

Moscona, A. 1956. Development of heterotypic combinations of dissociated embryonic chick cells. *Proc. Soc. Exptl. Biol.* **92**:410–416.

Moscona, A. 1957. The development *in vitro* of chimeric aggregates of dissociated embryonic chick and mouse cells. *Proc. Natl. Acad. Sci.* **43**:184–193.

Moscona, A. 1961. Effect of temperature on adhesion to glass and histogenetic cohesion of dissociated cells. *Nature* **190**:408–409.

Moscona, A. A. 1965. Recombination of dissociated cells and the development of cell aggregates, pp. 489–529. *In* B. M. Willmer (ed.). Cells and Tissues in Culture. Academic Press, New York.

Moscona, A. A. 1971. Embryonic and neoplastic cell surfaces: Availability of receptors for concanavalin A and wheat germ agglutinin. *Science* **171**:905–907.

Moscona, M. H., and Moscona, A. A. 1963. Inhibitions of adhesiveness and aggregation of dissociated cells by inhibitors of protein and RNA synthesis. *Science* **142**:1070–1071.

Pessac, B., and Defendi, V. 1972. Cell aggregation: Role of acid mucopolysaccharides. *Science* **175**:898–900.

Rall, T. W., and Sattin, A. 1970. Factors influencing the accumulation of cyclic AMP in brain tissue, pp. 113–134. *In* P. Greengard and E. Costa (eds.). Role of Cyclic AMP in Cell Function. Raven Press, New York.

Roth, S., McGuire, E. J., and Roseman, S. 1971. An assay for intercellular adhesive specificity. *J. Cell. Biol.* **51**:525–535.

Schmidt, M. J., Palmer, E. C., Dettbarn, W.-D., and Robison, G. A. 1970. Cyclic AMP and adenyl cyclase in the developing rat brain. *Develop. Biol.* **3**:53–67.

Seeds, N. W. 1971. Biochemical differentiation in reaggregating brain cell culture. *Proc. Natl. Acad. Sci.* **68**:1858–1861.

Seeds, N. W. 1972. Reassembling the brain. *New Scientist* **54**:12–14.

Seeds, N. W. 1973. Biochemical differentiation in reaggregating brain cell culture. II. Monoamine oxidase, catechol-*O*-methyltransferase lactate dehydrogenase and S-100 protein. (Submitted for publication.)

Seeds, N. W., and Gilman, A. G. 1971. Norepinephrine stimulated increase of cyclic AMP levels in developing mouse brain cell cultures. *Science* **174**:292.

Seeds, N. W., and Vatter, A. E. 1971. Synaptogenesis in reaggregating brain cell culture. *Proc. Natl. Acad. Sci.* **68**:3219–3222.

Sidman, R. L., Green, M. C., and Appel, S. H. 1965. Catalog of the Neurological Mutants of the Mouse. Harvard University Press, Cambridge, Mass.

Silberstein, S. D., Shein, H. M., and Berv, K. R. 1972. Catechol-*O*-methyl transferase and monoamine oxidase activity in cultured rodent astrocytoma cells. *Brain Res.* **41**:245–248.

Steinberg, M. S. 1970. Does differential adhesion govern self-assembly processes in histogenesis? Equilibrium configurations and the emergence of a hierarchy among population of embryonic cells. *J. Exptl. Zool.* **173**:395–433.

Trinkaus, J. P., and Groves, P. W. 1955. Differentiation in culture of mixed aggregates of dissociated tissue cells. *Proc. Natl. Acad. Sci.* **41**:787–795.

Varon, S., and Raiborn, C. W., Jr. 1969. Dissociation, fractionation, and culture of embryonic brain cells. *Brain Res.* **12**:180–199.

Werner, I., Peterson, G. R., and Shuster, L. 1971. Choline acetyltransferase and acetylcholinesterase in cultured brain cells from chick embryos. *J. Neurochem.* **18**:141–151.

Wilson, S. H. Schrier, B. K., Farber, J. L., Thompson, E. J., Rosenberg, R. N., Blume, A. J., and Nirenberg, M. W. 1972. Markers for gene expression in cultured cells from the nervous system. *J. Biol. Chem.* **247**:3159–3169.

Wolf, M. K. 1970. Anatomy of cultured mouse cerebellum. Organotypic migration of granule cells demonstrated by silver impregnation of normal and mutant cultures. *J. Comp. Neurol.* **140**:281–298.

Woodward, D. J., Hoffer, B. J., Siggins, G. R., and Bloom, F. E. 1971. The ontogenetic development of synaptic junctions, synaptic activation and responsiveness to neurotransmitter substances in rat cerebellar purkinje cells. *Brain Res.* **34**:73–97.

Chapter 3

Differentiation and Interaction of Clonal Cell Lines of Nerve and Muscle

David Schubert,[1] A. John Harris, Stephen Heinemann,
Y. Kidokoro, James Patrick, and Joseph Henry Steinbach

The Salk Institute
San Diego, California

I. INTRODUCTION

Since some of the basic problems in neurobiology are ultimately biochemical in nature, it follows that clonal populations of neuronal cells will be required to define the underlying mechanisms. Initial progress in this direction was made by Harrison, who was able to maintain primary explants of nervous tissue for a limited time *in vitro* (Harrison, 1907). With the introduction of more sophisticated tissue culture technology, it became possible to observe nervous tissue *in vitro* for extended periods of time and to demonstrate functional interaction between individual cells within the population (Crain *et al.*, 1968). Although the viability of these cultures was adequate, the problem of cell heterogeneity was yet to be overcome; two independent directions were taken in search of a solution. One was the fractionation of cell populations from whole brain (Roots and Johnston, 1964; Varon and Raiborn, 1968), and the other consisted of the use of neoplastic tissue as a relatively pure source of nerve cells (Murray and Stout, 1947). These approaches were, however, faced with the common difficulty that the neuronal cells in the population did not divide, and the various fractionation schemes were unable to yield homogeneous collections of cells. Since the requirement for homogeneous or clonal populations of cells necessarily demands cell division, methods which yield dividing nerve cells are clearly required. This

[1]Address all correspondence to David Schubert, The Salk Institute, P.O. Box 1809, San Diego, California 92112.

problem is not unique to the nervous system but is common to the study of most differentiated functions in cell culture, for the maximally differentiated end cell usually does not divide *in vivo* (Grobstein, 1959). Perhaps the only way of circumventing this situation at present is by adapting neoplasms of differentiated cells or their immediate developmental precursors to continuous cell culture. Subsequent cloning then yields homogeneous populations of cells. This approach was successfully applied to the study of endocrine (Sato and Yasumura, 1966), hepatic (Thompson *et al.*, 1966), and endoreticular (Cohn, 1967) cell function and has since been extended to many other cell types. Among these is a mouse neoplasm, C1300, of apparently neuronal origin which has been established in continuous cell culture and characterized as a neuroblastoma (Augusti-Tocco and Sato, 1969; Schubert *et al.*, 1969). In addition to the above lines, Yaffe (1968) has established clonal myogenic cells, and it has recently been possible to induce and establish in clonal culture several more nerve cell lines (Carlisle *et al.*, 1973). The availability of clonal neural and myogenic cell lines thus presents a unique opportunity to study the two major classes of electrically excitable cells.

Before continuing with a description of these cell lines and their interactions, a brief statement should be made concerning the types of questions which one can expect to answer through their use and the advantages of clonal lines over primary cultures.

With respect to the first point, the problems which can be studied advantageously in clonal lines of electrically excitable cells are many. The more obvious ones are the following: (1) The ionic basis of electrical excitation in nerve and muscle has been described in detail. The problem remaining is the definition of the macromolecular membrane components involved in excitation and the mechanisms by which these components function. Since these mechanisms are likely to be complex, it follows that mutant cell lines blocked at various levels of membrane function may be needed to supplement detailed biochemical studies. Only clonal systems make this approach possible. (2) Very little is known about the initiation and stabilization of the more differentiated states of nerve and muscle, primarily because of the difficulty in obtaining homogeneous populations of cells. The use of clonal cell lines capable of differentiation will remove this difficulty. Again, this work can be expedited by the use of mutants. (3) Perhaps the greatest single problem in neurobiology is the elucidation of the mechanisms by which one cell is able to recognize and form a functional synapse with another, i.e., the problem of synaptic specificity. Because this problem is clearly biochemical in nature, it follows that the cellular heterogeneity characteristic of primary cultures severely limits their usefulness. Since a tropic effect suggestive of early stages of synapse formation between two clonal cell lines has been demonstrated (Harris *et al.*, 1971), and since several clonal lines of nerve and muscle are now available, it is likely that cell cultures can be successfully exploited in studies dealing with synaptic specificity. In summary, many of the unsolved problems in neurobiology are ultimately biochemical in nature and may require genetic analysis. Therefore, homogeneous populations of dividing cells will be required; only clonal lines fulfill these demands.

In spite of the obvious advantages of clonal cell lines over primary cultures, they are subject to a common criticism, for it has frequently been argued that since permanent cell lines are most readily derived from neoplasms they are necessarily aberrant. This is certainly true, but there is no reason to believe, unless proven otherwise, that they are abnormal in any respect other than cell division and the metabolic processes associated with this state. In any case, it is necessary to compare the function that is being studied in cell culture with that observed *in vivo*. If the functions appear similar, then it is very likely that the underlying mechanisms will be the same *in vivo* and in cell culture, and that the latter system can be successfully exploited to study these mechanisms. If there is some specific functional abnormality in the cultured cells, then two possibilities exist. Either there has been a stable genetic variation in the line, or the culture conditions are not adequate to allow the cells to express the given function. These two alternatives are usually not easily distinguishable, and both should be considered when interpreting data on cell lines, particularly if the observations are inconsistent with data from *in vivo* experimentation.

In the following paragraphs, an attempt will first be made to briefly describe the origins of the nerve and muscle lines, including an analysis of the source of the dissimilarities among the different neuroblastoma clones. This will be followed by an examination of results concerning the morphological, chemical, and electrophysiological differentiation of clonal neuroblast and myoblast cell lines, and finally by a quick perusal of the tropic interaction between these lines. At least the morphological differentiation of the neuroblastoma is reversible. Since this process in the myoblast line is reversible to a much lesser extent, a comparison will be made between these dissimilar differentiative processes.

II. ORIGIN OF CELL LINES

A. Neuroblastoma C1300

The mouse neoplasm C1300 arose spontaneously in the body cavity of the A strain of mouse about 30 years ago, and the tumor line was maintained by subcutaneous transfer in animals until it was adapted to cell culture (Augusti-Tocco and Sato, 1969; Schubert *et al.*, 1969). Once a number of clones were examined in detail, two abnormalities became obvious: (1) There was a great degree of heterogeneity among different clones with respect to morphology (the ability to form neurites), karyotype, enzyme levels, and overall growth characteristics (Schubert *et al.*, 1971*a*; Amano *et al.*, 1972). (2) There was similar extreme morphological heterogeneity within a single clone when cells were allowed to extend neurites on tissue culture dishes. The latter observation is readily explained, since it has been established that neurite formation is dependent on, and primarily controlled by, the interaction between the cell and the surface on which it is grown (see below). It is likely that microheterogeneities on the surface of the culture dish dictate the cell morphology. For example, if a cell settles on a spot where it can attach firmly, it will tend to flatten and extend neurites, while another cell may attach on a less adhesive spot on the dish and remain in a more rounded condition. It should be noted that clonal lines of melanocytes and fibroblasts also show a great deal of morphological heterogeneity, probably for the same reasons.

The hypothesis that morphological variability is a result of culture dish microheterogeneity has received strong support from the following experiment: Cells were plated under conditions where more than 99 % of the population extended neurites. About 40 cells which did not extend neurites were then cloned *in situ* and subsequently assayed for the ability to form neurites. All of the clones were able to form neurites with the same efficiency as the original clone.

A large number of clones have been derived from the C1300 tumor which have different properties. The heterogeneity between these clones can be explained by one of three alternatives: (1) The original neoplastic event occurred in several different cells at the same time. Such an event could, for instance, be mediated through a virus which transformed several cells simultaneously. These cells would then have to be propagated in the original tumor line, none having a selective advantage such as a faster generation time. (2) Since nerve and glial cells undergo a series of developmental events, possibly from a common precursor, it is conceivable that the original neoplasm was derived from such a cell. This cell, when subjected to culture conditions, could give rise to several types of more differentiated cells. (3) The original neoplastic event took place in a unique cell, but somatic cell variation and mutation occurred during the subsequent thousands of cell generations in the tumor. In this case, the result would be a collection of cells in the tumor with a heterogeneous set of properties, but all originally derived from the same cell.

On the basis of data discussed below on the mouse neuroblastoma C1300 and by virtue of previous observations with a similar relationship between other neoplasms and tissue culture lines derived from them (Schubert *et al.*, 1968; Horibata and Harris, 1970), it appears that the third alternative is the most plausible.

The first alternative suggests that several lines arose at once and were all maintained in the tumor for 30 years. This is unlikely for several reasons. Since the spontaneous induction of a neuronal tumor is itself an extremely rare event, the probability of two or more such events occurring simultaneously approaches zero. If several neoplastic events did occur, they would have to be temporally very close together, for an advantage of a few generations between two cell lines with equal generation times would lead to a preponderance of the first-occurring cell in the tumor. Similarly, if all cells in the population did not have identical generation times, the stem cell with the fastest division time would eventually become the overwhelmingly predominant cell type. Since there are literally dozens of stem lines within the C1300 tumor line, it is thus unlikely to be a tumor of multiple cell origin. Also arguing against this hypothesis is the observation that there are a number of basic traits which all of the different clones have in common (see below).

The second hypothesis, that the tumor arose in a less differentiated precursor cell which in turn gave rise to a collection of more differentiated cell types, appears to be equally untenable. As described below, the different clones have a number of properties in common which are independent of their growth conditions and thus their state of differentiation. Among these properties is the possession of an electrically excitable membrane, which places the whole population of cells in the neuroblast category. It is unlikely that one stem cell could, under conditions of rapid division and in the apparent absence of any external influence, give rise to a collection of *unique* cells (clones) with stable properties. However, if neuroblastoma cells are developmentally primitive, they may, under the proper external influence, be induced to interact with a variety of cell types. Evidence for such interactions has been presented (Harris *et al.*, 1971).

The third and certainly the simplest alternative is that a single neoplastic event took place, initially producing a tumor of homogeneous cell type. Through the thousands of cell generations which followed, an extensive alteration and rearrangement of the genetic material within the population took place. This resulted in an extremely heterogenous population of cells which is evidenced by the wide range of karyotypes among clones (Amano *et al.*, 1972). A completely analogous example has been described in mouse myelomas, where it was possible, using marker chromosomes, to follow the detailed lineage of different stem lines within the tumor and of clones in tissue culture (Schubert *et al.*, 1968; Horibata and Harris, 1970). Thus the results described by Amano *et al.* (1972), which show that different clones of neuroblastoma C1300 have vastly different levels of tyrosine hydroxylase, choline acetylase, and acetylcholinesterase, and different karyotypes, are most simply explained by assuming that the original neoplastic cell expressed all of the enzymatic activities and had some given karyotype, for example, tetraploid. During subsequent tumor passage, the karyotypic changes were so great that some of the activities were lost in some stem lines, due to either chromosome loss or mutation, while other activities were enhanced by a gene dosage effect due to gene or chromosome duplication. Some activities which are found in all clones, such as acetylcholinesterase and an electrically excitable membrane, are presumably linked to functions whose loss would be lethal. Other markers not associated with neural function, such as the histocompatibility locus H_2^d, have been lost in some clones (J. Patrick, unpublished observation).

Many combinations of enzyme activities and karyotype have been observed by Amano *et al.* (1972). Although it was suggested by these authors that there is some regulatory function which dictates that the cell be of either the adrenergic or cholinergic type, this alternative has not been proven, and the above considerations indicate that this is not the most likely of the several possible interpretations of the available data. A similar argument may be made against any interpretation of cell hybridization data, unless extreme care is taken in following the fate of the chromosomes of the parental lines. The problem of distinguishing between regulatory events and chromosomal rearrangement or loss is one of the major obstacles in somatic cell genetics and should not be underemphasized. As mentioned previously, however, these problems do not negate the use of these cell lines for experiments involving the various functional aspects of the cells, for it is unlikely that the mechanisms involved are different from the *in vivo* situation.

B. Myoblast

The selection and characterization of the clonal myoblast line L6, which was used exclusively in the studies outlined below, has been described in detail (Yaffe, 1968; Richler and Yaffe, 1970) and will be only briefly outlined here. L6 was established by transferring cells from primary cultures of new-born rat thigh muscle for two passages in the presence of methylcholanthrene and subsequently cloning the dividing cells in the population. This cell line has a diploid karyotype indistinguishable from that of primary culture myoblasts and is capable of fusing to form multinucleate striated fibers which are often observed to contract. Thus the myoblast appears to be much more of a minimal-deviation cell line than the neuroblastoma, an observation consistent with its mode of isolation and the arguments presented above.

III. MORPHOLOGICAL DIFFERENTIATION

A. Neuroblastoma

As indicated above, when cells from the mouse tumor C1300 are adapted to tissue culture and cloned, there is a great heterogeneity among the clones with respect to morphology, growth characteristics, and enzymatic activities. Since a detailed description of several clones is clearly impossible here, the following discussion will be limited to summarizing the characteristics of one clone, called C1.

Clone C1 was derived from an agar cloning procedure and judged pure with respect to karyotype, which is tetraploid (Schubert *et al.*, 1969). Its growth characteristics have remained constant for several years; subclones of C1 are indistinguishable from the parental line. When grown in medium containing 10% fetal calf serum in plastic petri dishes, the cells grow as round cells in suspension culture and do not attach to the surface of the dish. When transferred to plastic tissue culture dishes (which are similar to petri dishes except that they have been chemically treated to enhance cell adhesion), the cells attach to the surface and extend neurites. In 10% serum, this process is relatively asynchronous and only about half of the cells extend neurites. Since this form of induced neurite formation appeared to offer a unique opportunity to study the development of neuronal properties in a mammalian cell, the parameters involved in this process were examined in detail.

Three independent conditions were found which influence neurite extension: (1) Cells grown in the presence of 5-bromodeoxyuridine (BUdR) in normal serum concentrations extend neurites synchronously (Schubert and Jacob, 1970). (2) A dialyzable compound(s) secreted by the neuroblastoma and other cell lines induces neurite formation (Schubert et al., 1971a). (3) Media containing low concentrations of serum induce neurite formation, serum-free media being the most effective (Seeds *et al.*, 1970; Schubert *et al.*, 1971a). The latter process is both the most temporally efficient and the most readily applied of the three methods of inducing neurite formation. Thus when exponentially growing cells in suspension culture are plated in tissue culture dishes in the absence of serum, the following series of morphological events take place: (a) within 5 min the cells attach to the dish (Fig. 1A); (b) after 15 min the cells become extensively flattened, and hundreds of spinelike processes extending from the circumference of the cell are observed (Fig. 1B) (it is likely that these spines are derived from the small processes approximately 1 μ in diameter and a few microns in length observed by electron microscopy on the round cells; Schubert *et al.*, 1969); and (c) neurite formation starts at about 2 hr (Fig. 1C) and continues for several days (Fig. 1D). The data presented in Fig. 2 show that the change in neurite formation as a

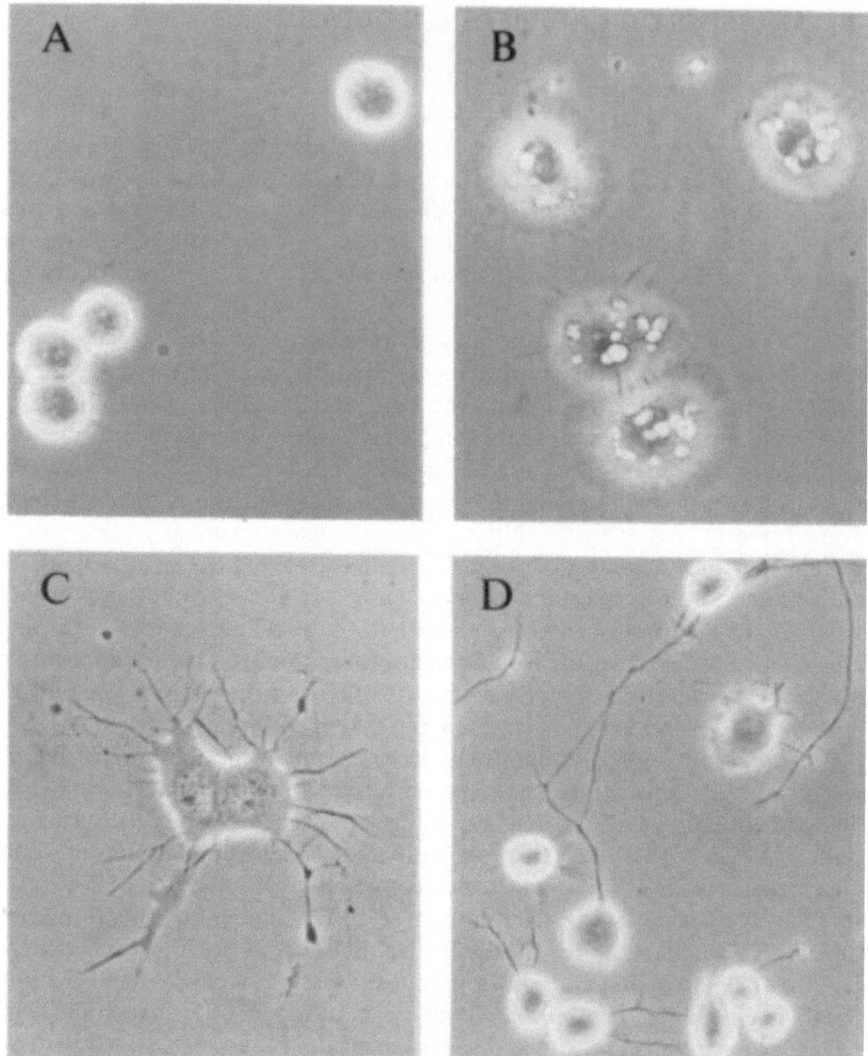

Fig. 1. Morphological differentiation of neuroblastoma C1300. Cells were plated in serum-free medium in 60-mm tissue culture dishes at 2×10^5 cells per plate. Phase photomicrographs were taken at various times after plating. Time after transfer to tissue culture dish: (A) 5 min, (B) 15 min, (C) 5 hr, (D) 24 hr. (From Schubert *et al.*, 1971a.)

function of serum concentration is a property of the whole population of cells and not of a limited number of cells within the population. A series of curves similar to those shown in Fig. 2 can also be generated by the use of BUdR or conditioned media (Schubert and Jacob, 1970; Schubert *et al.*, 1971a).

Since it was necessary to quantitate the data from this type of experiment, a morphological criterion was employed to distinguish the round cell from the more differentiated cell containing neurites. This criterion was the existence of one or more elongate processes (neurites) extending from the perikaryon which were greater than 40 μ in length. This minimum neurite length was chosen to exclude the many fine spinelike processes up to 10 μ in length around the circumference of cells plated in tissue culture dishes in low-serum medium (Fig. 1B). The term "differentiation" has been applied to this event only to imply that a process has taken place which leads from a less morphologically complex cell, the neuroblastoma round cell, to a more complex cell, as defined by a number of parameters. The word "differentiation," as used in this particular case, clearly does not imply a state of terminal differentiation in the classical sense (Grobstein, 1959) but only a state of increased morphological complexity (see discussion in Section VI).

On the basis of the above studies, it can be concluded that the neuroblastoma clone C1 is induced to differentiate (extend neurites) by enhancing the interaction between the cell and the surface of the culture dish on which

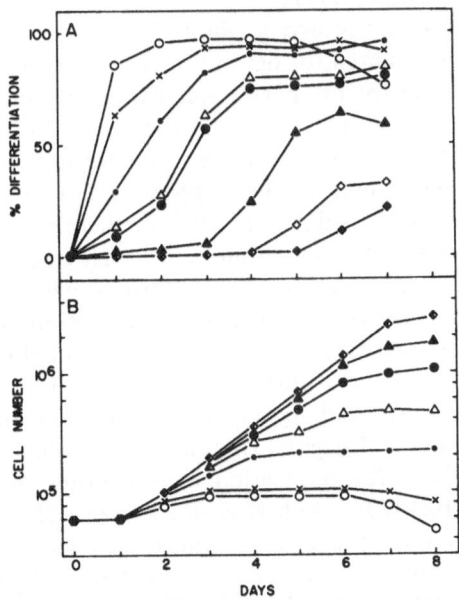

Fig. 2.   Relationship between differentiation and serum concentration. Exponentially growing cells in petri dishes (where the cells are unable to attach to the surface) were plated on tissue culture dishes at various serum concentrations. Viable cell number and percent differentiation were determined. (A) Percent differentiation plotted as a function of time; (B) viable cell number per dish plotted as a function of time. Open circles, serum-free media; cross marks, 0.5% serum; dots, 1% serum; open triangles, 2% serum; filled circles, 3% serum; filled triangles, 5% serum; open diamonds, 10% serum; filled diamonds, 20% serum. (From Schubert *et al.,* 1971*a.*)

it is grown. Thus decreasing the serum in the growth medium strengthens the electrostatic interaction between the cell surface and the culture dish through the removal of serum proteins which neutralize this interaction. This form of induced differentiation can be blocked by a number of different nonserum proteins, probably because they alter the net cell surface charge (Sherbet *et al.*, 1972). A similar serum effect has been described for other cell lines (Witkowski and Brighton, 1972). BUdR is also known to induce the flattening of a number of cell types (Bischoff and Holtzer, 1970), clearly by increasing the affinity between the cell and culture dish surfaces. It has been argued that the same interactions are responsible for the BUdR-induced differentiation of the neuroblastoma and that BUdR functions by metabolically altering the cell surface (Schubert and Jacob, 1970). It has since been demonstrated that cells induced to differentiate with BUdR contain a cell-surface glycoprotein which is not detectable in undifferentiated cells (Brown, 1971). Low molecular weight metabolites which enhance differentiation probably function in a similar manner, for a small molecule like actinomycin D can greatly increase the interaction between cells and the culture dish in the absence of protein synthesis (Schubert *et al.*, 1971a).

The fact that a relatively strong affinity between the cell and the surface of the culture dish is required for neurite extension argues that similar interactions are prerequisite for the phenotypic expression of neurite formation but says nothing about the mechanism of the induced differentiation. Since some of the conditions which induce neurite formation (e.g., serum-free medium) also inhibit cell division, there appear to be two alternatives. Either the interaction *per se* induces differentiation, or there is a causal relationship between cell division and differentiation in the sense that the cessation of cell division induces neurite extension. The following evidence strongly argues that there is no causal relationship between cell division and differentiation: (1) The inhibition of DNA synthesis does not induce differentiation under conditions where the cells are able to express the differentiated phenotype (Schubert and Jacob, 1970; Schubert *et al.*, 1971a). (2) Conditions have been defined which permit a nearly maximum rate of cell division where the majority of the cells in the population have neurites over 40 μ in length (Schubert and Jacob, 1970; Schubert *et al.*, 1971a). (3) Cells plated in conditioned medium from stationary-phase cultures differentiate but do not divide, presumably because of the depletion of a nondialyzable growth-promoting factor in the serum (Holley and Kiernan, 1968). In contrast, cells plated in dialyzed conditioned medium from the same culture neither divide nor differentiate (Schubert *et al.*, 1971a).

On the basis of the available data (Schubert *et al.*, 1969; Harris and Dennis, 1970; Schubert and Jacob, 1970; Schubert *et al.*, 1971a), the following model can be constructed for the control of the reversible differentiation in clone Cl of mouse neuroblastoma C1300 (Fig. 3): (a₁) When cultured in

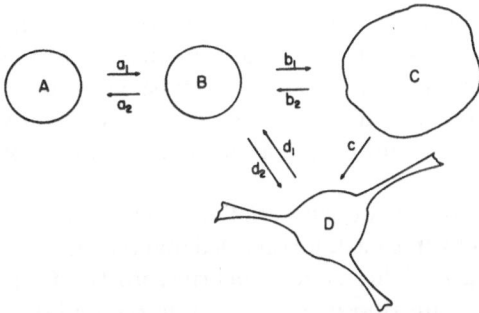

Fig. 3.   Schematic representation of morphological differentiation. (A) Cells in suspension culture; (B) cells attached to a surface with the same morphology as cells in suspension culture; (C) cells attached to a surface with extremely flattened morphology; (D) cells on a surface with neurites extended. (From Schubert *et al.*, 1971*a*)

plastic tissue culture dishes, the cells attach to the substrate. (a_2) High protein or cell concentrations can reverse this process. (b_1) If cells are plated in tissue culture dishes in the absence of serum, the cells rapidly become extremely flattened. This property is inherent in the undifferentiated cell and does not require protein or RNA synthesis. (b_2) Cell flattening is reversed by serum or various proteins. (c) In the continued absence of serum, the cells begin to extend neurites within a few hours after plating. This process, defined here as differentiation, is accompanied by a change in macromolecular synthesis and enzyme activity, and in the acetylcholine sensitivity of the neurites. Neurite formation requires protein synthesis but apparently not RNA and DNA synthesis. (d_2) A variety of conditions can induce the attached neuroblastoma cells to extend neurites without going through the morphological flattened stage. For example, both BUdR and 0.5% serum induce differentiation without preliminary flattening. (d_1) Differentiation is reversible, for both the regression of neurites and the initiation of cell division can be induced by serum, and neurite extension is reversed in serum-free medium by various proteins.

Time-lapse cinemicroscopy shows that when plated in serum-free medium the cells initially extend and retract numerous filopodia at a great rate and actively move about the surface of the culture dish; nuclear rotation is frequently observed. After several hours, some of the filopodia become stabilized and are no longer retracted into the cell body. The cells then become less mobile, and the neurites grow rapidly for several days. These events appear to be completely analogous to those observed in primary cultures of neurons (Nakai, 1964).

The morphological changes observed during differentiation with the light microscope are correlated with dramatic changes observed at the electron microscopic level of resolution (Schubert *et al.*, 1969, 1971*a*). Cells grown in suspension were a homogeneous population of round cells having many small processes less than 1 μ in diameter projecting from their limiting membrane. Cellular organization was dominated by a diffuse system of endoplasmic reticulum and associated C-type virus particles. In addition, dense-core vesicles with uniformly staining contents slightly withdrawn from the limiting membrane and having a maximum diameter of 0.4 μ were found in the cytoplasm.

Electron microscopy of semiserial sections of neurites at 4 and 14 hr after plating in serum-free medium revealed that the microtubule organelle was completely lacking at 4 hr, even in neurites up to 100 μ in length. These neurites were filled with ribosomes, mitochondria, and occasional dense-core vesicles (Schubert *et al.*, 1971a). Only after 14 hr were microtubules observed. Even then they occurred in less than 10% of the neurites, some of which extended several hundred microns from the perikaryon. After several days, all of the cells in the population possessed long processes which may be classified as containing components which were mostly microfibrillar, mostly microtubular, or essentially perikaryon cytoplasm. The latter two types were the most frequently observed. Mitochondria, microtubules, glycogen, and dense-core vesicles were found in much greater abundance in neurites than in the perikaryon and were always included in a section of the end of a process if it was in contact with another cell (Schubert *et al.*, 1969). The nuclei of the differentiated cells were flattened and deeply indented, similar to nuclei in cultured rat neurons (Bunge *et al.*, 1965). Also in contrast to that of round cells, the endoplasmic reticulum of the differentiated cell was compact and not dominated by developing virus.

Since the above data clearly demonstrate that neurite extension can take place under conditions where no microtubules are present, it follows that neurite growth does not require this organelle. The data do not, however, rule out the possibility that a unique microtubule system associated with the plasma membrane is involved in neurite extension. These results suggest that microtubule polymerization may aid in the stabilization of elongate processes but that neurite growth *per se* is due to activity within the growth cone. Similar suggestions have been made on the basis of studies with primary cultures of nervous tissue (Yamada *et al.*, 1970; Handel, 1971). It should be pointed out, however, that neurites lacking microtubules have not been reported in primary cultures, presumably because these cells were derived from relatively mature neurons which contained extensive microtubule networks *in vivo*.

B. Myoblast

Clones of the myoblast cell line L6 differentiate into mature muscle fibers in a manner analogous to that of primary rat and chicken myoblast cultures (Richler and Yaffe, 1970). Mononucleate myoblasts divide with a generation time of approximately 20 hr until they become confluent. At that time, cell fusion is initiated, and fusion is essentially complete within 2–3 days (Fig. 4). The fused myotubes are initially unstriated and frequently are observed to contract spontaneously; striations appear in the cultures about 1 week after fusion.

Electron microscopy (Humphreys and Schubert, 1973) reveals that myoblasts are associated with each other through typical gap junctions, which are probably responsible for the electrical coupling between cells. Myoblast cytoplasm is filled with free ribosomes, distended rough endoplasmic reticu-

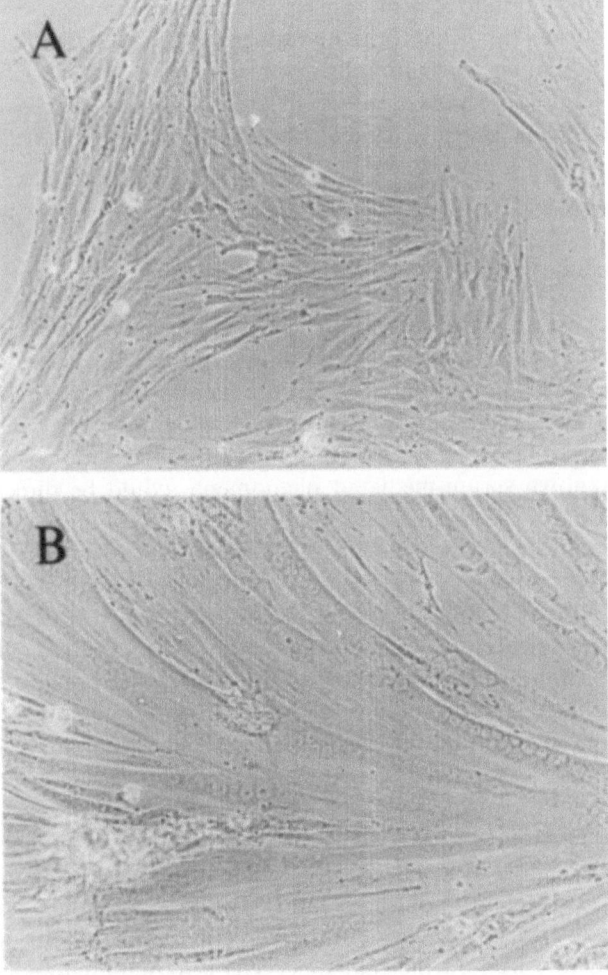

Fig. 4. Morphological differentiation of myogenic cell line. (A) Exponentially growing myoblasts; (B) multinucleate myotubes 3 days after the initiation of cell fusion.

lum, and mitochondria. Large quantities of 60-Å-diameter filaments are found in the cell cortex, while 100-Å filaments and, rarely, myofilaments, are seen in the cytoplasm.

Myoblasts usually fuse into myotubes with central nuclei. Concomitant with fusion, free ribosomes associate into large polysomes and thick myosin filaments appear in a random orientation near them; thin actin filaments are also randomly oriented throughout the cytoplasm. The first filaments to become longitudinally aligned and to form a lattice with actin hexagonally surrounding the myosin are those which have migrated to the cell surface. A few microtubules are observed near the myofilaments at this time. The transverse tubule system and sarcoplasmic reticulum develop simultaneously and are easily distinguishable in myotubes before the myofilaments form sarcomeres. Sarcomere formation first occurs subjacent to the cell membrane, and a basal lamina is observed above striated muscle fibers. At this time, the nuclei are no longer centrally located but are lined up at the cell membrane.

IV. CHEMICAL DIFFERENTIATION

A. Neuroblastoma

When studying differentiation in a cell culture system, it is imperative that the number of variables possibly affecting the event approach unity as closely as possible. For example, if neuroblastoma cells are grown in high-serum medium and then changed to serum-free medium, cell attachment to the culture dish is enhanced and cell division is inhibited; both of these effects, plus any unknown serum-mediated phenomena, could be directly involved in the induction of differentiation. To avoid this type of ambiguity, all of the experiments concerning neuroblastoma differentiation described here were carried out by making use of the fact that clone Cl attaches to and differentiates on tissue culture dishes but not on plastic petri dishes. By varying the culture dish surface only, it is possible to hold the variables of cell division and serum constant. In this experimental situation, it has been established that a surface-mediated stimulus induces changes in the biosynthetic pattern of the neuroblastoma in addition to the observed morphological alterations.

To examine these changes, exponentially growing cells were plated in low serum under identical growth conditions except that one set of cells was plated on tissue culture dishes where they attached and differentiated, while the other was plated on petri dishes where there was no attachment or morphological differentiation. Leucine-H^3 or C^{14} was then added to the separate sets of cultures and the cultures were incubated for 4 hr, thus labeling the protein synthesized during that time. The differentiated and round cells, labeled with H^3 and C^{14}, respectively, were then mixed and lysed, and the labeled material was electrophoresed on acrylamide gels. The ratios of leucine-H³ to leucine-C¹⁴ across the gels were examined, and it was established that there were discrete differences in the spectrum of leucine-containing macromolecules synthesized by the morphologically differentiated cell and its round-cell precursor (Schubert *et al.*, 1971*a*). In a similar experiment, it was shown that the same surface-mediated interaction induces specific changes in macromolecular synthesis during BUdR-induced differentiation (Schubert and Jacob, 1970).

In addition to the quantitative changes in macromolecular synthesis, it has been demonstrated that the specific activity of acetylcholinesterase in the neuroblastoma is dependent on the conditions of growth (Blume *et al.*, 1970; Kates *et al.*, 1971). However, by employing the type of experimental design where the surface was the only variable, it was established that the major factor responsible for the increase in esterase activity was aging and cell death (Schubert *et al.*, 1971*b*). Thus exponentially growing cells were plated under identical growth conditions on tissue culture dishes which permitted differentiation and on agar-coated dishes which prohibited cell attachment. Cell number, percentage of differentiated cells, protein per cell, and the specific activity of acetylcholinesterase were then followed as a function of time. The data presented in Fig. 5 show that there is a faster initial increase in the specific activity of acetylcholinesterase in cells extending neurites than in

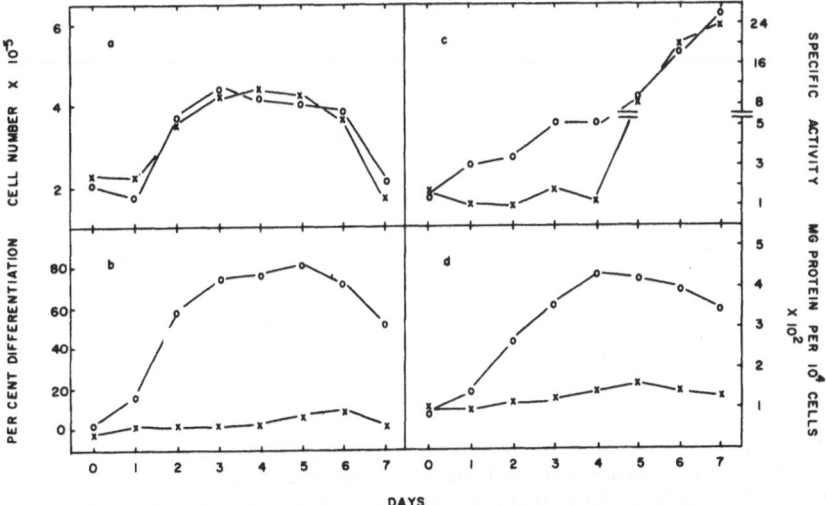

Fig. 5. Induction of acetylcholinesterase activity in neuroblastoma cells. Exponentially growing cells were plated on tissue culture (circles) or agar-coated (cross marks) dishes at 2×10^5 cells per plate in media containing 1 % fetal calf serum. Acetylcholinesterase activity was determined at *p*H 8 using acetylthiocholine as substrate. (a) Viable cell number $\times$ 10^{-5} per 60-mm dish; (b) percentage of the cells in the population with neurites greater than 40 μ long; (c) specific activity of acetylcholinesterase, Δ OD_{440}/min/mg protein; (d) mg protein/10^4 cells $\times$ 10^2. (From Schubert *et al.*, 1971*b*.)

the round-cell population; cell number and viability were identical in both populations. Since there was approximately a fourfold increase in the amount of protein per cell after 4 days in the population possessing neurites (Fig. 5d), it follows that there was about a twentyfold difference in enzyme activity per cell between the two populations. This strongly supports the hypothesis that attachment to a surface, and not the cessation of cell division, exerts a strong influence on the control of protein synthesis in differentiating neuroblasts. These results do not, however, establish that acetylcholinesterase is controlled during neurite formation by a mechanism other than neurite growth *per se*. For if most of this enzyme is membrane bound, then the observed increase in esterase accompanying neurite formation may result simply from the increased ratio of membrane surface area to cytoplasm.

The increase in acetylcholinesterase activity can be divided into two phases. In the first phase, the relatively slow increase is correlated with

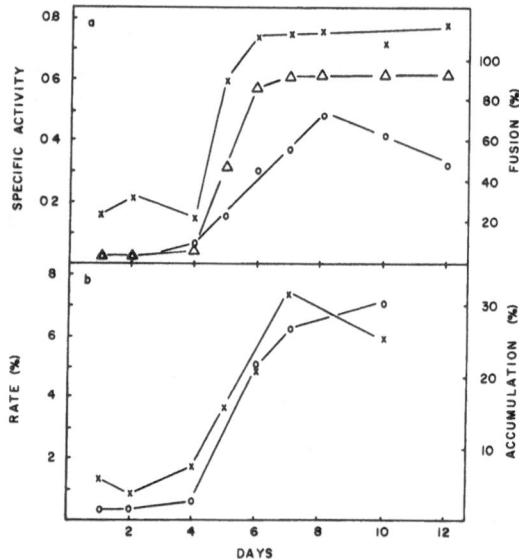

Fig. 6.   Enzyme and myosin heavy chain synthesis, and cell fusion during myogenesis. (a) Myoblasts were assayed for myokinase and creatine phosphokinase during the process of cell fusion. The relative specific activities are represented as Δ OD_{340}/min/mg protein. Cross marks, specific activity of myokinase; open circles, specific activity of creatine phosphokinase; triangles, percent of total nuclei in fused fibers. (b) Rate of synthesis and accumulation of myosin heavy chain as a function of time. Cells were either pulse labeled or continuously labeled with leucine-C^{14}, and the percent of total trichloroacetic acid precipitable counts incorporated into myosin heavy chain was determined as described elsewhere (Schubert *et al.*, 1973). Cross marks, rate of heavy chain synthesis; circles, heavy chain accumulation.

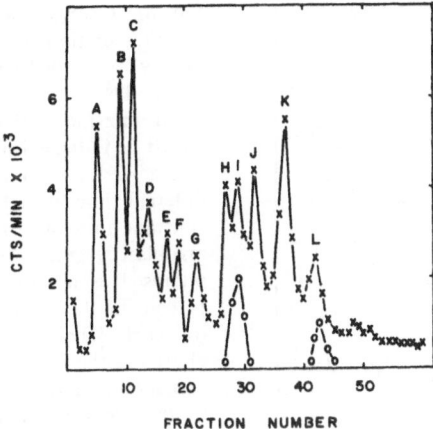

Fig. 7.   Secreted proteins from myotubes. Cells were labeled for 24 hr with leucine-H³, and the secreted proteins were reduced and alkylated and coeletrophoresed on 6% acrylamide gels containing 0.1% sodium dodecylsulfate with leucine-C¹⁴-labeled IgG as markers. (Electrophoresis was from left to right.) Cross marks, H³ secreted protein; Circles, C¹⁴-IgG heavy (50,000 mol. wt.) and light (23,000 mol. wt.) chains. (From Schubert *et al.*, 1973.)

neurite formation and the concomitant increase in protein per cell; the latter more rapid increase in specific activity is accompanied by a loss of viable cells (Fig. 5a) and a general deterioration of the cells in culture. This later rapid increase in esterase activity is not a result of neuroblast differentiation, for the rate of induction is equal in attached cells with neurites and the round-cell suspension culture. It follows that unless culture conditions are properly controlled, an increase in acetylcholinesterase activity in the neuroblastoma is nothing more than an expression of cellular geriatrics or unfavorable growth conditions.

B.   Myoblast

The enzymatic changes accompanying myoblast fusion and muscle differentiation in the myoblast clone L6 have been thoroughly studied by Richler and Yaffe (1970). In agreement with their data, Fig. 6a shows that there is an increase in the specific activity of both myokinase and creatine phosphokinase which parallels the fusion of mononucleate myoblasts into multinucleate myotubes. It has also been established that myoblasts synthesize myosin heavy chains and that both the rate of synthesis as defined by pulse-labeling experiments and the accumulation of myosin heavy chain increase following the initiation of cell fusion (Fig. 6b; Schubert *et al.*, 1973).

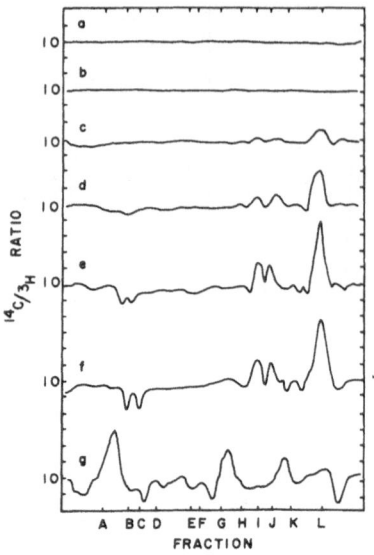

Fig. 8. Changes in rates of specific protein secretion during differentiation. Cells were labeled with leucine-C[14] or leucine-H[3] for 8 hr on some of the days when enzyme activities were determined as indicated in Fig. 6. Secreted leucine-C[14]-labeled proteins from the different times were then mixed with a constant amount of leucine-H[3]-labeled myoblast secreted protein and electrophoresed as described in Fig. 7. The percent of the total isotope in the gel for each label was determined and plotted as the ratio of C[14]-labeled protein at each point during differentiation to the constant H[3]-labeled myoblast protein. The positions of the 12 secreted proteins are indicated on the abscissa and the ratios on the ordinate. Each hatchmark on the ordinate represents a deviation of 0.2 from the ratio of 1 on which each curve is centered. Ratio plots (a) through (f) were obtained from cells labeled on days 1, 2, 4, 5, 6, and 8 in Fig. 6. Ratio plot (g) was derived from intracellular material of C[14]-labeled myotubes (day 8, Fig. 6) and H[3]-labeled myoblasts (day 2, Fig. 6). (From Schubert *et al.*, 1973)

In addition to the expected changes in enzyme activity and myosin synthesis, it has been shown that there is at least a quantitative change in the rates of protein secretion during differentiation. Figure 7 shows an acrylamide electrophoresis pattern of proteins secreted by fused cells; the pattern is qualitatively the same in myoblasts. Of the 12 resolved secreted proteins, only three have been characterized. It has been established that proteins B, C, and D are collagen α-chains (Schubert *et al.*, 1973). The collagen chains were identified on the basis of their high content of proline, glycine, and alanine, their susceptibility to collagenase digestion, and their similarity to collagen α-chains secreted by fibroblasts. It is likely that the proteins secreted by these cells are utilized in the construction of the basement membrane material associated with the myotubes. Collagen fibers are also frequently observed on myotubes (Schubert *et al.*, 1973). When cells are pulse labeled for 8 hr with leucine-C[14] during various stages of differentiation, and the secreted material is compared by acrylamide gel electrophoresis with leucine-H[3] protein secreted from myoblasts, there is at least a quantitative change in the rates of secretion of several proteins (Fig. 8; Schubert *et al.*, 1973).

V. ELECTRICAL DIFFERENTIATION

A. Neuroblastoma

The availability of cell culture lines with electrically excitable membranes makes possible a large number of experiments which may be expected to clarify such problems as the differentiation of excitable membranes and the molecular events responsible for excitation. In these studies, as with all work on cellular differentiation in culture, care must be taken to use proper culture conditions when a comparison between differentiated and undifferentiated cells is attempted. In addition, extreme caution must be exerted in the experimental procurement and analysis of electrophysiological data, for, due to the extreme fragility of the cells, high resistance electrodes must be used which can lead to electrical artifacts, especially when a bridge circuit is employed. It has been unequivocally demonstrated that differentiated neuroblastoma cells possess excitable membranes (Nelson et al., 1969; Harris and Dennis, 1970) and are sensitive to acetylcholine (Harris and Dennis, 1970). In addition, data have been presented from which it was concluded that there is a temporal sequence of development of discrete electrical membrane properties in the neuroblastoma (Nelson et al., 1969; Minna et al., 1972). These conclusions were based on electrophysiological recording from a population of neuroblastoma cells exhibiting various stages of neurite formation and from similar populations of hybrid cell lines. Four classes of responses were observed, including passive responses, delayed rectification, partial responses, and action potentials. On this basis, it was suggested that these events may represent different stages of neuroblast differentiation (Nelson et al., 1969, 1971; Minna et al., 1972). It is, however, possible to test this developmental hypothesis by a direct experiment. Thus, if it were established that neuroblastoma round cells, growing for many generations in suspension culture where they are unable to differentiate, exhibit active membrane responses, it would follow that there is no developmental sequence of the action-potential mechanism in these cells. The following experiments demonstrate that undifferentiated cells are capable of generating action potentials.

Cells were grown for at least 20 generations in medium containing 20% fetal calf serum on petri dishes or agar-coated culture dishes which completely inhibited cell attachment and subsequent differentiation. To record from the cells, they were transferred from the suspension culture to tissue culture dishes, still in medium containing 20% serum. Under these conditions, the cells settle to the bottom of the dish and loosely attach to it; they do not flatten nor do they initiate neurite formation until after a week in culture (Schubert et al., 1971a). Immediately after transferral from suspension to the tissue culture

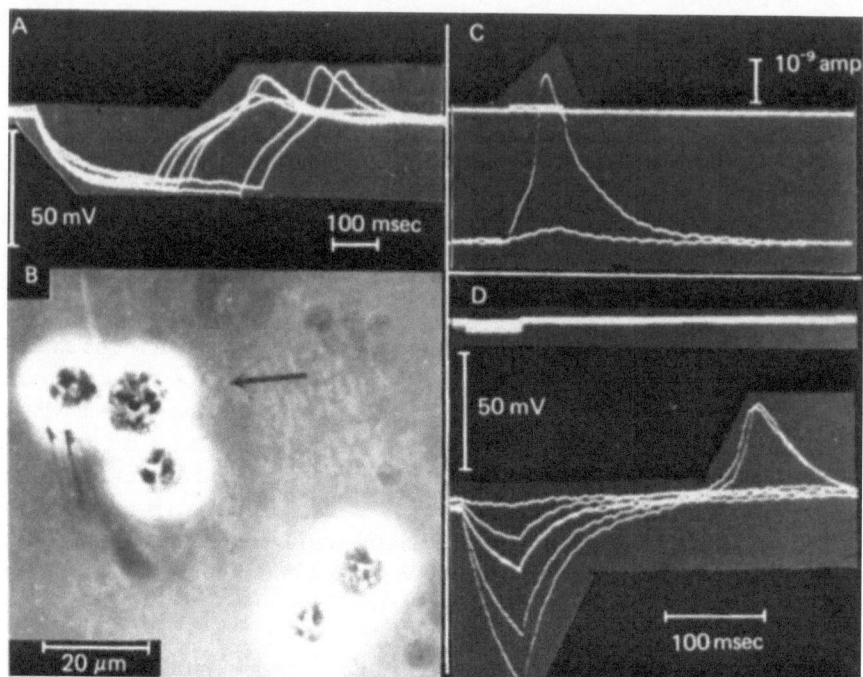

Fig. 9. Electrical activity of neuroblastoma round cell. Neuroblastoma clones were grown for over 20 generations in suspension culture where they were completely inhibited from attaching. Cells were then transferred to tissue culture dishes in the same medium where they become loosely associated with the culture dish surface. The cells were then immediately assayed for their ability to generate an action potential. Upper traces show the amount of current applied. (A) Anode-break response of cell identified by arrow in (B). The clone used was N12, and the cell had a resting potential of -50 mV. The duration of the hyperpolarizing current was 200 msec at less than 1×10^{-10} amp. (B) Arrow points to clone N12 cell recorded from in A. (C) Action potential evoked by depolarization of clone C1A recorded from the same experimental situation as clone N12. The resting potential of this cell was -60 mV. (D) Action potential in same cell as C evoked by anode-break excitation. Calibration of current, voltage, and time applies to both C and D.

dishes, the cells were assayed for electrical activity. Figure 9 shows that the undifferentiated round cell is capable of generating an action potential, either by anode-break excitation (A and D) or by a depolarizing current (C). The all or none property of the action potential is clearly demonstrated in Fig. 9C, where the peak potential overshoots zero membrane potential by 15 mV. These cells are not, however, sensitive to the iontophoretic application of acetylcholine. These results have been repeated with several clones, including C1, C1A, N4, N12, and N18 (the last three clones are described by Amano *et al.*, 1972). Thus the round cell, under conditions where any past history of differentiation has been eliminated, is electrically excitable. These data rule out the possibility that the ability to generate an action potential is acquired during differentiation of the neuroblastoma *in vitro* and strongly suggest that alternative explanations for the various types of responses observed in the cells must be sought.

Due to the experimental situation, false negative results can be generated through any of the following situations: (1) Culture conditions and the general state of health of the culture can affect the responses that one observes. It has been repeatedly observed in our laboratory that slight changes in culture conditions, such as *p*H shifts or varying serum concentrations, drastically affect the ability to record from cells, as evidenced by lower resting

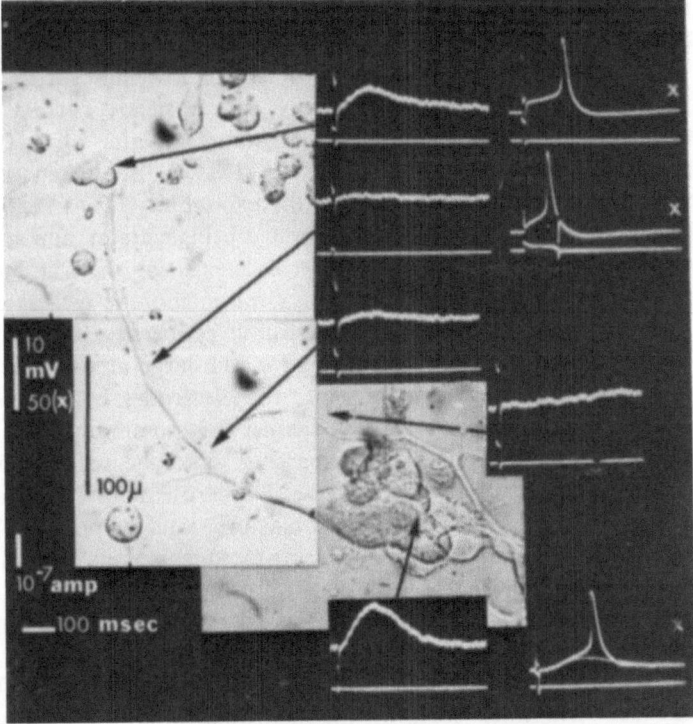

Fig. 10.   Distribution of acetylcholine sensitivity over the suface of a differentiated neuroblastoma cell with one process, 3 weeks after plating. Sensitivity to acetylcholine is restricted to the cell body, where acetylcholine application evoked an action potential (lower right), and to the neurite growth cone. Extracellular electrical stimulation of the axon or its tip gave rise to an action potential which propagated back to the cell body (two top right traces; points of stimulation as for acetylcholine application). Calibration for voltage, current, and time is given at the lower left; "50(X)" means 50 mV and applies to records marked with X. (From Harris and Dennis, 1970.)

potentials and difficulty in obtaining stable penetrations. The fact that some electrophysiological work has been carried out under conditions of serum starvation may explain the diversity of observed responses (Minna *et al.*, 1971, 1972). (2) The electrophysiological technique that is employed can lead to artifacts. All the published work on neuroblastoma has been done by penetrating the cell with a single electrode and using a bridge circuit to both pass current and record voltage changes. The fact that neuroblastoma cells are extremely fragile and easily damaged makes it necessary to use high-resistance electrodes. The long time constant of the potential change in these electrodes can mask the membrane response, with the result that an electrically active membrane can look like a passive membrane and will be classified as such. Another problem is that many times the cell is damaged during penetration. The resting potential might be lowered, the action potential mechanism could be inactivated, and a normally excitable cell would again be recorded as having a passive membrane.

In an attempt to get around the problem of low and variable resting potentials, a number of workers routinely pass a steady current into the cell to artificially hyperpolarize the cell to a standard value of -60 to -80 mV (Nelson *et al.*, 1969, 1971; Minna *et al.*, 1971, 1972). They then pass pulses of current through the electrode to test for excitability. These experiments have all been done with a single electrode and a bridge circuit, and are subject to the criticism that the electrode may not be measuring the true membrane potential, resulting in false negative assays for membrane excitability. The authors took care to select electrodes with ohmic properties, but it is possible that inside the cell and during the passage of the large amounts of current required to hyperpolarize the membrane, the electrodes behave in a nonohmic manner. The only valid control against this possibility is to use two electrodes and show that the current-passing electrode records the same voltage changes as the recording electrode. Numerous two-electrode experiments in our laboratory with both neuroblastoma and myoblast cells have, in fact, shown that the current-passing electrode does not consistently follow the recording electrode.

These considerations make it imperative that the results of single electrode recordings be confirmed by placing two electrodes into the cell; one for passing current, the other for measuring voltage changes. This is particularly true when new cell lines such as the neuroblastoma–L-cell hybrids are characterized with respect to the excitability of their membranes, (Minna, et *al.*, 1971, 1972).

Once the neuroblastoma cells become more morphologically differentiated, it is possible to map the distribution of acetylcholine sensitivity over their surface (Harris and Dennis, 1970). Cells with neurites were either uniformly sensitive or the sensitivity was localized to the cell body and the growth cone area (Fig. 10). The temporal sequence of the restriction of sensitivity has not been established. However, it is likely that dividing round cells in suspension culture are initially insensitive to acetylcholine, that cells in the early stages of neurite formation are uniformly sensitive, and that acetylcholine sensitivity retracts to the cell body and growth cone in the mature cell.

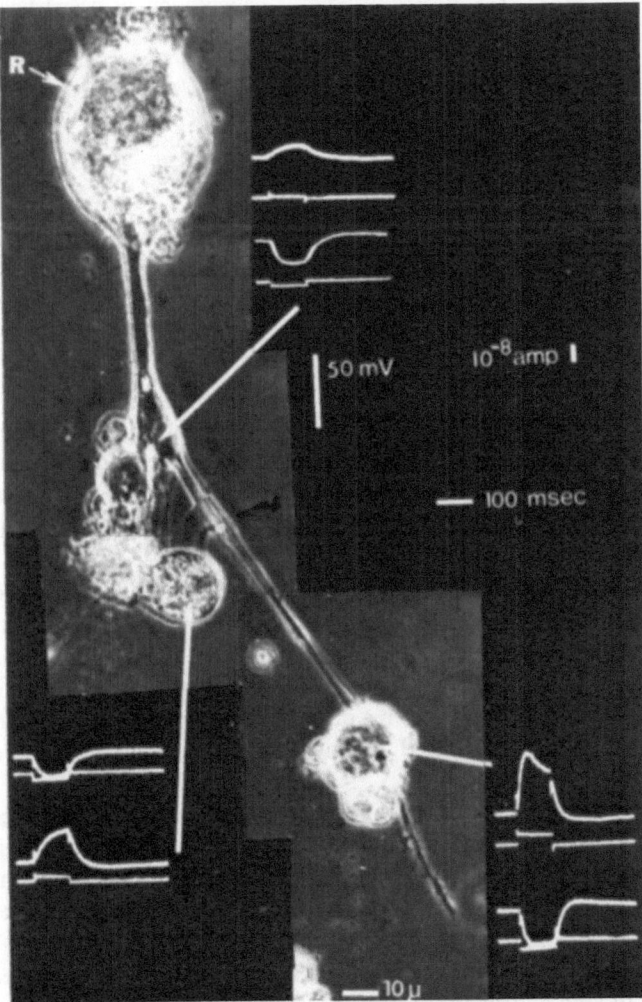

Fig. 11.   Electrical coupling between neuroblastoma cells. Cells were plated on tissue culture dishes for 3 weeks in medium containing 20% serum. Electrical coupling was demonstrated by recording from one cell (marked by R) and passing current through each of two other cells. The three cells were coupled through electrotonic junctions. The upper right records were taken by injecting current into a part of the process.

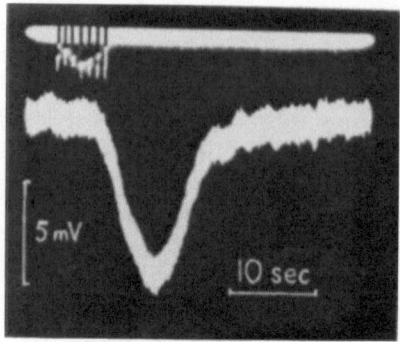

Fig. 12. Hyperpolarizing response to acetylcholine in exponentially dividing myoblasts. The change in the membrane potential (lower trace) was monitored with an intracellular electrode following the iontophoretic application of acetylcholine to myoblasts. The upper trace shows the amount of current repeatedly applied to the acetylcholine electrode (approximately 2×10^{-8} amp with a duration of 100 msec).

Although no electrophysiological evidence for chemical synapses between neuroblastoma cells has been found, electrical coupling between two or more cells has been demonstrated (Fig. 11).

B. Myoblast

In contrast to the lack of electrical differentiation in the neuroblastoma cell lines, it has been established that the myoblast clone L6 undergoes a clearly defined sequence of differentiation with respect to electrical excitability, acetylcholine sensitivity, and acetylcholine receptor synthesis (Kidokoro, 1973; Harris *et al.*, 1971; Patrick *et al.*, 1972).

Exponentially dividing myoblast cells have a resting potential of approximately -65 mV. They can be classified as electrically excitable, since a small action potential may be observed at the moment of cessation of a hyperpolarizing current pulse. They do not, however, show delayed rectification as examined by a long depolarizing current pulse; their steady-state current–voltage relation is linear in the region of the resting membrane potential (Kidokoro, 1973).

The myoblasts respond to the iontophoretic application of acetylcholine with a long-lasting hyperpolarizing response (Fig. 12), which is in contrast to the depolarizing response observed in fused cells with two or more nuclei. The myoblast cells are also electrically coupled to their nearest neighbors by electrotonic junctions (Fig. 13).

Once the cells initiate fusion, they acquire the ability to generate action potentials having a large amplitude when excited by anode-break stimulation. These action potentials are observed in binucleate cells. Action potentials in myotubes have a longer duration than those in rat skeletal muscle *in vivo* and have a plateau which is similar to the action potential in cardiac muscle. In addition, delayed rectification develops in myotubes (Kidokoro, 1973).

The long-lasting hyperpolarizing response to applied acetylcholine is lost when myoblasts fuse. In binucleate cells, it is less common to find this response, and a faster, depolarizing response is usually seen. The change is not sudden or complete, for hyperpolarizing responses have been seen in cells with as many as ten nuclei. In addition, some cells may show both a fast depolarizing response and a slow hyperpolarizing one. In older myotubes, only fast depolarizing responses are observed.

With further time in culture, action potentials and contraction of myotubes occur spontaneously. Cells with spontaneous action potentials do not necessarily spontaneously contract (Fig. 14), but contractions are always associated with spontaneous electrical activity. Once myotubes acquire striations, the action potential has a shorter duration and becomes more similar to that observed *in vivo*.

Also associated with cell fusion in myoblast cultures is the appearance of membrane receptors for acetylcholine as defined by the binding of I^{125}-labeled α-neurotoxin (Patrick *et al.*, 1972). This reagent, when suitably employed, binds specifically to the acetylcholine receptor. In these experiments, the binding specificity was rigorously defined by the following criteria: (1) The kinetics of toxin binding exactly paralleled that of receptor inactivation assayed by the iontophoretic application of acetylcholine. (2) Toxin binding was inhibited approximately 50% by K_m quantities of several receptor

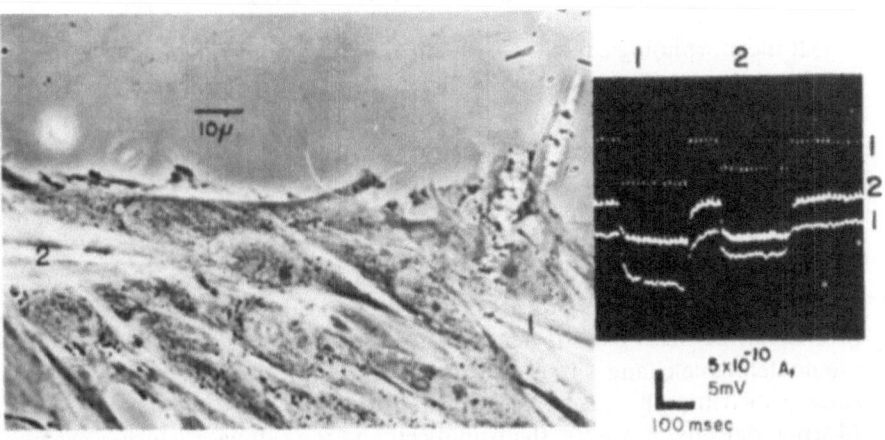

Fig. 13. Electrical coupling between myoblasts. Electrodes were inserted into two adjacent myoblasts. Current pulses were passed through each using a bridge circuit. The figure shows that current passed between the cells in either direction. The exact coupling coefficient cannot be evaluated, since the bridges became unbalanced on penetration. The current was passed through electrode 1 first, then electrode 2. Calibration bars: 10 μ, 100 msec, 5 mV, 5 × 10⁻¹⁰ amp.

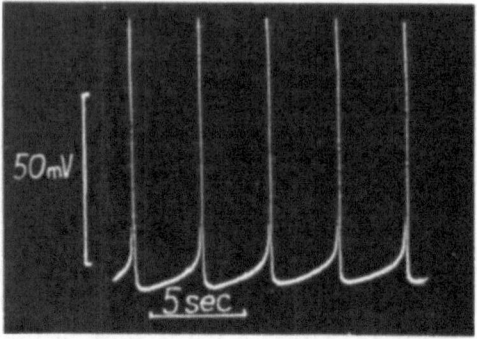

Fig. 14. Spontaneous action potentials in a myotube. A nonstriated myotube was impaled and the spontaneous action potentials were monitored. The cell did not contract spontaneously.

agonists and antagonists. (3) Toxin did not bind to a variety of nonexcitable cell culture lines nor to myoblasts. A time course for the appearance of acetylcholine receptors in myoblast cultures is presented in Fig. 15. The appearance of acetylcholine receptors is temporally related to the onset of the fusion and increases at a rate approximating that of the fusion process.

VI.   DIFFERENTIATION AND CELL CULTURE

If the morphological and biochemical behavior of the neuroblastoma and myoblast cultures described above were to be compared, it would be generally agreed that the change observed in the myoblast cultures is an example of differentiation in the classical sense (Grobstein, 1959). There would, however, be some disagreement as to whether or not the neuroblastoma is capable of differentiating in cell culture. The affirmation of myoblast differentiation is based on the facts that the process is apparently irreversible and that there are large changes, both qualitative and quantitative, in enzymatic and electrical activities. In contrast, the process of neurite extension by the neuroblastoma is reversible, the observed enzymatic changes are only quantitative, and there are no definable changes in the electrical properties of the cells except for the surface distribution of acetylcholine sensitivity (Harris and Dennis, 1970). Morphologically, however, the round cell and the cell with neurites are quite distinct, for only the latter has a network of microtubules.

A comparison of the two cell lines clearly presents problems which must be faced when studying cells which change in a manner analogous to that of neuroblasts and myoblasts as a function of time in culture. The first problem is simply one of semantics: should the term "differentiation" be applied to reversible processes, such as neurite formation, which occur in cell culture? The second is one of definition: if the word "differentiation" is acceptable, what set of criteria should be met before it is employed?

With respect to the first question, it is clear that if the old embryological dicta—that dividing cells do not differentiate and that cytodifferentiation is irreversible—are accepted, then the word "differentiation" cannot be applied to a process such as neurite formation in the neuroblastoma. More appropriate, perhaps, would be the word "modulation," coined by Weiss (1939) to indicate changes in cell properties which persist only as long as the initiating external influence, and reverse when it is withdrawn. Recently, however, the classical criteria for cytodifferentiation have been challenged, for several situations, both *in vivo* and *in vitro*, have been defined where highly differentiated cells are capable of reinitiating DNA synthesis (for review, see, e.g., Cameron and Jeter, 1971). Moreover, once a cell has been extracted from its normal environment to cell culture, it is difficult to predict how the maximally differentiated state of the cell will be expressed and, of perhaps more importance, what conditions are required to induce this state. Superimposed on these difficulties is the possibility that processes of cytodifferentiation which are normally irreversible *in vivo* may be reversible in cell culture. For example a neuroblast may extend and retract neurites *in vivo* until a stable synaptic contact is made with another cell, at which time it would become in-

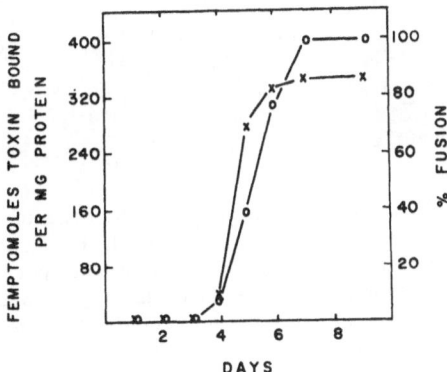

Fig. 15. Development of acetylcholine receptors during myogenesis. Myoblasts were plated on 60-mm tissue culture dishes at 5×10^4 cells per plate. At the indicated times, the number of toxin-binding sites, DNA content, protein content, and the percent of the nuclei in fused fibers were determined. No increase in the amount of DNA per plate was seen after the fifth day in culture. Circles, Percent of total nuclei in multinucleate cells; cross marks, femptomoles toxin bound/mg protein. Day 1 of the figure represents the third day after the cells were plated.

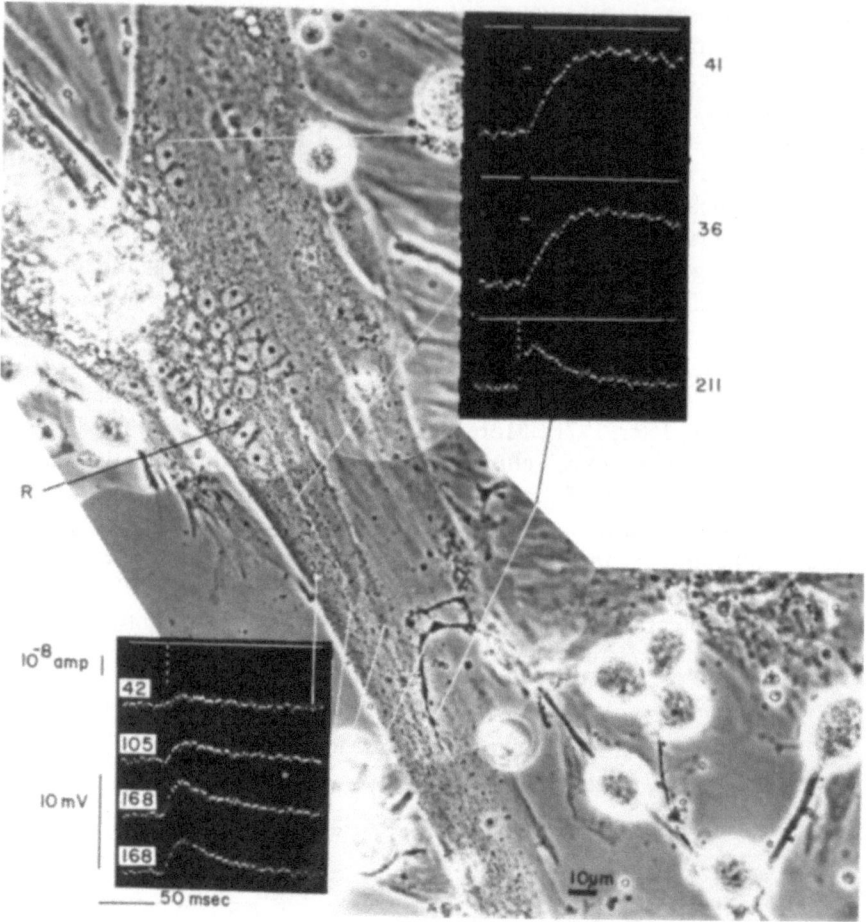

Fig. 16. Localization of acetylcholine sensitivity to the point of contact of a neuro-blastoma cell on a muscle fiber, 4 days after mixing the cells. The number corresponding to each point refers to acetylcholine sensitivity in mV/nC. An action potential could be evoked by a 1-msec pulse of acetylcholine applied to the contact region, whereas at other points on the muscle a 10-msec pulse was required for production of an easily measured depolarization. (From Harris *et al.*, 1971.)

capable of further division. If the same cell were placed in a tissue culture environment lacking the second target cell, it would never become stabilized with respect to division. It follows, however, that the process of differentiation, defined as the progression from a state of relative simplicity (neuroblast) to one of relative complexity (cell with neurites), is essentially the same in both cases. There is no reason, if the process is clearly delineated experimentally, why the term "differentiation" cannot be applied to both. Thus in a cell culture system it may be necessary to define "differentiation" as a process directed toward a given end but not necessarily reaching that final stage of ultimate functional complexity and specialization.

With respect to the second question, there is no ambiguity as to the criteria which must be met if the term "differentiation" is to be used in a clonal cell system. Clearly, the first requirement is that a series of well-defined changes toward a state of greater functional complexity and specialization, either morphological, biochemical, or electrophysiological, take place as a function of time in culture. In addition, this change must be qualitative in the sense that all of the cells within the culture respond to the given stimulus in a similar manner. This is an important point, for it is possible to induce cell flattening and neurite formation in a small fraction of the neuroblastoma cells within a population by processes which kill the majority of the cells. Similar morphological changes have been observed in fibroblast cultures following X-ray killing (Puck and Marcus, 1956). Clearly, such phenotypic alterations are not qualitative and cannot be defined as differentiative in nature.

Since BUdR, low-serum medium, and conditioned medium induce qualitative changes in the neuroblastoma round cell which lead to a more complex cell, at least at the morphological level, it follows that the term "differentiation" is applicable to this system.

VII. TROPIC INTERACTION BETWEEN NEUROBLASTOMA AND MYOBLAST CELL LINES

In an attempt to develop a clonal cell culture system where both the electrophysiology and biochemistry of synapse formation could be studied, neuroblastoma cells were allowed to differentiate on cultures of fused muscle, and the areas of nerve–muscle contact were examined electrophysiologically. Figure 16 shows that these cells interact in a manner analogous to the early events seen in normal synapse formation (Harris *et al.,* 1971). Thus when myotubes, which are normally uniformly sensitive to acetylcholine, are contacted by a neuroblastoma neurite, there is, after a given period of time, a discrete localization of acetylcholine sensitivity to the point of contact. This interaction is specific in the sense that fibroblasts and at least one other neuronal cell line do not induce localization, while another neuronal line besides C1300 does cause up to a thousandfold restriction of acetylcholine sensitivity. Although no unequivocal evidence for chemical synapse formation between neuroblastoma and muscle has yet been obtained, electrical junctions between the two cell lines have been demonstrated. This system thus provides an excellent model to analyze the mechanisms underlying the tropic effects of nerve on muscle.

VIII. SUMMARY

On the basis of the above data, it can be concluded that clonal tissue culture lines of neuroblastoma C1300 and a rat myoblast can differentiate in cell culture to cells morphologically and functionally resembling mature neurons and striated muscle fibers, respectively. It has been established that a strong interaction between the cell and the surface of the culture dish is the determining factor in neuroblastoma differentiation, defined here in terms of neurite extension and a quantitative change in macromolecular synthesis. Neuroblastoma differentiation is sometimes associated with an increase in the specific activity of acetylcholinesterase, but this increase is *primarily* due to aging and cell death, not neurite extension. Since the exponentially dividing neuroblastoma round cell is electrically excitable and can generate overshooting action potentials equivalent to the most differentiated cells, it follows that there is no developmental acquisition of the action-potential mechanism. The differentiated cell does, however, show a topographical distribution of acetylcholine sensitivity over its surface, and cells within the population are sometimes coupled by electrotonic junctions.

In contrast to the neuroblastoma, clonal myoblast cells undergo a clearly defined sequence of differentiation. The fusion of mononucleate myoblasts into multinucleate myotubes is accompanied by an increase in the specific activities of creatine phosphokinase and myokinase, a quantitative change in the rates of secretion of several proteins, and an increase in both the rate of synthesis and accumulation of myosin heavy chain. Myoblasts are electrically excitable, since a small action potential is generated by anode-break stimulation. Once myoblasts fuse, they acquire the ability to generate overshooting action potentials and, unlike the myoblasts, show delayed rectification. Myoblasts respond to the iontophoretic application of acetylcholine with a long-lasting hyperpolarizing response, while a depolarizing response is observed in fused cells with two or more nuclei. The acquisition of the depolarizing response is accompanied by an increase in acetylcholine receptors as defined by the specific binding of α-neurotoxin. Finally, it has been established that the neuroblastoma can induce the localization of acetylcholine sensitivity on the muscle in a manner reminiscent of the early stages of synapse formation.

IX. REFERENCES

Amano, T., Richelson, E., and Nirenberg, M. 1972. Neurotransmitter synthesis by neuroblastoma clones. *Proc. Natl. Acad. Sci.* 69:258–263.

Augusti-Tocco, G., and Sato, G. 1969. Establishment of functional clonal lines of neurons from mouse neuroblastoma. *Proc. Natl. Acad. Sci.* 64:311–315.

Bischoff, R., and Holtzer, H. 1970. Inhibition of myoblast fusion after one round of DNA synthesis in 5-bromodeoxyuridine. *J. Cell Biol.* **44**:134–150.

Blume, A., Gilbert, F., Wilson, S., Farber, J., Rosenberg, R., and Nirenberg, M. 1970. Regulation of acetylcholinesterase in neuroblastoma cells. *Proc. Natl. Acad. Sci.* **67**: 786–792.

Brown, J. C. 1971. Surface glycoprotein characteristic of the differentiated state of neuroblastoma C-1300 cells. *Exptl. Cell Res.* **69**:440–443.

Bunge, R., Bunge, M., Peterson, E., and Murray, M. 1965. An electron microscope study of cultured rat spinal cord. *J. Cell Biol.* **24**:163–191.

Cameron, I. L., and Jeter, J. R. 1971. Relationship between cell proliferation and cytodifferentiation in embryonic chick tissues, pp. 191–222. *In* I. L. Cameron, G. M. Padilla, and D. Zimmerman (eds.). Developmental Aspects of the Cell Cycle. Academic Press, New York.

Carlisle, W., Culp, W., Heinemann, S., Patrick, J., Schubert, D., Steinbach, J. H., and Tarikas, H. 1973. Induction and establishment neuronal and glial cell lines. (In preparation.)

Cohn, M. 1967. Natural history of the myeloma. *Cold Spring Harbor Symp. Quant. Biol.* **32**:211–220.

Crain, S. M., Peterson, E. R., and Bornstein, M. B. 1968. Formation of functional interneuronal connections between explants of various mammalian central nervous tissue during development *in vitro*, pp. 13–31. *In* G. E. W. Wolstenholme and M. O'Connor (eds.). Growth of the Nervous System. A CIBA Foundation Symposium. J. & A. Churchill Ltd., London.

Grobstein, D. 1959. Differentiation of vertebrate cells, pp. 437–496. *In* J. Brachet and A. Mirsky (eds.). The Cell, Vol. 1. Academic Press, New York.

Handle, M. A. 1971. Effects of experimental degradation of microtubules on the growth of cultured nerve fibers. *J. Exptl. Zool.* **178**:523–532.

Harris, A. J., and Dennis, M. J. 1970. Acetylcholine sensitivity and distribution on mouse neuroblastoma cells. *Science* **167**:1253–1255.

Harris, A. J., Heinemann, S., Schubert, D., and Tarikas, H. 1971. Trophic interaction between cloned tissue culture lines of nerve and muscle. *Nature* **231**:296–301.

Harrison, R. G. 1907. Observations on the living developing nerve fiber. *Anat. Rec.* **1**:116–118.

Holley, R. W., and Kiernan, J. A. 1968. "Contact inhibition" of cell division in 3T3 cells. *Proc. Natl. Acad. Sci.* **60**:300–304.

Horibata, K., and Harris, A. W. 1970. Mouse myelomas and lymphomas in culture. *Exptl. Cell Res.* **60**:61–77.

Humphreys, S., and Schubert, D. 1973. Morphological differentiation of a myogenic cell line. (In preparation.)

Kates, J. R., Winterton, R., and Schlessinger, K. 1971. Induction of acetylcholinesterase activity in mouse neuroblastoma tissue culture cells. *Nature* **229**:345–347.

Kidokoro, Y. 1973. Development of action potentials in a clonal skeletal myoblast cell line. *Nature New Biol.* **241**:158–159.

Minna, J., Nelson P., Peacock, J., Glazer, D., and Nirenberg, M. 1971. Genes for neuronal properties expressed in neuroblastoma × L cell hybrids. *Proc. Natl. Acad. Sci.* **68**:234–239

Minna, J., Glazer, D., and Nirenberg, M. 1972. Genetic dissection of neural properties using somatic cell hybrids. *Nature New Biol.* **235**:225–231.

Murray, M. R., and Stout, A. P. 1947. Distinctive characteristics of the sympathicoblastoma cultivated *in vitro*. *Am. J. Pathol.* **23**:429–435.

Nakai, J. 1964. The movements of neurons in tissue culture, pp. 337–385. *In* R. D. Allen and N. Kamiya (eds.). Primitive Motile Systems in Cell Biology. Acdemic Press, New York.

Nelson, P., Ruffner, W., and Nirenberg, M. 1969. Neuronal tumor cells with excitable membranes grown *in vitro*. *Proc. Natl. Acad. Sci.* **64**:1004–1010.

Nelson, P. G., Peacock., J. H., Amano, T., and Minna, J. 1971. Electrogenesis of mouse neuroblastoma cells *in vitro*. *J. Cell. Physiol.* **77**:337–352.

Patrick, J., Heinemann, S. F., Lindstrom, J., Schubert, D., and Steinbach, J. H. 1972. Appearance of acetylcholine receptors during differentiation of a myogenic cell line. *Proc. Natl. Acad. Sci.* **69**:2762–2766.

Puck, T. T., and Marcus, P. I. 1956. Action of X-rays on mammalian cells. *J. Exptl. Med.* **103**:653–666.

Richler, C., and Yaffe, D. 1970. The *in vitro* cultivation and differentiation capacities of myogenic cell lines. *Develop. Biol.* **23**:1–22.

Roots, B., and Johnston, P. V. 1964. Neurons of ox brain nuclei: Their isolation and appearance by light and electron microscopy. *J. Ultrastruct. Res.* **10**:350–361.

Sato, G. H., and Yasumura, Y. 1966. Retention of differentiated function in dispersed cell culture. *Trans. N.Y. Acad. Sci.* **28**:1063–1079.

Schubert, D., and Jacob, F. 1970. 5-Bromodeoxyuridine induced differentiation of a mouse neuroblastoma. *Proc. Natl. Acad. Sci.* **67**:247–254.

Schubert, D., Munro, A., and Ohno, S. 1968. Immunologlobulin biosynthesis I. A myeloma variant secreting light chain only. *J. Molec. Biol.* **38**:253–262.

Schubert, D., Humphreys, S., Baroni, C., and Cohn, M. 1969. *In vitro* differentiation of a mouse neuroblastoma. *Proc. Natl. Acad. Sci.* **64**:316–323.

Schubert, D., Humphreys, S., de Vitry, F., and Jacob, F. 1971a. Induced differentiation of a neuroblastoma. *Develop. Biol.* **25**:514–546.

Schubert, D., Tarikas, H., Harris, A. J., and Heinemann, S. 1971b. Induction of acetylcholine esterase activity in a mouse neuroblastoma. *Nature New Bio.* **233**:79–80.

Schubert, D., Tarikas, H., Humphreys, S., Heinemann, S., and Patrick, J. 1973. Protein synthesis and secretion in a myogenic cell line. *Develop. Biol.* **33**:18–37.

Seeds, N. W., Gilman, A. G., Amano, T., and Nirenberg, M. W. 1970. Regulation of axon formation by clonal lines of a neural tumor. *Proc. Natl. Acad. Sci.* **66**:160–167.

Sherbet, G. V., Lakshmi, M. S., and Rao, K. V. 1972. Characterization of ionogenic groups and estimation of the net negative electric charge on the surface of cells using natural *p*H gradients. *Exptl. Cell Res.* **70**:113–123.

Thompson, E. G., Tomkins, G. M., and Curran, J. F. 1966. Induction of tyrosine α-keto glutarate transaminase by steroid hormones in a newly established tissue culture cell line. *Proc. Natl. Acad. Sci.* **56**:296–303.

Varon, S., and Raiborn, C. W. 1968. Dissociation, fractionation, and culture of embryonic brain cells. *Brain Res.* **12**:180–199.

Yaffe, D. 1968. Retention of differentiation potentialities during prolonged cultivation of myogenic cells. *Proc. Natl. Acad. Sci.* **61**:477–483.

Yamada, K. M., Spooner, B. S., and Wessells, N. K. 1970. Axon growth: Roles of microfilaments and microtubules. *Proc. Natl. Acad. Sci.* **66**:1206–1212.

Weiss, P. 1939. Principles of Development. Holt, New York.

Witkowski, J. A., and Brighton, W. D. 1972. Influence of serum on attachment of tissue cells to glass surfaces. *Exptl. Cell Res.* **70**:41–48.

Chapter 4

Biochemical Characterization of a Clonal Line of Neuroblastoma

G. Augusti-Tocco, E. Parisi, and F. Zucco

Laboratorio di Embriologia Molecolare
C.N.R., Arco Felice
Naples, Italy

and

L. Casola and M. Romano

Istituto Internazionale di Genetica e Biofisica
C.N.R.
Naples, Italy

I. INTRODUCTION

Study of the molecular mechanism of differentiation has been hampered by, among other difficulties, the complexity of the systems investigated, where several changes occur at the same time and overlap each other. The possibility of selecting a homogeneous cellular population in which only a limited step of cellular maturation occurs may provide a useful system for studying cell differentiation.

Neuroblastoma cultures seem to fit this requirement. Clonal lines derived from a transplantable mouse neuroblastoma (Jackson C1300) express in culture several functional properties characteristic of neurons (Augusti-Tocco and Sato, 1969; Nelson *et al.*, 1969; Schubert *et al.*, 1969; Augusti-Tocco *et al.*, 1970; Olmsted *et al.*, 1970; Augusti-Tocco, 1971; Amano *et al.*, 1972). These cells can undergo maturation in culture, as shown by outgrowth of neurites in cells grown in monolayer culture; neurites are absent in the tumor and in suspension cultures.

The immature cells growing in suspension or as a tumor in the mouse already express several neurospecific functions; e.g., specific enzymes (Augusti-Tocco and Sato, 1969) and the mechanism for action potential (Augusti-Tocco et al., 1970) are present. The outgrowth of neurites occurring in monolayer cultures with the appearance of neurotubular structures may well represent the next step of neuronal maturation, even though these cells cannot be considered completely mature neurons because of their failure to form synapses in the culture conditions used up to now.

This situation resembles the sequence of events occurring during neuronal maturation: neuroblasts (round cells) give rise to multipolar neurons, which in turn form synapses when reaching the appropriate target cells. At present, it is not known what is the degree of expression of neurospecific functions at the various maturational steps, e.g., when the action-potential mechanism becomes active in the neuronal differentiation and whether the various neurospecific markers appear at the same time during maturation. Work on neuroblastoma suggests that the expression of various neurospecific markers is controlled independently. This has been shown for choline acetylase and acetylcholinesterase (Amano et al., 1972; Siman-Tov and Sachs, 1972) and for acetylcholinesterase and 14–3–2 protein (Augusti-Tocco et al., 1973). It might be true also for the action-potential mechanism and formation of synapses, although one should bear in mind that the inability of the cells in culture to form synapses might depend on irreversible metabolic alterations due to the neoplastic nature of the lines studied.

If neurite outgrowth represents one of the many sequential steps occurring during embryonic development, neuroblastoma cultures can be used as a model for the study of the molecular events underlying neuronal differentiation.

TABLE I

Protein and Nucleic Acid Composition of Mouse Neuroblastoma Clone NB41A3[a]

	$\mu g/10^6$ cells		
	DNA	RNA	Protein
Suspension	34	30	570
Monolayer	36	56	620

[a] 1–2×10^6 cells were washed with PBS (phosphate-buffered saline) and homogenized in RSB (reticulocyte standard buffer; Penman, 1966). Aliquots were taken for protein assay according to the method of Lowry et al. (1951). Another aliquot was used for nucleic acid determinations. RNA and DNA were precipitated by 5% TCA (trichloroacetic acid), and the precipitate was washed twice with 5% TCA. RNA was then hydrolyzed with 0.3 N KOH at 37°C overnight. DNA was precipitated by 5% PCA (perchloric acid), and after centrifugation RNA was assayed in the supernatant by the orcinol method (Mejbaum, 1939) and DNA in the precipitate by the diphenylamine method (Giles and Myers, 1965).

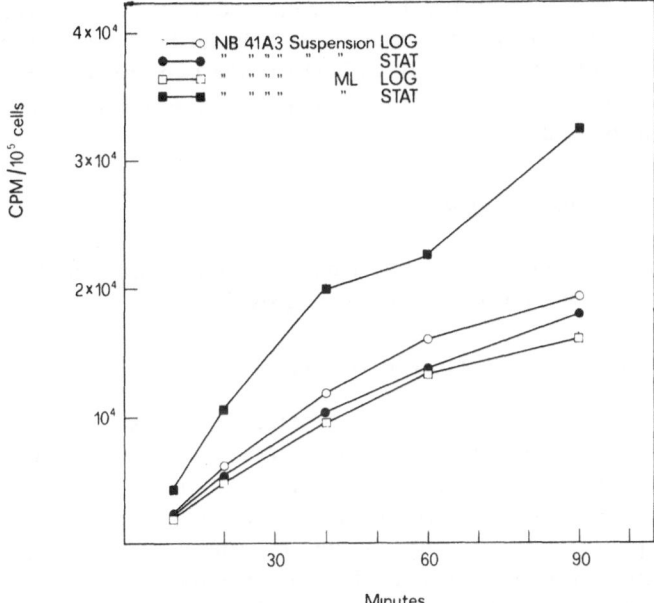

Fig. 1. Rates of incorporation of uridine-C¹⁴ into acid-insoluble material. Monolayer and suspension cells were incubated with 2.5 μc/ml uridine-C¹⁴ in Hank's solution. Incubation was stopped by washing the cells with cold Hank's solution containing 10^{-3} M uridine. Cells were suspended in RSB, and BSA (bovine serum albumin) and TCA to 5% final concentration were added. The precipitate was washed twice with 5% TCA, and then RNA was hydrolyzed in 0.3 N KOH at 37°C overnight. 5% final PCA was added, and radioactivity incorporated into RNA was measured in the supernatant. Scintillation fluid was 4 g/liter PPO (2,5-diphenyloxazole) and 50 mg/liter POPOP [p-bis-2-(5-phenyloxazolyl)benzene] in toluene containing 5% Bio-Solv solubilizer (BBS–3, Beckman).

At the molecular level, differentiation can be equated with the synthesis of specific proteins. Since ribonucleic acid (RNA) plays a major role in the control of protein synthesis, maturation is likely to be preceded by some changes in the RNA biosynthetic process of the cell.

In this chapter, we describe some changes in the pattern of RNA and protein biosynthesis occurring at the time of neurite outgrowth.

II. NUCLEIC ACID AND PROTEIN CONTENT

Deoxyribonucleic acid (DNA), total RNA, and total proteins were measured in cells growing in monolayer and suspension cultures. Table I shows that DNA per cell remains constant in the two conditions of growth. On the other hand, total RNA per cell is doubled in the monolayer with respect to the suspension culture. Protein content does not change when the cells are passed from suspension to monolayer culture. However, subcellular distribution of proteins seems to be different in the two growth conditions; the soluble proteins are 37% and 27% of total protein, respectively, in monolayer and suspension cells.

III.   RNA BIOSYNTHESIS

Uridine incorporation was studied in suspension and monolayer cultures in logarithmic and stationary phases of growth.

A.   Uridine Incorporation into RNA

Figure 1 shows that uridine incorporated into RNA continues increasing throughout the time period studied. The amount of incorporated uridine per cell is the same in suspension cells in both logarithmic and stationary phases, and in monolayer cells in logarithmic phase. When monolayer cells go into the stationary phase of growth, uridine incorporation into RNA increases. The difference in uridine incorporation between monolayer and suspension cells in stationary phase is not due to a difference in pool sizes of RNA precursors. Table II shows that the specific activity of uridine-5'-triphosphate (UTP) does not change.

B.   Sedimentation Pattern on Sucrose Gradient of Newly Synthesized RNA

1.   Uridine-Labeled RNA

RNA in neuroblastoma cells in monolayer and suspension cultures was labeled with uridine-C^{14} and run on sucrose gradient. Sedimentation profiles are shown in Figs. 2 and 3. RNA extracted after a 10-min pulse of uridine-

TABLE II

Specific Activity of Uridine-5'-Triphosphate[a]

		cpm/pmole	
Incubation time	=	20 min	90 min
Suspension		27.7	64.2
Monolayer		26.9	74.5

[a]Cells in stationary phase were incubated with uridine-C^{14} and the radioactivity in UTP was measured after thin layer chromatography of the acid-soluble extract. The cellular concentration of UTP had been previously measured by P^{32}-labeling (Colby and Edlin, 1970).

C^{14} is polydisperse, and no clear peak of radioactivity is observed. This polydisperse RNA remains present at all incubation times studied, although ribosomal RNA synthesis becomes predominant. A peak of preribosomal RNA (45S) appears after 30 min of labeling. At these short incubation times, the overall pattern of radioactivity on the gradient is essentially similar for monolayer and suspension cells. Processing of 45S preribosomal RNA goes through a number of maturation steps, similar to the ones described in HeLa cells (Penman, 1966). In fact, at 90 and 120 min of incubation, a second peak of radioactivity appears in the 30S–32S region.

In contrast to the situation described in other types of cells, in neuroblastoma cells a discrete peak of labeled 45S is still present after 4 hr of labeling. The radioactivity in 45S as compared to the total radioactivity in the two ribosomal RNAs is markedly higher in suspension than in monolayer cells.

It is worth noting that at all times of incubation a certain amount of radioactivity is pelleted in the sucrose gradient, in spite of numerous phenol extractions and DNase (deoxyribonuclease) treatment. This radioactivity is alkali and RNase (ribonuclease) sensitive, and its amount varies with the time of incubation and the type of cells.

2. Methionine-Labeled RNA

Methylation of RNA was studied by labeling cells for 20 min with radioactive methionine (Fig. 4). After sucrose gradient analysis of phenol-extracted RNA, radioactivity is found in the 45S region. The peak of radioactivity found in the light region of the gradient (4S) is most likely due to methionyl transfer RNA. Similar to what occurs in other cell types (Weinberg et al., 1967), Hn (heterogeneous) RNA is not methylated.

3. Adenosine-Labeled RNA

Poly A (polyriboadenylic acid) sequences associated with heterogeneous nuclear RNA were recently described in several cell lines (Edmonds et al., 1971; Darnell et al., 1971; Lee et al., 1971). Poly A synthetase was also found in nervous tissue (Dravid et al., 1971). For these reasons, we investigated the synthesis of poly A sequences associated with rapidly labeled RNA in neuroblastoma cells. Poly A was determined, after adenosine-H^3 labeling, as radioactivity resistant to low concentration of RNase at low ionic strength (Darnell et al., 1971). In Table III, the RNase resistance of uridine- and adenosine-labeled RNA after a 20-min pulse is compared. Uridine-labeled RNA is completely digested by RNase, while roughly 5% of the adenosine-labeled RNA is resistant. This material is alkali sensitive. Adenosine-labeled RNA was also run on sucrose gradient (Fig. 5) to investigate the distribution of RNase-resistant material. Total acid-insoluble radioactivity is polydispersed (Fig. 5,

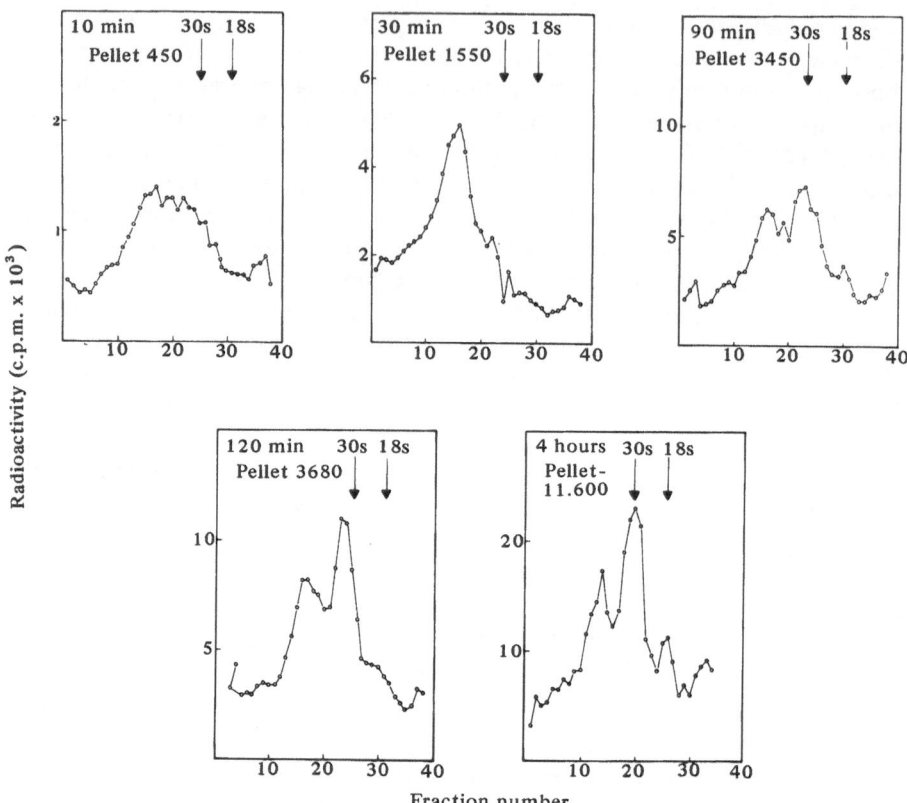

Fig. 2. Sucrose gradient analysis of uridine-C14-labeled RNA of neuroblastoma cells growing in monolayer. Cells in stationary phase were incubated with 5 μc/ml uridine-C14 in in Hank's solution for different times. Phenol-extracted RNA (Scherrer and Darnell, 1962) was layered on a 15–30% sucrose gradient in SDS (sodium dodecylsulfate) buffer (Penman, 1966) and centrifuged at 21,000 rpm in the SW25.3 Spinco rotor at 24°C for 16 hr. Gradients were analyzed for optical density, and radioactivity in RNA was measured in each fraction after TCA precipitation and filtration on millipore. Filters were counted in Bray's scintillation fluid. The gradient pellet was suspended in SDS buffer, TCA-precipitated, and filtered as above. The arrows indicate the position of optical density peaks.

upper part), as seen after uridine labeling (Figs. 2 and 3). As shown in the lower part of Fig. 5, RNase-resistant material is present in all regions of the gradient. However, unlike the total radioactivity, it is predominant in the upper half of the gradient. As already described for uridine-labeled RNA, the gradient pellet contains a certain amount of radioactivity. This radioactivity is partially resistant to RNase.

If RNA is subjected to RNase treatment and then run on sucrose gradient, all the radioactivity sediments at the top of the gradient.

4. Polysomal Patterns

Polysomal patterns were investigated in monolayer and suspension cells. Sucrose sedimentation analysis was performed on a postmitochondrial fraction after detergent treatment of the homogenate. Polysomes of different sizes are present, and no clear differences in their distribution are observed between the two types of cells (Fig. 6). However, a different ratio of polysomes and monosomes in the two types of cells indicates that in monolayer cells a larger fraction of the ribosomes are clustered into polysomes. RNase treatment prior to sucrose sedimentation causes the disappearance of all polysomes and gives a single peak of monosomes.

As judged by the ultraviolet-absorbing material on the gradient, monolayer cells show a high content of ribosomal particles. This may account for the higher RNA content in monolayer cells (Table I).

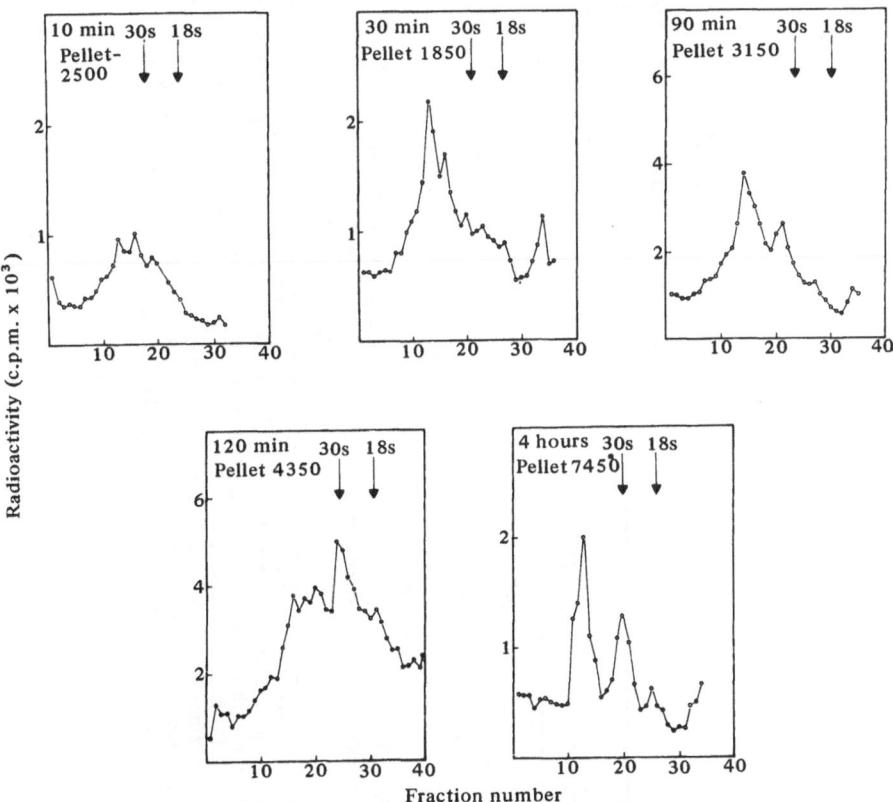

Fig. 3. Sucrose gradient analysis of uridine-C^{14}-labeled RNA of neuroblastoma cells growing in suspension. See Fig. 2.

TABLE III

RNase Resistance of Rapidly Labeled RNA[a]

Cell line	Label	Treatment of RNA	Acid-precipitable material (cpm)	Percent resistance
NB41A3 suspension	Uridine-C^{14}	None	5,290	
		Ribonuclease digestion	0	0
	Adenosine-H^3	None	83,325	
		Ribonuclease digestion	4,600	5.50
NB41A3 monolayer	Uridine-C^{14}	None	25,850	
		Ribonuclease digestion	29	0.11
	Adenosine-H^3	None	106,040	
		Ribonuclease digestion	5,870	5.55

[a]Cells in stationary phase were labeled for 20 min with either uridine-C^{14} (5 μc/ml in Hank's solution, specific activity 62 mc/mmole) or adenosine-H^3 (400 μc/ml in Hank's solution, specific activity 16 c/mmole). RNA was extracted at pH 5.5 (Scherrer and Darnell, 1962). An additional extraction at pH 9.0 was carried out on the remaining phenol phase. RNA in the combined aqueous phases, after ethanol precipitation, was subjected to DNase (deoxyribonuclease) treatment (10 μg/ml DNase for 1 hr at 0°C in 10^{-2} M tris, pH 7.4, 10^{-3} M $MgCl_2$) followed by a further phenol extraction and ethanol precipitation. RNA was then dissolved in 10^{-2} M tris, pH 7.4, 10^{-3} M $MgCl_2$. An aliquot was precipitated with 5% TCA in the presence of BSA and filtered on millipore. Another aliquot was treated with RNase A (2 μg/ml) and RNase T (50 units/ml) in 0.5 × SSC (0.15 M NaCl, 0.015 M sodium citrate) at 37°C for 30 min followed by TCA precipitation (Darnell *et al.*, 1971).

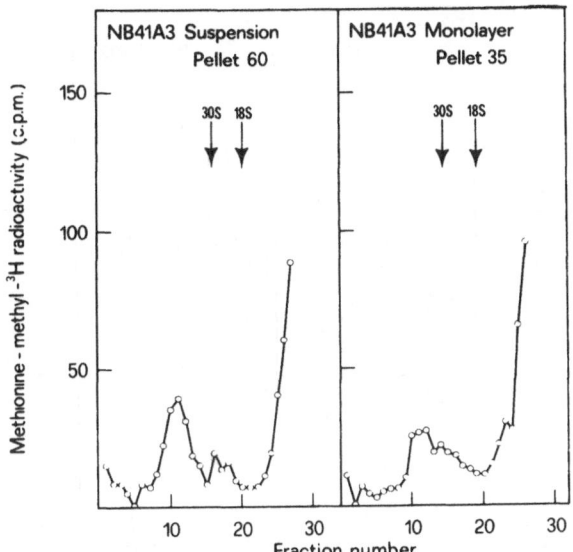

Fig. 4. Methylation of rapidly labeled RNA. Cells in stationary phase were labeled for 20 min with methionine-H³ (66 μc/ml in Hank's solution, specific activity 125 mc/mmole). RNA extraction and sucrose gradient centrifugation were as in uridine-labeling experiments.

5. Ribosomal RNA Decay

The kinetics of ribosomal RNA decay were compared in monolayer and suspension cells by pulse-chase experiments with radioactive methionine. The use of this precursor minimizes reutilization of the label and allows a more accurate estimate of RNA turnover (Weber, 1972).

Figure 7 shows that methionine-labeled ribosomal RNA decays with a half-life of 20 hr in both suspension and monolayer cells.

IV. PROTEIN BIOSYNTHESIS

A. Uptake and Incorporation of Leucine

Uptake of leucine-C¹⁴ and incorporation into protein was studied in monolayer and suspension cells, in logarithmic and stationary phases of growth.

As shown in Fig. 8A, the uptake of leucine does not change with the phase of growth in either condition of culture.

Leucine uptake by monolayer and by suspension cells does not show any significant difference in the first 2 hr of incubation. Beyond this time, uptake

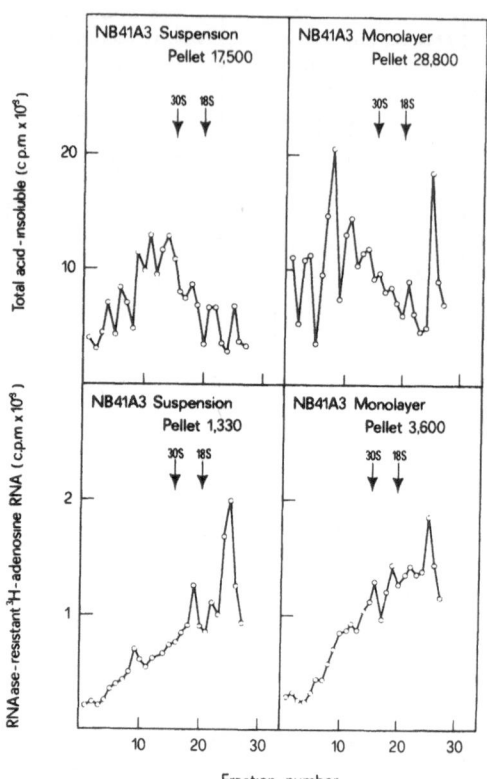

Fig. 5. Sucrose gradient analysis of adenosine-H³-labeled RNA. Cells were labeled with adenosine-H³ as described in Table III. Phenol-extracted RNA (see Table III) was analyzed on sucrose gradient as described in Fig. 2. Gradient fractions were divided into two 150-μl aliquots, and to each aliquot 50 μl of 2 × SSC was added. To one set of samples RNase (10 μg/ml) was added, and all samples were incubated at 37°C for 30 min. TCA-insoluble radioactivity was measured in both sets of samples as described in Fig. 2. Top traces show total acid-insoluble radioactivity, bottom traces show RNase-resistant radioactivity.

by monolayer cells does not increase further, while uptake by suspension cells continues to increase throughout the time interval studied.

Similarly, as shown in Fig. 8B, in the first hour leucine incorporation is the same in monolayer and suspension cultures; at longer incubation times, incorporation continues to increase in suspension cells and it remains constant in monolayer cells from 2 hr on.

This leveling off of leucine incorporation in monolayer cells depends on the plateau attained by the leucine uptake after long incubation time. The rate of incorporation measured as percentage of leucine entered into the cells appears to be very similar, if not the same, in monolayer and suspension cells.

Fig. 6.   Polysomal patterns of neuroblastoma cells. (A) Polysome profile
of suspension cells (8 × 10⁶ cells); (B)
polysome profile of suspension cells
after RNase treatment (8 × 10⁶ cells);
(C) polysome profile of monolayer cells
(4 × 10⁶ cells); (D) polysome profile
of monolayer cells after RNase treatment (4 × 10⁶ cells). Cytoplasmic
extracts were prepared from cells in
stationary phase. Cells were allowed to
swell in RSB at 0°C for 10 min and then
homogenized. One-tenth volume of a
detergent mixture (10% deoxycholate
and 10% Tween 40 1:2) was added to
the homogenate, which was then centrifuged at 2000 rpm in the International

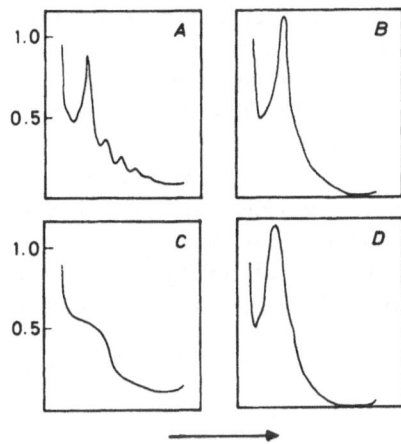

centrifuge. The supernatants were divided into two aliquots, and one was
treated with RNase (1 µg/ml) at 0°C for 10 min. Sedimentation analysis of
polyribosomes was performed on 15–30% sucrose gradient in RSB. The gradients
were centrifuged for 70 min at 40,000 rpm in the SW41 Spinco rotor at 4°C.
The optical density profiles were recorded continuously through an ISCO UV
recorder. Direction of sedimentation is indicated by the arrow.

B.   Analysis of Proteins by Polyacrylamide Gel Electrophoresis

The data reported in the previous section indicate that, unlike RNA
synthesis, the rate of protein synthesis of neuroblastoma cells is not affected
by the growth conditions. It was therefore necessary to investigate whether
qualitative differences were present. A qualitative comparative analysis of
labeled protein synthesized by the two cell types was undertaken by sodium
dodecylsulfate–polyacrylamide gel electrophoresis. Cell surface seems to be
mainly involved in the morphological change observed between suspension
and monolayer cultures. Therefore, this study was limited to insoluble proteins as the most likely to be involved in this change.

Cultures in logarithmic or stationary phase were labeled with either
leucine-C¹⁴ or leucine-H³ for 24 hr, and samples of the insoluble proteins
of monolayer and suspension cells were run together on SDS gels.

The proteins synthesized in logarithmic and stationary phases of growth
appear to be different on the basis of their molecular weight. In logarithmic
phase (Fig. 9), the radioactivity is rather uniformly spread throughout the gel,
while in stationary phase (Fig. 10) there is a prevalence of radioactivity in the
region of the gel where standard proteins of molecular weight 20,000–50,000
migrate (fractions 15–50).

The ratio of the two isotopes in each gel fraction is shown in Figs. 9 and 10 to make more clear the comparison of the distribution of radioactivity between suspension and monolayer cells.

Very little difference is seen in the comparison of cells in logarithmic phase (Fig. 9). However, in stationary phase, when neurite outgrowth is predominant, the ratio of radioactivity incorporated by the two cell types shows a significant difference (Fig. 10). Changes in the spectrum of protein synthesized by cells when growing neurites have been reported (Schubert and Jacob, 1970; Schubert *et al.*, 1971). In these experiments, neurite outgrowth was induced by either 5-bromodeoxyuridine (BUdR) or serumless medium. It is therefore difficult to explain the different types of changes observed.

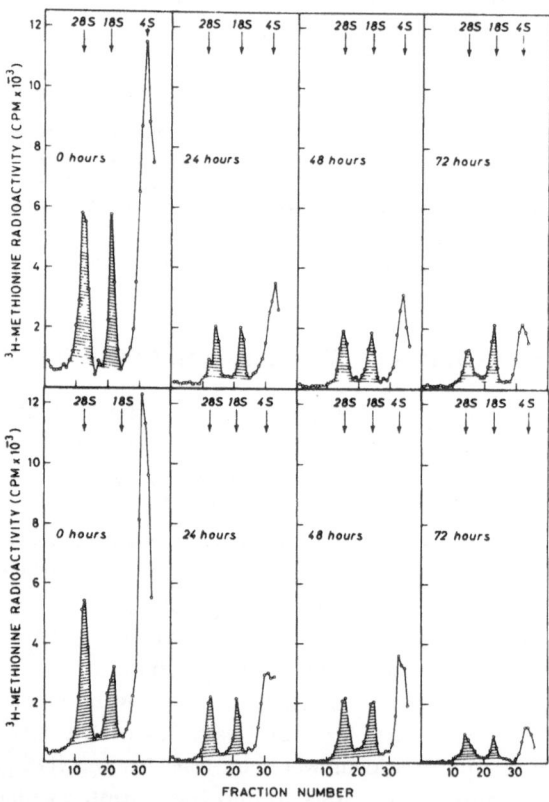

Fig. 7.   Ribosomal RNA decay. Cells in stationary phase were incubated for 28 hr with 15 μc/ml of methylmethionine-H^3(4 c/mmole) in F10 medium in the presence of adenosine, guanosine, and thymidine (2.5×10^{-5} M). At the end of the incubation, the radioactive medium was removed, the cells were repeatedly washed, and incubation was continued in medium containing 2×10^{-2} M cold methionine. At the times indicated in the figure, cells were collected. RNA extraction and sucrose gradients were performed as described in Fig. 2. Upper part, suspension cells; lower part, monolayer cells.

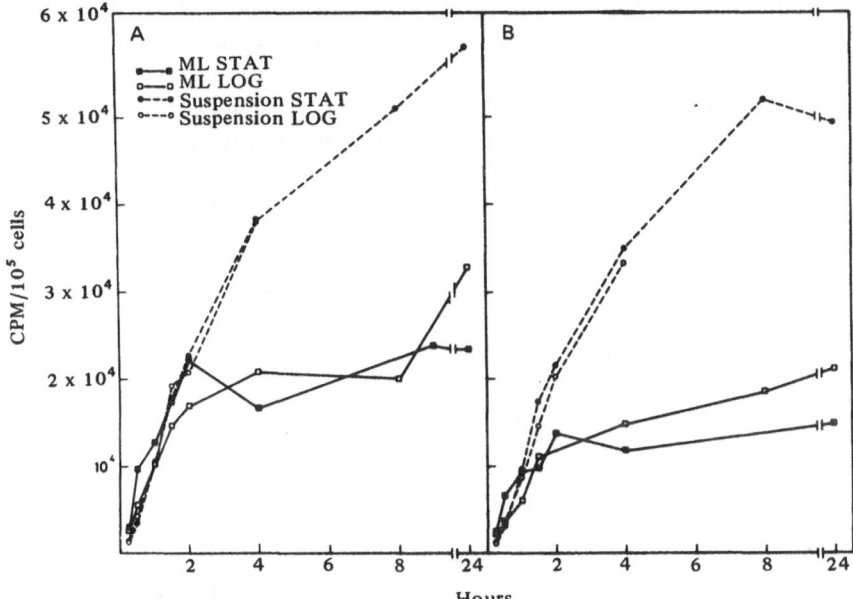

Fig. 8.   Uptake and incorporation of leucine-C^{14}. Monolayer and suspension cultures in logarithmic and stationary phases of growth were incubated with F10 medium (Ham, 1963) (minus leucine) containing 0.1 µc/ml leucine-C^{14}, specific activity 262 mc/mmole. The serum added to the medium had been exhaustively dialyzed against PBS. (A) Uptake was measured by filtering the cells on GFA (Whatman) filters. The cells were repeatedly washed with PBS containing 10^{-3} M leucine. The filters were dried and counted in 4 g/liter PPO and 50 mg/liter POPOP in toluene. (B) Incorporation was measured on TCA-insoluble material, after repeated washings with 5% TCA on GFA filters. The filters were counted as in A.

V.   GLYCOPROTEINS OF THE CELL SURFACE

In the previous paragraphs, we have reported the variations of RNA and protein biosynthesis accompanying neurite outgrowth in neuroblastoma cells. As already mentioned, maturation in these cultures is brought about by factors acting on the cell surface, i.e., cell attachment and flattening in tissue culture dishes, as opposed to growth as round cells in suspension culture.

Alterations of cell surface, morphologically shown by variation of cell attachment to glass, are caused by virus transformation (Buck *et al.*, 1970). Biosynthesis of surface glycoproteins has been shown to be involved in this process (Buck *et al.*, 1970; Warren *et al.*, 1972).

A comparative analysis of surface glycoproteins synthesized in monolayer and suspension cultures therefore seemed of interest.

Cells were labeled with glucosamine-H³ or glucosamine-C¹⁴, and surface glycoproteins, removed by mild trypsination of cells, were analyzed as described (Buck *et al.*, 1970).

Figure 11 shows the pattern of elution from a Sephadex G50 column of glycopeptides obtained by pronase digestion of glycoproteins. The patterns of elution of glycopeptides from monolayer and suspension cells (Fig. 11A) are very similar. However, the slowest-migrating peak from suspension cells

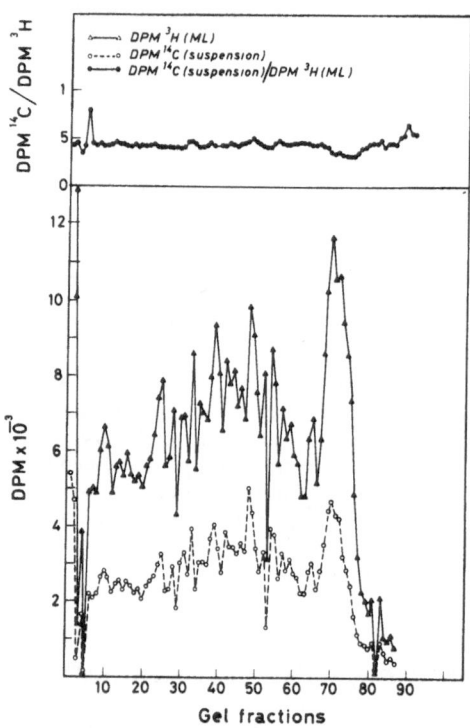

Fig. 9. Polyacrylamide gel electrophoresis of insoluble proteins of neuroblastoma cells in logarithmic phase of growth. Exponentially growing monolayer and suspension cultures were incubated for 24 hr with F10 containing either 5 μc/ml leucine-H³, specific activity 360 mc/mmole, or 2.5 μc/ml leucine-C¹⁴, specific activity 262 mc/mmole. Serum was dialyzed as in Fig. 8. Cells were homogenized in 0.01 M phosphate buffer, *p*H 7.6, and centrifuged at 40,000 rpm in the 40 Spinco rotor for 90 min. Pellets were solubilized in 0.01 M phosphate buffer, *p*H 7.4, 1% SDS, 1% mercaptoethanol at 100°C for 30 sec. Samples from the two pellets were mixed and run on 12-cm SDS–polyacrylamide gels, as described (Weber and Osborne, 1969). Acrylamide concentration was 6%. Gels were cut in slices 1.27 mm thick. Slices were left overnight at room temperature in 0.25 ml NCS solubilizer (Nuclear Chicago) and counted with 10 ml of 4 g/liter PPO, 50 mg/liter POPOP in toluene. Counting efficiency was 76% for C¹⁴ and 52% forH³.

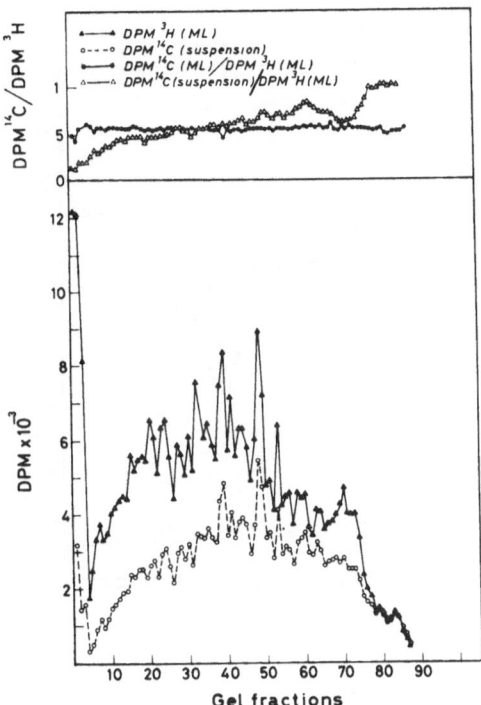

Fig. 10.   Polyacrylamide gel electrophoresis of insoluble protein of neuroblastoma cells in stationary phase of growth. Monolayer and suspension cultures in stationary phase were incubated with leucine-H³ and leucine-C¹⁴ as described in Fig. 9.

moves slightly faster. Suspension cells also appear to synthesize relatively more of the glycopeptides migrating ahead of this peak. Differences in the biochemical composition of neuroblastoma cell surface have been reported after bromodeoxyuridine treatment (Brown, 1972). Figure 11B shows that in cochromatography of monolayer cells labeled with either glucosamine-H³ or glucosamine-C¹⁴ the peaks of H³ and C¹⁴ radioactivity are coincident and the ratio C¹⁴/H³ remains constant throughout the column. In various experiments, the pattern of radioactivity on Sephadex G50 shows some variations, as may be seen by comparing parts A and B of Fig. 11. This may depend on minor differences in the trypsin treatment from one experiment to another.

VI.   DISCUSSION

Very little is known about the biochemical aspects of embryonic development of the nervous system. The cellular heterogeneity of nervous tissue

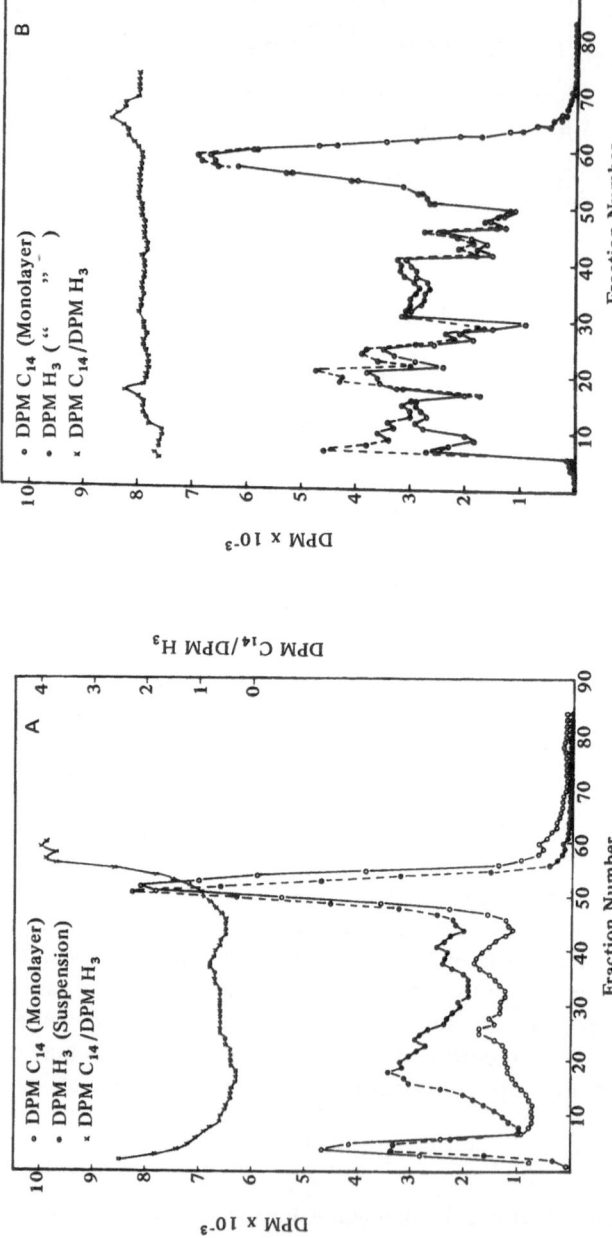

Fig. 11. Sephadex G50 profiles of labeled glycopeptides. Cells, 3 days after plating, were incubated with 1 μc/ml glucosamine-H[3] (1.3 c/mmole) or glucosamine-C[14] (7.05 mc/mmole) in complete F10 medium for 72 hr. Trypsinization of the cells, pronase digestion of the trypsinates, and Sephadex column were as described (Buck *et al.*, 1970), except that SDS and mercaptoethanol were omitted in the elution buffer of the Sephadex column. Fractions of the Sephadex column were counted in Bray's scintillation fluid. Counting efficiency was 65% for C[14] and 47% for H[3].

further complicates the study of biochemical events accompanying cellular maturation.

Neuroblastoma cultures appear to be a useful and simple system for this kind of study.

We have focused our attention on protein and RNA biosynthesis, with the aim of characterizing the metabolism of these macromolecules at the time of the morphological maturation observed in culture, i.e., neurite outgrowth.

The first interesting observation is the higher RNA content found in monolayer as compared to suspension cultures (Table I). An increase of RNA content occurs during neuroblast differentiation in chick cerebral hemispheres (Jacob, 1971) and in rabbit brain as fetal maturation proceeds (DeKaban et al., 1971). These findings may be related to the well-known appearance of Nissl bodies during the maturation of neuroblasts into neurons (Lumsden, 1968). Electron microscopy has shown that Nissl bodies are aggregates of ribonucleoprotein particles either free in the cytoplasm or attached to the endoplasmic reticulum (Lumsden, 1968).

The experiments summarized in Fig. 1 show that uridine incorporation into RNA is higher in monolayer than in suspension cells. Since the rate of RNA synthesis depends on the specific activity of the immediate precursor pool (uridine triphosphate, in this case), which is the same in suspension and monolayer cells (Table II), the higher uridine incorporation indicates that the rate of RNA synthesis increases when neuroblastoma cells are induced to change from immature to mature morphology.

The following considerations support the conclusion that the higher rate of RNA synthesis in monolayer cells determines the accumulation of ribosomal RNA in these cells:

1. The general pathway of biosynthesis of ribosomal RNA is substantially different in monolayer and suspension cells. The rate of synthesis and processing of 45S seems higher in monolayer cells (Figs. 2 and 3), as judged by the higher rate of uridine incorporation into RNA and by the faster disappearance of 45S preribosomal RNA in these cells.

2. The turnover of ribosomal RNA in monolayer and suspension cells is the same (Fig. 7).

The biological meaning of the increase of ribosomal RNA content in mature neurons may lie with mechanisms concerned with neurite outgrowth. Although not completely proven, neurites seem to contain a certain amount of ribosomal RNA (Casola et al., 1969; Bondy, 1972) which derives from the neuronal soma by axoplasmic flow.

Sucrose gradient analysis of uridine-labeled RNA summarized in Figs. 2 and 3 shows that both monolayer and suspension cells also synthesize heterogeneous (Hn) RNA.

Hn RNA, sedimenting faster than 45S, seems to be present in higher amount in suspension cells, as indicated by the high level of radioactivity associated with the gradient pellet in suspension cells after a 10-min pulse.

Rapidly labeled RNA, isolated after incubation with adenosine-H^3, is partially resistant to RNase, showing the presence of poly A sequences bound to RNA. Adenosine-labeled RNA of the two cell types does not show any difference in the percentage of RNase resistance (Table III) and in the distribution of RNase-resistant material on sucrose gradient (Fig. 5). Although the biological role of poly A in animal cells is yet unknown, it is worth mentioning that neuroblastoma cells appear to contain a considerably higher level of poly A than other cell lines studied (Edmonds *et al.*, 1971).

Protein biosynthesis also appears to be, to some extent, different in suspension and monolayer cells, although in the cell line studied no changes were observed in the protein content per cell and in the rate of protein synthesis.

As far as qualitative differences in the synthesized proteins are concerned, suspension cells synthesize relatively more protein of lower molecular weight, as shown by the higher ratio of radioactivity in the lower part of the gel in suspension *vs.* monolayer cells. It is worth noting that monolayer cells in logarithmic phase (Fig. 9) (where neurite outgrowth is less prominent than in stationary phase) also synthesize more protein of lower molecular weight.

Cochromatography of labeled glycopeptides from monolayer and suspension cells (Fig. 11A) suggests that the surface glycoproteins of the two cell types do differ to some extent. Such a difference might be due to a change in the biochemical composition of the cell surface. Otherwise, the attachment of cells to the culture dish may determine conformational changes of the membrane proteins and cause an increased or decreased exposure of surface components to trypsin.

In the first instance, it must be considered that the observed variation of isotope ratio in the various regions of the column could occur if the radioactivity in the glycoprotein fraction were present in more than one sugar and if these sugars had different pool size in the two cell types. Nevertheless, preliminary experiments have shown that after acid hydrolysis of the glycoprotein fraction followed by paper chromatography only glucosamine is labeled. The observed difference in glycopeptides may not be due to cell membrance constituents but to extracellular products. In fact, intercellular interactions in the two conditions of growth differ considerably. Cells in suspension cultures grow in aggregates, in which cells are kept together by some extracellular material. This material may not be produced by cells growing in monolayer.

In conclusion, the results reported above demonstrate that in culture conditions which promote neurite outgrowth several metabolic changes occur. They can be summarized as follows: (1) changes in the cell surface (either in the biochemical composition or in the molecular structure, (2) changes in the spectrum of protein synthesized, (3) accumulation of ribosomal RNA caused by a higher rate of RNA synthesis, and (4) different rates of synthesis of Hn RNA.

The observation that changes in RNA and protein biosynthesis are mediated through an effect on the cell surface (attachment to the culture dish) appears of particular interest in light of the role of the cell surface in development (Furshpan and Potter, 1968; Sidman, 1972; Goldschneider and Moscona, 1972).

VII. REFERENCES

Amano, T., Richelson, E., and Nirenberg, M. 1972. Neurotransmitter synthesis by neuroblastoma clones. *Proc. Natl. Acad. Sci.* **69**:258–263.

Augusti-Tocco, G. 1971. *In* F. A. Morris, P. G. Nelson, and F. H. Ruddle (eds.). Contributions of clonal systems to neurobiology; *Neurosci. Res. Bull.*, Vol. 11

Augusti-Tocco, G., and Sato, G. H. 1969. Establishment of functional clonal lines of neurons from mouse neuroblastoma. *Proc. Natl. Acad. Sci.* **64**:311–315.

Augusti-Tocco, G., Sato, G. H., Claude, P., and Potter, D. D. 1970. Clonal cell lines of neurons, pp. 109–120. *In* H. A. Padykula (ed.) Control Mechanisms in the Expression of Cellular Phenotypes. Academic Press, New York.

Augusti-Tocco, G., Casola, L., and Grasso, A. 1973. Neuroblastoma cells and 14-3-2, a brain specific protein. Submitted for publication.

Bondy, S. C. 1972. Axonal migration of various ribonucleic acid species along the optic tract of the chick. *J. Neurochem.* **19**:1769–1776.

Brown, J. C. 1972. Surface glycoprotein characteristic of the differentiated state of neuroblastoma C–1300 cells. *Exptl. Cell Res.* **69**:440–442.

Buck, C. A., Glick, M. C., and Warren, L. 1970. A comparative study of glycoproteins from the surface of control and Rous sarcoma virus transformed hamster cells. *Biochemistry* **9**:4567–4576.

Casola, L., Davis, G. A., and Davis, R. E. 1969. Evidence for RNA transport in rat optic nerve. *J. Neurochem.* **16**:1037–1041.

Colby, C., and Edlin, G. 1970. Nucleotide pool levels in growing, inhibited, and transformed chick fibroblast cells. *Biochemistry* **9**:917–920.

Darnell, J. E., Wall, R., and Tushinski, R. J. 1971. An adenylic acid–rich sequence in messenger RNA of Hela cells and its possible relationship to reiterated sites in DNA. *Proc. Natl. Acad. Sci.* **68**:1321–1325.

DeKaban, A. S., Patton, V. M., and Cain, D. F. 1971. Structural and biochemical maturation of the cerebral pallium in rabbit fetuses: morphogenesis and lipids. *J. Neurochem.* **18**:2451–2459.

Dravid, A. R., Pete N., and Mandel, P. 1971. An enzyme system in rat brain nuclei incorporating AMP into polyadenylate. *J. Neurochem.* **18**:299–300.

Edmonds, M., Vaughan, M. H., and Nakazato, H. 1971. Poly-adenylic acid sequences in the heterogeneous nuclear RNA and rapidly-labeled polyribosomal RNA in Hela cells: possible evidence for a precursor relationship. *Proc. Natl. Acad. Sci.* **68**:1336–1340.

Furshpan, E. J., and Potter, D. D. 1968. Low-resistance junctions between cells in embryos and tissue culture, pp. 95–127. In A. A. Moscona, and A. Monroy, (eds.). Current Topics of Developmental Biology, Vol. 3. Academic Press, New York.

Giles, K. W., and Myers, A. 1965. An improved diphenylamine method for the estimation of DNA. *Nature* **206**:93.

Goldschneider, I., and Moscona, A. A. 1972. Tissue-specific cell-surface antigens in embryonic cells. *J. Cell Biol.* **53**:435–449.

Ham, R. G. 1963. An improved nutrient solution for diploid Chinese hamsters and human cell lines. *Exptl. Cell Res.* **29**:515–526.

Jacob, M. 1971. RNA metabolism and differentiation of the central nervous system. *In* Abstracts 7th FEBS Meeting, Varna, p. 70.

Lee, S. Y., Mendecki, J., and Brawerman, G. 1971. A polynucleotide segment rich in adenylic acid in the rapidly-labeled polyribosomal RNA component of mouse sarcoma 180 ascites cells. *Prod. Natl. Acad. Sci.* **68**:1331–1335.

Lowry, O. H., Rosebrough, N. F., Farr, A. L., and Randall, R. G. 1951. Protein measurement with the Folin phenol reagent. *J. Biol. Chem.* **193**:265–275.

Lumsden, C. E. 1968. Nervous tissue in culture, pp. 67–140. *In* G. H. Bourne (ed.) The Structure and Function of Nervous Tissue. Academic Press, New York.

Mejbaum, W. 1939. Über die Bestimmung kleiner Pentosemengen, insbesondere in Derivaten der Adenylsäure. *Hoppe-Seylers Z. Physiol. Chem.* **258**:117–120.

Nelson, P., Ruffner, W., and Nirenberg, M. 1969. Neuronal tumor cells with excitable membranes grown *in vitro*. *Proc. Natl. Acad. Sci.* **64**:1004–1010.

Olmsted, J. B., Carlson, K., Klebe, R., Ruddle, F., and Rosenbaum, J. 1970. Isolation of microtubule protein from cultured mouse neuroblastoma cells. *Proc. Natl. Acad. Sci.* **65**:129–136.

Penman, S. 1966. RNA metabolism in the Hela cell nucleus. *J. Molec. Biol.* **17**:117–130.

Scherrer, K., and Darnell, J. E. 1962. Sedimentation characteristics of rapidly labeled RNA from Hela cells. *Biochem. Biophys. Res. Commun.* **7**:486–490.

Schubert, D., and Jacob, F. 1970. 5-Bromodeoxyuridine-induced differentiation of a neuroblastoma. *Proc. Natl. Acad. Sci.* **67**:247–254.

Schubert, D., Humphreys, S., Baroni, C., and Cohn, M. 1969. *In vitro* differentiation of a mouse neuroblastoma. *Proc. Natl. Acad. Sci.* **64**:316–323.

Schubert, D., Humphreys, S., de Vitry, F., and Jacob, F. 1971. Induced differentiation of a neuroblastoma. *Develop. Biol.* **25**:514–546.

Sidman, R. L. 1972. Cell interactions in developing mammalian central nervous system, pp. 1–13. *In* L. G. Silvestri (ed.). Cell Interactions. North-Holland, Amsterdam and London.

Siman-Tov, R. and Sachs, L. 1972. Enzyme regulation in neuroblastoma cells. *Europ. J. Biochem.* **30**:123–129.

Warren, L., Critchley, D., and Macpherson, I. 1972. Surface glycoproteins and glycolipids of chicken embryo cell transformed by a temperature-sensitive mutant of Rous sarcoma virus. *Nature* **235**:275–278.

Weber, K., and Osborn, M. 1969. The reliability of molecular weight determinations by dodecylsulfate–polyacrylamide gel electrophoresis. *J. Biol. Chem.* **244**:4406–4412.

Weber, M. J. 1972. Ribosomal RNA turnover in contact inhibited cells. *Nature* **235**:58–61.

Weinberg, R. A., Loening, U., Williems, M., and Penman, S. 1967. Acrylamide gel electrophoresis of Hela cell nucleolar RNA. *Proc. Natl. Acad. Sci.* **58**:1088–1095.

Chapter 5

Regulation of Neuronal Enzymes in Cell Culture

Roger N. Rosenberg

Department of Neurosciences and Pediatrics and University Hospital
University of California at San Diego School of Medicine
La Jolla, California

I. INTRODUCTION

In 1907, Ross G. Harrison published a report, "Observations on the Living Developing Nerve Fiber," the first published account of the maintenance and growth of neural tissue *in vitro*. He explanted a small portion of neural tube from a frog embryo and demonstrated the development of an axis cylinder from perikaryon over clotted lymph. The great importance of this experiment was that (1) it indicated that neuronal morphological differentiation could be continued and studied for prolonged periods *in vitro* and (2) it provided unambiguous data to support the Cajal neuron doctrine, as the evolving naked fibers in his cultures were processes of neuronal units and not syncytial in origin. Since Harrison's paper, a voluminous body of literature has accumulated documenting the development of explants *in vitro* from central and peripheral nervous systems. This has been comprehensively reviewed by Murray (1965) and includes the following topics: cellular morphology and movements, neurite outgrowth, neurophysiological properties, neurosecretion, effect of drugs and nerve growth factor, the electron microscopic appearance of long-term cultured neurons, maintenance of and new synapse formation *in vitro*, myelination *in vitro*, axoplasmic flow, and experimental allergic encephalomyelitis and neuritis studied *in vitro*. The quantitative biochemical characterization of neuronal differentiation *in vitro* has been developed more recently and is the subject of this chapter.

These investigations were supported by a research grant from the American Cancer Society, Inc., New York, N.Y. (6–444–946–58605).

The development of highly sensitive radioisotopic microassays for enzymes involved in neurotransmitter biosynthesis has allowed characterization of enzyme activities in small amounts of neural tissue during stages of differentiation in cell culture. It has become possible with these new techniques to move beyond morphological and histochemical descriptive characterizations of *in vitro* neuronal differentiation. The enzymology of neurotransmitter synthesis and degradation in cell culture has opened an exciting new chapter in the quantitative understanding of developmental processes in the nervous system. The cell culture system provides a highly dynamic approach to the study of neuronal differentiation, as rates of cell growth, cell density, and growth environment can be varied at will to study their effects on specific enzymatic events.

Dissociated newborn Balb/C mouse brain and the cloned C1300 Ajax mouse neuroblastoma are two distinctly different cell culture systems which have provided interesting quantitative enzymatic information about the differentiation of nervous system tissue. The Balb/C mouse brain approach allows dissociated neurons, glia, fibroblasts, histiocytes, and blood vessel endothelial cells to interact as single cells and re-form into a monolayer on a petri dish or into an aggregate of mixed cells in a suspension–rotation culture. The cell culture of mouse neuroblastoma utilizes a pure population of cloned, transformed neuroblasts and allows the study of enzymatic and morphological development of neurons devoid of the effect by any other cell type. This chapter will concern itself with describing recent experiments which demonstrate the regulation of neuronal marker enzymes as cells in culture are made initially to become undifferentiated, then allowed to divide rapidly, and finally observed to develop differentiated neuronal properties.

II. DISSOCIATED PRIMARY MOUSE BRAIN CULTURES

A. Monolayer Cultures

Newborn Balb/C mouse brain was cultured as single cells after serial trypsin dissociations (Schrier *et al.*, 1970, Wilson, *et al.*, 1972). Ten million viable brain cells as determined by exclusion of nigrosin stain were placed in 150-mm petri dishes and incubated in 10% CO_2, 90% air, 100% humidity, 37°C in Dulbecco's modified Eagle's medium with 10% fetal calf serum and 50 units/ml penicillin and 10 μg/ml streptomycin. The ontogeny of the cultures was followed by assays of cell number, DNA and protein content, and activities of three enzymes considered to be markers of neuronal differentiation.

Choline-*O*-acetyltransferase (CAT) (E.C. 2.3.1.6) and acetylcholinesterase (AChE) (E.C. 3.1.1.7), two important enzymes in acetylcholine
metabolism, and glutamic acid decarboxylase (GAD) (E.C. 4.1.1.15), responsible for the synthesis of the inhibitory neurotransmitter γ-aminobutyric
acid (GABA), were chosen for characterization. CAT, AChE, and GAD
activities were assayed according to the methods of Wilson *et al.* (1972) and
Schrier *et al.* (in press). Protein was assayed by the method of Lowry *et al.*
(1951). Enzyme activities per milligram of protein were measured for three
enzymes approximately every 3 days in culture for a 2-week period (Schrier
et al., 1970; Wilson *et al.*, 1972).

Single-cell populations were obtained from intact newborn Balb/C
mouse brains by serial exposure to 0.25% trypsin in Puck's Ca^{2+},Mg^{2+}-free
D_1 salt solution, at 37°C, for three 15-min intervals. This yielded about
100×10^6 viable brain cells per gram wet weight of brain, or 7.4×10^6 cells
from the dissociation of a single mouse brain. The dissociation yielded 21%
of the DNA present in an intact brain as measured quantitatively by fluoro-

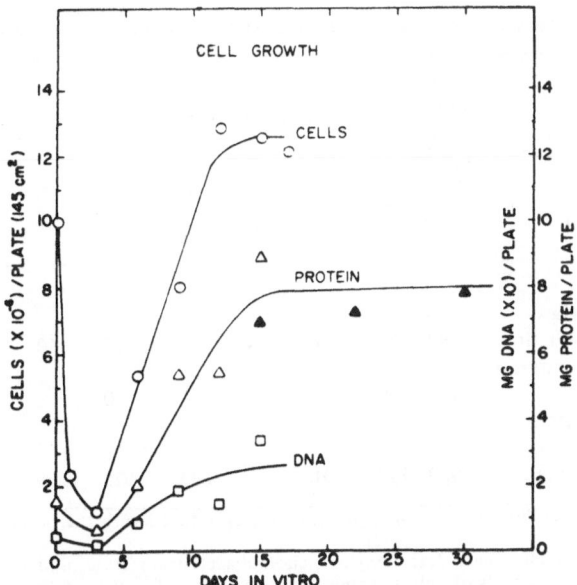

Fig. 1.   Growth characteristics of newborn mouse brain cells in culture. The day 0 values
represent the DNA and protein content of the initially plated cells. On day 0, 10^7 viable
cells were placed in each dish. Circles represent the cell count, triangles the protein content,
and squares the DNA content per plate. The filled triangles indicate the protein content
for an extended time period. (From Schrier *et al.*, 1970, and Wilson *et al.*, 1972. Reproduced with the permission of *J. Biol. Chem.*)

metric measurement, and if this represented about 21 % of the total number of cells then the Balb/C newborn mouse brain contains about 35×10^6 cells.

As shown in Fig. 1, about 10 % of the initially plated cells remained viable by day 3 in culture, and it was the rapid division of these surviving cells which produced a monolayer of about 12×10^6 cells after 2 weeks in culture. There was a parallel rise in total plate protein and DNA content during the growth period.

Aliquots of the freshly dissociated newborn mouse brain cells were assayed for CAT, AChE, and GAD activities and compared to newborn mouse brain homogenate, cultured nonneuronal brain cells, and cultured nonbrain cells (Table I). The remainder of the freshly dissociated cells were placed in culture, and enzyme assays were performed every 3 days. The range and sensitivity of assays, enzyme stability and product recovery, and assay conditions are described in Tables II–IV.

A summary of the changes in enzyme activities as the cultures grew and

TABLE I

Enzyme Specific Activities in Newborn Mouse Brain and Cultured Cells[a]

Determination	Newborn mouse brain homogenate	Cultured cells							Newborn mouse brain cells
		Brain, nonneuronal				Nonbrain			
		C6	C12	CHB	RC179	L929	Hela	3T3-S	
Glutamate decarboxylase									
By CO_2 production	487	79	71	84	43	55	13	8	93
By γ-Aminobutyrate production	496	8	5	1	3	0.2		6	86
Choline acetyltransferase	75	9			2	10	3	5	16
Acetylcholinesterase	25,900	732	701		280	625	299	102	1120

From Schrier et al, (1970) and Wilson et al. (1972). Reproduced with the permission of J. Biol. Chem.

[a]Specific activities of glutamate decarboxylase, choline acetyltransferase, and acetycholinesterase were determined on extracts of cultured cells. An uncentrifuged homogenate of newborn Balb/C mouse brain was used for comparison. The maximum content of homgenate protein in the assays was 237 µg for mouse brain homogenates, 110 µg for C6, 906 µg for $C2_1$, 852 µg for CHB, 258 µg for RG179, 1306 µg for L929 (B82 clone), 939 µg for HeLa, 533 ug for 3T3-S (Swiss mouse 3T3), and 580 µg for mouse brain cells cultured 30 days. Formation of γ-aminobutyric acid was determined in assays with ʟ-glutamate-U-C^{14} as substrate, followed by electrophoresis and chromatography. All determinations on cultured cells were 7–20 days after confluency. Glutamate decarboxylase activity shown for C6 represents the highest activity (at 31.5 mg of cell protein per 150-mm dish) found among four separate points on a growth cruve.

TABLE II

Range and Sensitivity of Assays

Assay	Source of homogenate	Incubation time (min)	Radioactive product	Usual range and sensitivity, amount of C^{14} or H^3 product per reaction (pmoles)	Average amount of C^{14} or H^3 product/min/mg protein (pmoles)
Acetylcholinesterase	Neuroblastoma clone N18	10	Acetate-H^3	1,000⎱ 14,000⎰	75,000
			Acetate-C^{14}	75⎱ 14,000⎰	75,000
Choline acetyltransferase	Mouse brain (age 35 days)	10	Acetylcholine-C^{14}	5⎱ 700⎰	1,500
Glutamate decarboxylase	Mouse brain (newborn)	10	$C^{14}O_2$	20⎱ 3,000⎰	150
Catechol-O-methyltransferase	Neuroblastoma clone N18	20	3-Methoxy-4-hydroxybenzoic acid-C^{14}	10⎱ 1,200⎰	75

From Wilson *et al.* (1972). Reproduced with the permission of *J. Biol. Chem.*

differentiated is seen in Fig. 2. It is of great interest that each of the marker enzymes selected followed a different pattern of induction of activity. The "signal" for induction of CAT was present as the cells were rapidly dividing and persisted into the postconfluent phase. Although there were increasing amounts of acetylcholine being synthesized as the cultures approached and became confluent, there remained persistent low levels of AChE activity. Apparently, the "signal" for its induction was independent of the concentrations of acetylcholine present under these culture conditions or the AChE activity expressed was adequate to hydrolyze available acetylcholine. GAD activity, i.e., synthesis of GABA, remained low during the period of rapid cell division, and only with confluency and restricted cell division was there induction of GABA formation. GAD activity in brain cultures was at least tenfold higher than in nonneuronal cell cultures.

The morphological appearance of the cultures changed dramatically during this 2-week culture period. At first, cells were rounded-up and appeared as nonspecific undifferentiated cells. During the first week in culture, cells developed processes and several cell types were recognizable only as being polygonal or spindle shaped, but no characteristic cell resembling a neuron could be identified. By day 9 in culture, phase-dark large multipolar

TABLE III

Enzyme Stability and Product Recovery[a]

Modification	Choline acetyltransferase (%)	Acetyl-cholinesterase (%)	Glutamate decarboxylase (%)	Catechol-O-methyltransferase (%)
Enzyme stability				
Complete reaction	100	100	100	100
Minus enzyme	2	9	8	9
Enzyme frozen and thawed				
three times	98	99	109	108
Enzyme held at 1 C for 2–3 hr	100	100	116	104
Enzyme held at 100 for 10 min	2	9	8	8
Reaction incubated at 1 C				
Product recovery	9	31	10	7
Radioactive product added				
instead of substrate	95	110	94	83

From Wilson *et al.* (1972). Reproduced with the permission of *J. Biol. Chem.*
[a]The amounts of radioactive product formed (picomoles) per complete reaction corresponding to 100% were 610, 1x,300, 630, and 114 for choline acetyltransferase, acetylcholinesterase, glutamate decarboxylase, and catechol-O-methyltransferase reactions, respectively. Product recovery was tested by adding the following compounds to reactions in place of radioactive substrate; choline acetyltransferase assay, 28 nmoles of acetylcholine iodide -x-C^{14} (1.53 × 10 dpm); acetylcholinesterase, 208 nmoles of sodium acetate-C^{14} (8.05 × 10^6 dpm; glutamate decarboxylase, 35 nmoles of $NaH^{14}CO_3$ (3.97 × 10^5 dpm; catechol-O-methyltransferase, 0.133 nmole of 3-methoxy-4-hydroxybenzoic acid-C^{14} (3.4 × 10^8 dpm) and 0.015 nmole of 4-methoxy-3-hydroxybenzoic acid-C^{14} (350 dpm).

cells could be seen (Fig. 3), and during the next 2 weeks many more phase-dark cells became evident with the elaboration of many long, complex-appearing neurites (Fig. 4), suggesting circuit formation. A culture maintained for 42 days and then stained with a Bodian protargol silver stain which has high affinity for neuronal processes contained many cells which stained positively and looked like characteristic neurons (Fig. 5).

Thus the monolayer culturing of mixed, dissociated newborn Balb/C mouse brain cells resulted in the organization of a new network of cells. Most important is that this approach provided simultaneous direct morphological and enzymatic data of neuronal redifferentiation *in vitro* and that changes in activities of enzymes concerned with acetylcholine and GABA metabolism were selective.

B. Suspension–Rotation Cultures

Recently, a suspension-rotation brain cell culture system derived from embryonic dissociated mouse brain was developed by Seeds (1971) and Seeds and Gilman (1971). Dissociated cells from embryonic mouse brain reaggregated in suspension–rotation cultures, and between days 4 and 14 in culture there were significant increases in specific activities of CAT, AChE, and GAD. Also within hours of rotation culturing, an aggregate of cells was produced which was capable of producing a four- to sixfold increase in the intracellular level of cyclic AMP (adenosine-3′,5′-monophosphate) due to a brief incubation with 10^{-4} M norepinephrine or isoproterenol (Seeds and Gilman, 1971). The cyclic AMP response to these sympathomimetic agents did not occur with freshly dissociated brain nor in cultures 15 hr old, but was present in 9-day cultures. This response could be considered to be a developmental event, as a similar nonresponsiveness was observed in brains of newborn rats and appeared only after 4 days of age.

Synaptogenesis has been observed to occur in dissociated embryonic brain cells which reassociate in rotation culture to form aggregates (Seeds and Vatter, 1971). Synapse formation was not evenly distributed within the aggregate but rather was found in groups, making a direct comparison difficult of the number of synapses made between 12- and 33-day-old rotation

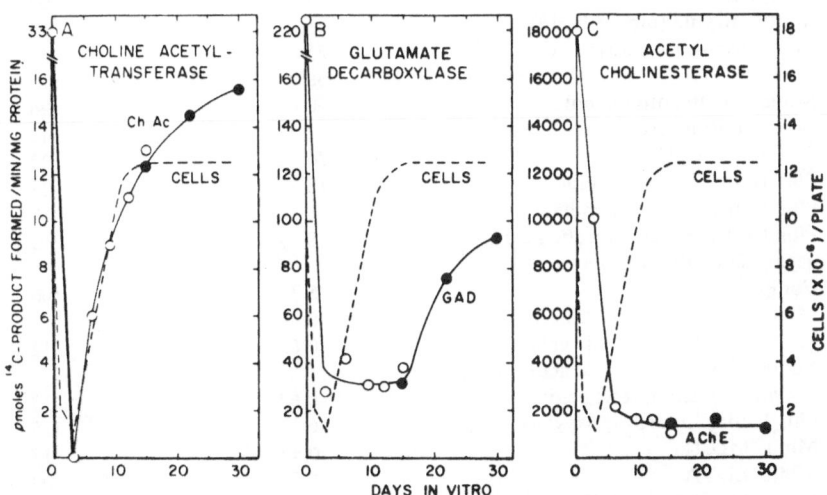

Fig. 2.   The specific activities of CAT, GAD, and AChE plotted against the time that cells were in culture. Initially, 10^7 viable newborn Balb/C mouse brain cells were placed in each 150–mm petri culture dish. These enzymes were assayed according to the methods described in Tables II–IV and in the text. The day 0 points represent the specific activity of the enzyme in the initially plated cells. The dashed line represents the cell count. Open circles represent the activity of the culture mg protein min, and filled circles represent the same activity for an extended time period. (From Schrier *et al.*, 1970, and Wilson *et al.*, 1972. Reproduced with the permission of *J. Biol. Chem.*)

TABLE IV

Assay Conditions[a]

Modification	Amount of radioactive product formed per (pmoles) minute	Percentage
Choline acetyltransferase		
Complete	64	100
Minus enzyme (mouse brain)	2	3
Minus choline	2	3
Minus NaCl	40	62
Minus Triton X100	61	94
Plus 2 mM MgCl^2	59	91
Acetylcholinesterase		
Complete	1130	100
Minus enzyme (neuroblastoma)	105	9
Minus Triton X100	750	66
Minus NaCl	1140	101
Minus EDTA	1160	102
Minus EDTA, plus 1 mM MgCl^2	1130	100
Plus 10^{-5} M BW 284C51	135	12
Glutamate decarboxylase		
Complete	63	100
Minus enzyme (mouse brain)	5	8
Minus pyridoxal phosphate	55	87
Minus EDTA	68	110
Minus 2-mercaptoethanol	60	96
Minus Triton X100	87	140
Plus 1 mM MgCl^2	76	120
Plus 10 mM iodoacetamide	18	29
Plus 10 mM hydroxylamine	8	12
Plus 1 mM amino-oxyacetic acid	8	12
Catechol-O-methyltransferase		
Complete	5.7	100
Minus enzyme (neuroblastoma)	0.48	9
Minus dihydroxybenzoic acid	0.69	12
Minus dihydroxybenzoic acid, plus 1 mM p-hydroxyphenylacetic acid	0.67	13
Plus 1 mM p-hydroxyphenylacetic acid	6.5	115
Minus MgCl$_2$	0.98	17
Minus EDTA	5.7	100
Minus MgCl$_2$ and EDTA	3.0	52
Plus 0.5% (v/v) Triton X100	6.6	115
Plus 1 mM 2-mercaptoethanol	7.9	140
Plus 0.25 mM dihydroxymethoxybenzoic acid	1.3	23
Plus 1 mM tropolone	0.94	17

From Wilson *et al.* (1972) Reproduced with the permission of *J. Biol. Chem.*
[a]Each reaction contained the following: 40, 15, 366, and 60 μg of homogenate protein for the choline acetyltransferase, acetycholinesterase, glutamate decarboxylase, and cathechol-O-methyltransferase reactions, respectively. Enzyme specific activities, in the order stated above were 1480, 64,400, 140, and 88 pmoles of product/min/mg protein. Glutamate decarboxylase was measured by method (a) with glutamic acid-1-C^{14} as substrate.

aggregates. However, between days 12 and 33 *in vitro*, it was estimated that there was a fivefold increase in the number of synapses, increased numbers of vesicles per synapse, and increased electron density adjacent to the post-synaptic membrane. These observations by Seeds and Vatter are indeed important, as they provide a model system *in vitro* for approaching for the first time directly the molecular events involved in synapse formation and for approaching the question of whether cell–cell interaction is highly specific and under genetic control or more flexible and random.

In summary, the sequence of events occurring during neural differentiation of primary dissociated brain cells in rotation–suspension or monolayer culture includes (1) morphological dedifferentiation with loss of cell processes and formation of nonspecific-appearing cells; (2) cellular attachment to a flat surface or cell–cell aggregation in rotation culture; (3) establishment of a confluent monolayer of cells or an enlarging clump of aggregated cells in rotation; (4) emergence after a variable latent period of morphologically recognizable neurons; (5) expression of biochemically differentiated neuronal functions, i.e., increased specific activities of CAT, AChE, and GAD, for the synthesis and hydrolysis of acetylcholine, and formation of GABA from glutamate, respectively; (6) neurotransmitter induction of $3',5'$-cyclic AMP; and (7) *de novo* formation of synapses in culture.

III. NEUROBLASTOMA C1300 AJAX MOUSE CELLS IN CULTURE

The distinct advantage of culturing cloned neuroblastoma over culturing dissociated whole brain in suspension–rotation or monolayer cultures is that it is a cell line of pure neuroblasts devoid of nonneural cells. Although neuroblastoma C1300 cells are tumor cells and have been in culture for 5000–8000 cell generations, they have retained many properties of differentiated *in vivo* mammalian neurons, including possessing (1) CAT (Augusti-Tocco and Sato, 1969; Rosenberg *et al.*, 1971), AChE (Blume *et al.*, 1970), tyrosine hydroxylase (Augusti-Tocco and Sato, 1969), and catechol-*O*-methyl-transferase (Blume *et al.*, 1970); (2) neurites containing microtubules, neurofilaments, and dense-core vesicles (Schubert *et al.*, 1969); (3) catechol formation (Schubert *et al.*, 1969); and (4) membranes capable of generating action potentials in response to electrical stimulation or acetylcholine (Nelson *et al.*, 1969).

The C1300 neuroblastoma cell line derived from the Ajax mouse was originally adapted to cell culture by Augusti-Tocco and Sato (1969). They demonstrated that the monolayer cell cultures of neuroblastoma were capable of metabolizing acetylcholine and also possessed tyrosine hydroxylase.

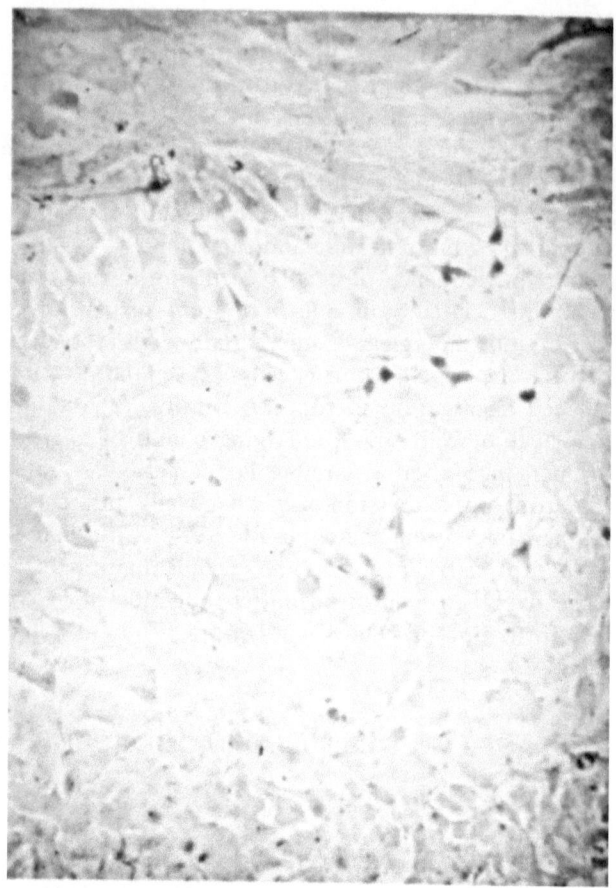

Fig. 3. Photomicrograph of a culture 9 days *in vitro*. There is a layer of flat, polygonal-shaped cells, and there are occasional phase-dark pyramidal-shaped cells with multipolar processes which morphologically resemble neurons. ×50. (From Schrier *et al.*, 1970, and Wilson *et al.*, 1972. Reproduced with the permission of *J. Biol. Chem.*)

Human neuroblastoma also has been cultured *in vitro* and has been shown to contain enzymes concerned with norepinephrine synthesis and degradation. Here then is a powerful system for studying neuronal differentiation of enzymes needed for neurotransmitter metabolism.

Blume *et al.* (1970) demonstrated that AChE activity in neuroblastoma cells could be regulated and that enzyme activity was inversely related to the rate of cell division. The specific activity of mouse neuroblastoma AChE increased 25-fold when the rate of cell division was restricted, while catechol-

O-methyltransferase (E.C. 2.1.1.6) did not change significantly (Fig. 6.)
Thus when cultures were confluent, when cell division was restricted, and
when neurite formation was evident, the highest levels of AChE activity per
milligram of protein were present. The rate of cell division could be regulated
by adjusting the serum concentration. By removing fetal calf serum during
the growth period, cell division ceased and AChE activity was significantly
and rapidly induced. Readdition of serum to the culture medium resulted in a
brisk reestablishment of cell division and a reduction in AChE activity
(Fig. 7).

This inverse relationship of cell growth to the activity of a neurotransmitter enzyme was also shown by Rosenberg *et al.* (1971) using CAT. Rapid cell
growth was associated with lower enzyme activity than when cellular division
was restricted. Thymidylate synthetase, the enzyme which converts de-
oxyuridylate to thymidylate, was utilized as an enzymatic marker for cell
division in this study, and its activity was out of phase with CAT, i.e., highest

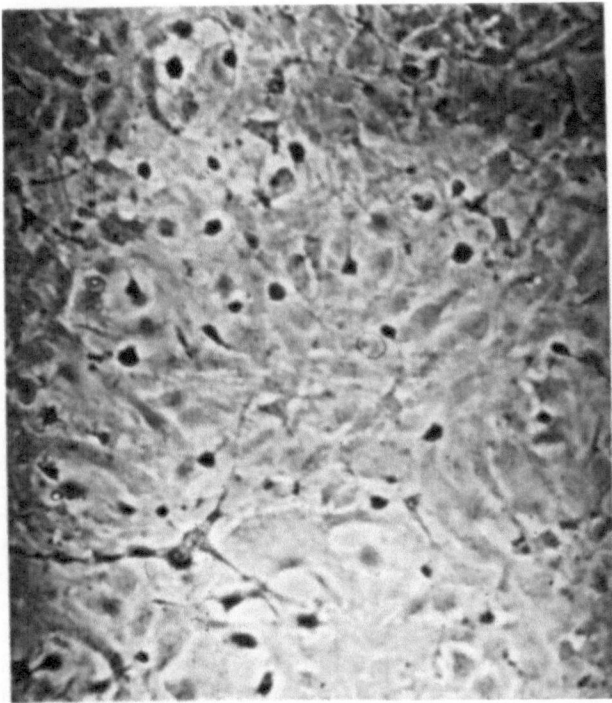

Fig. 4.   Photomicrograph of a 25-day-old culture. The increased number of phase-dark
pyramidal-shaped neuron–like appearing cells is evident compared to that in Fig. 3. Note
one large multipolar-appearing phase-dark cell with long discrete neurites. ×35. (From
Schrier *et al.*, 1970, and Wilson 1972. Reproduced with the permission of *J. Biol. Chem.*)

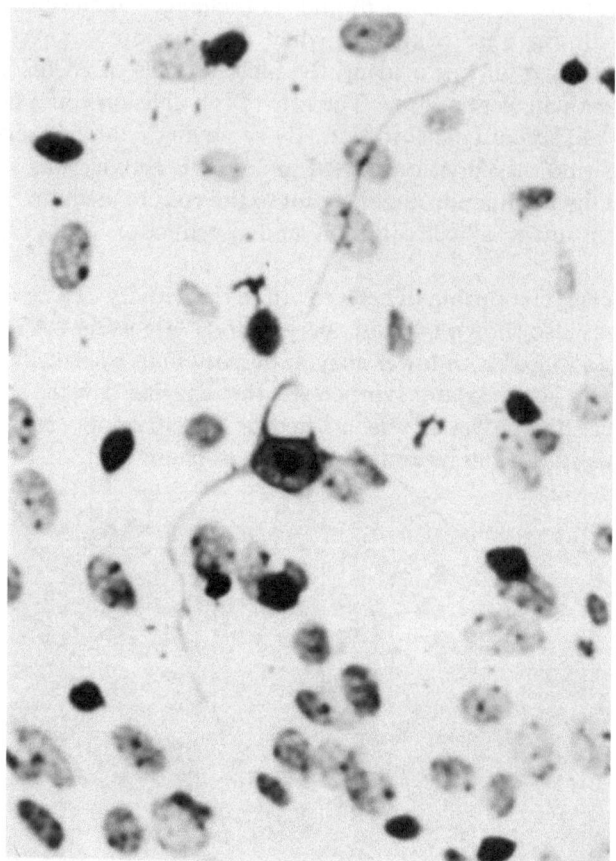

Fig. 5. By day 43 in culture, many phase-dark cells are evident containing long processes, as seen in the cell illustrated in Fig. 4. A neuron-like appearing cell is shown here after staining of the culture with a modified Bodian protargol silver stain which has affinity for neurites of neurons. The cell demonstrates long neurites by this technique, which suggests that it is a neuron, and its uniqueness is readily appreciated by comparing it to surrounding cells. Note the pyramidal-shaped soma and a large central nucleus which also suggests that it is a neuron. ×420. (From Schrier *et al.*, 1970 and Wilson *et al.*, 1972. Reproduced with the permission of *J. Biol. Chem.*)

activity with rapid cellular division and lowest activity with confluency (Figs. 8 and 9). These experiments suggest that neurons are genetically programmed either to rapidly divide and induce enzymes essential for that process (thymidylate synthetase) or to become postmitotic and induce enzymes for neurochemical transmission (CAT, AChE).

Clones of neuroblastoma have been recently described (Amano *et al.*,

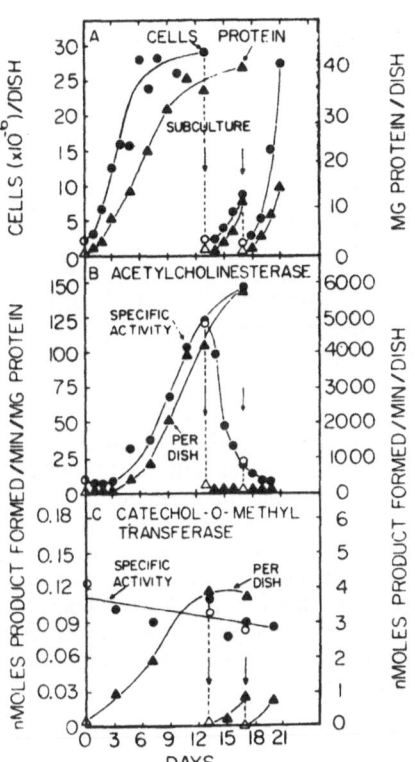

Fig. 6. Neuroblastoma cells in logarithmic growth were subcultured without trypsin. On days 13 and 17 of incubation, some of the cells were dissociated with trypsin (indicated by the vertical dashed lines). Filled and open symbols represent the values obtained before and after subculture, respectively. In A, cells/dish are shown by the filled circles and mg protein/dish by the filled triangles. More than 85% of the cells were viable throughout the experiment. In B, AChE specific activity is shown by the filled circles and AChE activity/dish by the filled triangles. In C, catechol-O-methyltransferase specific activity is shown by the filled circles and the activity/dish by the filled triangles. (From Blume et al., 1970. Reproduced with the permission of Proc. Natl. Acad. Sci.)

1972) which possessed high levels of either CAT, or tyrosine hydroxylase, or neither enzyme. Thus three types of clones of neuroblastoma cells were found to exist with respect to neurotransmitter synthesis: cholinergic, adrenergic, and clones which did not synthesize acetylcholine or catechols. All the clones contained AChE and apparently cannot be used as a specific marker of cholinergic neurons. Thus this elegant contribution by Amano et al. points out that at the single neuron level, despite thousands of generations in culture, distinct classes of neuroblastoma cells exist which have retained the genetic expression for a single neurotransmitter. Further, it was suggested that the expression of a gene required for the synthesis of one transmitter may restrict the expression of genes for alternate neurotransmitters. Thus a gene product of CAT might inhibit gene expression for tyrosine hydroxylase, and the simultaneous expression of both these genes might in turn inactivate them, with the formation of a cell with both low cholinergic and low adrenergic activities. These indeed are provocative concepts and important problems for future investigation.

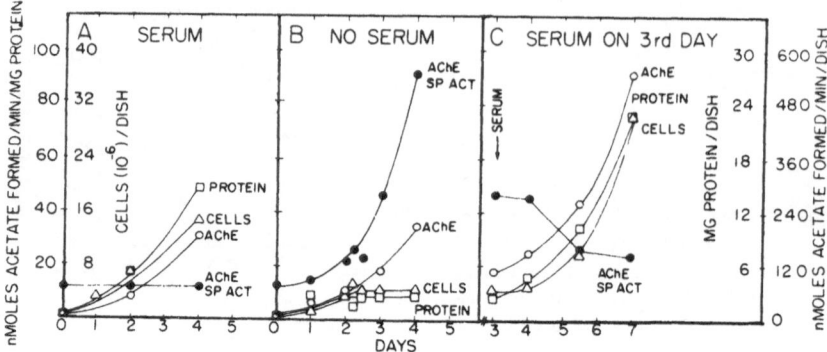

Fig. 7. The rate of cell division was regulated by adjusting the serum concentration. Neuroblastoma cells were incubated for 24 hr prior to 0 time in 150–mm dishes containing the medium described in the text (Dulbecco's modified Eagle's medium plus 10% fetal calf serum). At 0 time, the medium was removed and cells were washed once with growth medium; then fresh medium with or without 10% fetal calf serum was added as specified in A and B, respectively. Some cells were incubated for 3 days without serum, as shown in B; nondividing cells were then shifted up to the rapidly dividing state by addition of 10% fetal calf serum (C). The medium was changed, and fresh medium containing 10% fetal calf serum was added at 4 and 5.5 days. Symbols: filled circles, AChE specific activity: open circles, AChE activity/dish; open triangles, cells (10^6/dish); squares, mg protein/dish. (From Blume *et al.*, 1970. Reproduced with the permission of *Proc. Natl. Acad. Sci.*)

Neurite formation can also be regulated, as shown by Seeds *et al.* (1970), with length and rapidity of their development being inversely proportional to serum concentration in the growth medium. Seventy percent of cultured neuroblasts developed neurites in a few hours in the absence of serum compared to less than 10% of cells cultured for 70 hr in the presence of 10% fetal calf serum. Cycloheximide experiments using up to 1.8×10^{-4} M, a concentration which inhibits proline incorporation into protein by more than 97%, had little effect on neurite outgrowth. The antimitotic drugs vinblastine and colchicine inhibited neurite outgrowth completely at 10^{-7} and 10^{-6} M, respectively. Seeds *et al.* (1970) suggested that neurite formation depended on the assembly of microtubules from preformed protein subunits and did not require protein synthesis as long as the subunit pool was maintained.

IV. NEUROBLAST–GLIOBLAST BIOCHEMICAL RELATIONSHIPS

Neurobiologists have fixed their interests mainly on the neuron and less on the other major cell type in brain, the glial cell. Processes of astroglial cells *in vivo* are found extensively along the soma and axons of neurons and the endothelial cells of capillaries and thus are strategically positioned to provide transport of anabolites and catabolites between plasma and neuron and between neurons. The other important glial cell type, the oligodendroglia, synthesizes the axonal myelin sheath.

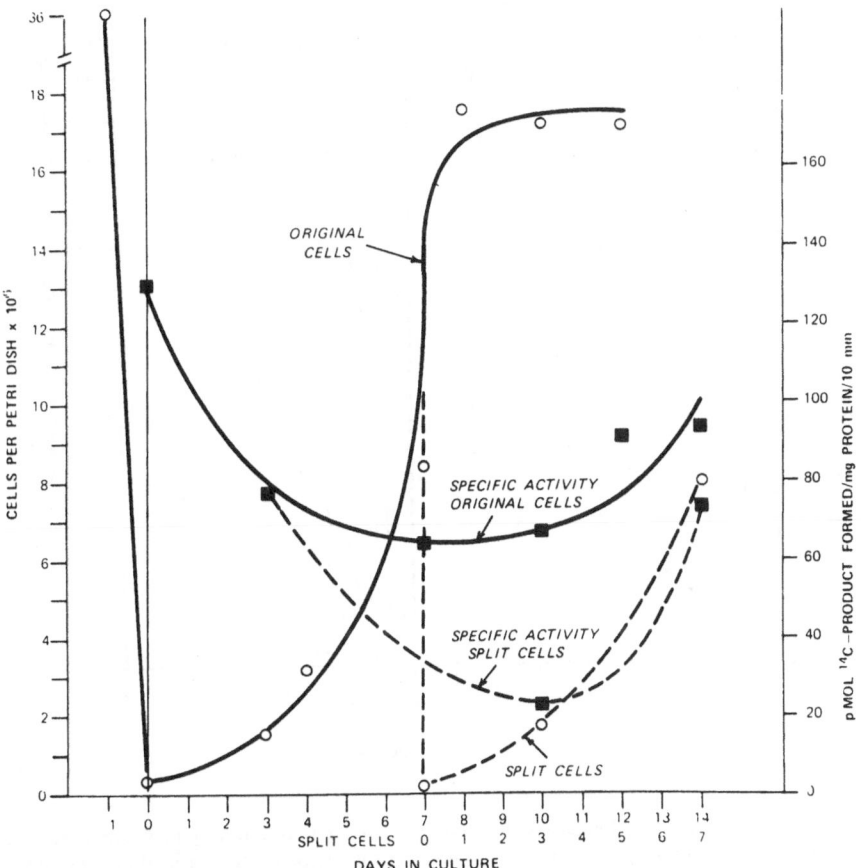

Fig. 8. The growth and number of cells present per petri dish are shown in relation to the specific activity of CAT. On day 7 of incubation, some of the cells were dissociated with trypsin (as indicated by the vertical dashed line). More than 90% of the cells were viable throughout the experiment. The rate of growth of cells incubated at day 0 of the experiment and not subcultured is shown by the solid line and open circles. Subcultured cell growth is shown by the dashed line and open circles. CAT specific acitvity of the cells incubated at day 0 and not subcultured is shown by the solid line and filled squares, and by the dashed line and filled squares for the subcultured cells. (From Rosenberg *et al.*, 1971. Reproduced with the permission of *Proc. Natl. Acad. Sci.*)

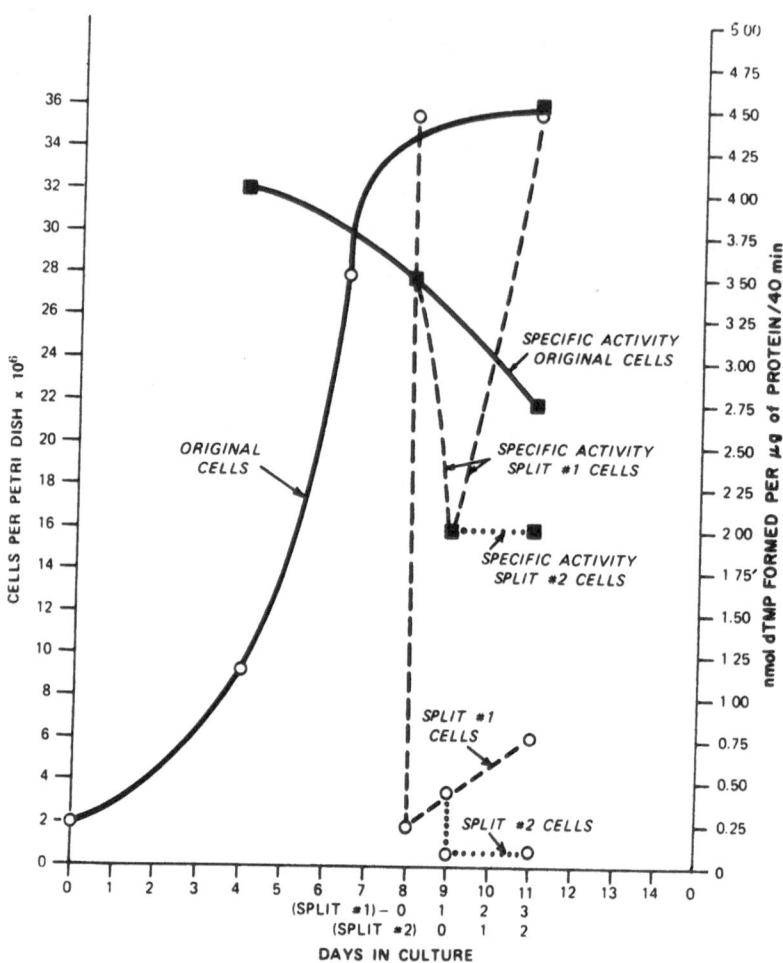

Fig. 9. Thymidylate synthetase specific activity is shown in relation to the growth rate and number of cells present per petri dish. Some cells were subcultured with trypsin on day 8 of incubation, and some of these subcultured cells were subcultured again 1 day later (as indicated by the vertical dashed lines). More than 90% of the cells were viable throughout the experiment. The rate of growth of the cells incubated at day 0 of the experiment and not subcultured is shown by the solid line and circles. The rate of growth of cells subcultured on day 8 of incubation is shown by the dashed line and circles, and the rate of growth of those cells subcultured again 1 day later is shown by the dotted line and circles. Thymidylate synthetase specific activities are shown as follows: solid line and squares, cells incubated on day 0 and not subcultured; dashed line and squares, cells subcultured on day 8 of incubation; dotted line and squares, cells subcultured again 1 day later. (From Rosenberg *et al.*, 1971. Reproduced with the permission of *Proc. Natl. Acad. Sci.*)

A. Cyclic AMP

Tumor glioblastoma cells have been grown in monolayer culture as a means of investigating various biochemical parameters which may be affected by neuroblasts or neurotransmitters to provide a better understanding of these events in the intact brain. Gilman and Nirenberg (1971) demonstrated a 200-fold induction in cyclic AMP in a clonal line of rat glial tumor cells (C6 cells) by norepinephrine. Clark and Perkins (1971) also showed a rapid increase in the concentrations of cyclic AMP in a tumor astrocyte cell line derived from a primary culture of a human glioblastoma multiforme by norepinephrine, epinephrine, and histamine. A similar 50- to 100-fold inductive effect by catecholamines on cyclic AMP formation occurred in primary monolayer cultures from embryonic rat brain, and there was a four- to sixfold increase in cyclic AMP in rotation–reaggregrated brain cultures by norepinephrine, suggesting that in these mixed cultures the induced cyclic AMP might be of glial origin (Seeds and Gilman, 1971).

B. Neurotransmitter Inactivation

Henn and Hamberger (1971) obtained enriched fractions of neurons and glia from rabbit brain and investigated accumulation of norepinephrine, serotonin, dopamine, and GABA. Both neurons and glia were able to concentrate monoamine transmitters about fourfold from an incubating medium containing 0.1–1 µM concentrations. Glial cell fractions were able to concentrate γ-aminobutyrate over a hundredfold from the medium as compared to only fourfold for the neuronal fraction. This suggests that glial cells in the intact brain might serve as an important buffer reservoir for inactivation of neurotransmitters which might otherwise increase in concentration in the synaptic cleft and that glia might be essential for maintenance of rapid, prolonged chemical neurotransmission.

C. Glucose Transport

Galambos postulated in 1961 that neuron–glia synapses occurred in addition to neuron–neuron synapses. A metabolic interrelationship between these two cell types was suggested by the finding by Gilman and Nirenberg (1971) that the neurotransmitter norepinephrine caused an increase in cyclic AMP in rat glioblastoma cells in culture. Further, it was known that glycogenolysis was increased by cyclic AMP due to an activation of a protein kinase which converts phosphorylase *b* to phosphorylase *a*, the active form of the enzyme. On the basis of these results, Newburgh and Rosenberg (1972) examined the effect of norepinephrine on the transport of glucose in cloned

TABLE V

Incorporation of Glucose-C^{14} into Glioblastoma Cells[a]

Substrate	Dpm (total in cells)					
	Preincubated with theophylline			No precincubation		
	Control	Norepinephrine	Percent inhibition of uptake	Control	Norepinephrine	Percent inhibition of uptake
D-Glucose-2-H^3	23,800 ±1,200[b]	21,800 ±950[b]	5	26,000 ±1,350[b]	16,700 ±1,280[b]	35
D-Glucose-1-C^{14}						
Expt. 1	31,60	2,340	26	3,400	1,590	52
Expt. 2	—	—	—	780	630	22
Expt. 3	1,100	800	27	1,160	810	30
Expt. 4	—	—	—	2,560	1,350	48
D-Glucose-2-C^{14}						
Expt. 1	4,600	4,150	10	5,950	2,340	60
Expt. 2	—	—	—	1,520	1,240	20
Expt. 4	—	—	—	5,900	4,350	26
D-Glucose-6-C^{14}						
Expt. 1	4,300	3,130	28	4,500	2,200	50
Expt. 2	—	—	—	1,480	1,200	20
Expt. 4	—	—	—	3,240	2,120	35

From Newburgh and Rosenberg (1972). Reproduced with the permission of *Proc. Natl. Acad. Sci.*

[a]The cells were incubated for 2 days in Dulbecco's modified Eagle's medium plus 10% fetal calf serum. Each 60-mm petri dish was initially inoculated with 3×10^6 cells in 3 ml of medium. The growth medium was removed and replaced with 2 ml of Earle's balanced salt solution containing the radioactive substrates. The cells were then incubated for an additional 30 min prior to filtering through a millipore filter by the procedure given in the text. When the cells were preincubated in the presence of theophylline, this was accomplished by replacing the growth medium with new growth medium containing 1×10^3 M theophylline and incubating for 1 hr. This latter medium was then removed, replaced with Earle's balanced salt solution containing the radioactive substrates, and incubated for 30 min. The radioactive medium contained D-glucose-2-H^3, 1.56×10^6 dpm, plus either D-glucose-1-C^{14}, 1.63×10^6 dpm, D-glucose-2-C^{14}, 3.36×10^5 dpm, or D-glucose-6-C^{14}, 2.24×10^5 dpm. Where indicated, the radioactive medium contained 0.017 mg/ml of norepinephrine, The incubations were at 37°C, 100% humidity, 90% air, and 10% CO_2.

[b]Standard error, $n = 3$.

glioblastoma cells (clone C6) isolated from a rat astrocytoma and in mouse neuroblastoma cells, clone C46, in cell culture. These cell lines were the gift of Dr. Gordon Sato.

Petri dishes (60 mm) were incubated with 3×10^6 cells for 2 days in Dulbecco's modified Eagle's medium (DMEM) with 10% fetal calf serum at 37°C in an atmosphere of 10% Co_2 and 90% air at 100% humidity. The medium was then changed to 2 ml of fresh DMEM or Earle's Balanced Salt solution containing the radioactive glucose desired and incubated for 30 min. For the studies with theophylline, the cells were incubated for 1 hr in the culture medium plus 1×10^{-3} M theophylline prior to adding the radioactive medium. Norepinephrine (0.017 mg/ml) was added where indicated. In the experiments in which cells were prelabeled with radioactive glucose, the cells were incubated for 2 hr in a radioactive medium, washed twice with a non-radioactive medium, and then incubated for 30 min in a nonradioactive medium. After the incubation, the cells were scraped from the petri dish, filtered through a millipore filter (HAWP 0.025, HA 0.45 μ, 25 mm), and washed twice with 0.32 M suerose, and the filter was counted in a Beckman scintillation counter.

For the studies of the effects of norepinephrine on the uptake of D-glucose-C^{14}, glioblastoma cells were grown for 2 days in DMEM plus 10% fetal calf serum. The growth medium was removed and replaced with the same medium of medium plus 1×10^{-3} M theophylline. After 1 hr, the medium was replaced with Earle's balanced salt solution containing various radio-labeled compounds, incubated for 30 min, and filtered. The results are shown in Table V. When the cells were not preincubated in theophylline, there was an inhibition by norepinephrine of from 20 to 50% of the incorporation of glucose. Less inhibition (10–30%) was found when the cells were preincubated in theophylline. If the cells were incubated as previously described except that Earle's balanced salt solution was replaced with DMEM plus 10% fetal calf serum plus the radioactive substrate, similar results were obtained (Table VI).

In another series of experiments, the cells were incubated for 2 hr in the presence of radioactive glucose and then washed, and the medium was changed to Earle's balanced salt solution. The cells were then incubated for 30 min in the presence of 1×10^{-3} M theophylline and norepinephrine. As shown in Table VII, norepinephrine caused an increase in the release of isotope from the cells as evidenced by the presence of less radioactivity in these cells. The evolution of $C^{14}O_2$ from specifically labeled glucose-C^{14} was determined. As shown in Table VIII, the addition of norepinephrine caused an increase in $C^{14}O_2$ evolution from glucose-1-C^{14}, glucose-2-C^{14}, and glucose-6-C^{14}.

The effect of norepinephrine on glucose metabolism in neuroblastoma cells was also studied. The cells were grown for 2 days in DMEM plus 10%

TABLE VI

Incorporation of Glucose-C^{14} into Glioblastoma Cells[a]

| | Dpm (total in cells) | | | | | |
| | Preincubated with theophylline | | | No preincubation | | |
Substrate	Control	Norepinephrine	Percent inhibition of uptake	Control	Norepinephrine	Percent inhibition of uptake
D-Glucose-2-H^3	13,100 ± 700[b]	8,100 ± 490[b]	38	11,250 ± 600[b]	9,000 ± 540[b]	21
D-Glucose-1-C^{14}						
Expt. 1	1,700	1,230	30	1,280	1,040	18
Expt. 2	1,350	690	50	—	—	—
Expt. 3	1,060	835	22	—	—	—
D-Glucose-2-C^{14}						
Expt. 1	1,310	940	28	1,970	1,300	34
D-Glucose-6-C^{14}						
Expt. 1	2,600	1,520	40	1,830	1,160	35
Expt. 2	670	320	51	—	—	—

From Newburgh and Rosenberg (1972). Reproduced with the permission of *Proc. Natl. Acad. Sci.*
[a]The conditions were the same as described in Table I except that the radioactive compounds were in Dulbecco's modified Earle's medium instead of Earle's balanced salt solution.
[b]Standard error, $n = 4$.

TABLE VII

Excretion of Radioactivity into the Medium from Glioblastoma Cells[a]

| | Dpm (total in cells) | | |
Substrate	Control	Norepinephrine	Increased excretion from cells
D-Glucose-2-H³	7420	4390	40
	±380[b]	±370[b]	
D-Glucose-1-C¹⁴			
Expt. 1	3240	2040	38
Expt. 2	2040	1410	30
Expt. 3	6650	3900	40
D-Glucose-2-C¹⁴			
Expt. 1	4270	2480	42
Expt. 3	7300	4800	34
D-Glucose-6-C¹⁴			
Expt. 1	2260	1790	22
Expt. 3	9000	7800	16

From Newburgh and Rosenberg (1972). Reproduced with the permission of *Proc. Natl. Acad. Sci.*
[a]The cells were grown under the same conditions as described in Table I. After 2 days, the growth medium was removed and replaced with Earle's balanced salt solution containing the radioactive substrates as in Table I. After 2 hr, the radioactive medium was removed, the cells were washed quickly, and 2 ml of Earle's balanced salt solution (nonradioactive) was added with or without norepinephrine. The cells were incubated for 30 min and then filtered.
[b]Standard error, $n = 3$.

TABLE VIII

The Effect of Norepinephrine on the Evolution of $C^{14}O_2$ from Glucose-C¹⁴, with Glioblastoma Cells[a]

| | Dpm/mg protein in $C^{14}O_2$ | |
Substrate	Control	Norepinephrine
D-Glucose-1-C¹⁴		
Expt. 1	950	1400
Expt. 2	3400	5600
D-Glucose-2-C¹⁴		
Expt. 2	1560	2750
D-Glucose-6-C¹⁴		
Expt. 1	860	970
Expt. 2	260	300

From Newburgh and Rosenberg (1972). Reproduced with permission of *Proc. Natl. Acad. Sci.*
[a]The cells were incubated for 2 days in Dulbecco's modified Earle's medium in 25-ml Ehrlenmeyer flasks containing a center well. The growth medium was then removed and replaced with Earle's balanced salt solution containing the radioactive substrates. To the center well was added 0.2 ml of 2 N KOH and a fluted filter paper. The flasks were then sealed with a rubber serum bottle stopper. After incubation at 37°C for 30 min, 1 ml of 1 N HCl was injected into the flask through the rubber stopper. The cells were incubated another 2 hr, and the filters and KOH were then removed and placed in a scintillation vial. The cells were scraped from the flasks for the protein determinations.

TABLE IX

Incorporation of Glucose-C[14] into Neuroblastoma Cells[a]

Substrate	Dpm (total in cells)	
	Control	Norepinephrine
D-Glucose-2-H[3]	7150	7400
	±550[b]	±600[b]
D-Glucose-1-C[14]	1140	1270
D-Glucose-2-C[14]	1400	1320
D-Glucose-6-C[14]	1440	1510

From Newburgh and Rosenberg (1972). Reproduced with permission of *Proc. Natl. Acad. Sci.*
[a]The conditions were the same as described in Table I except that neuroblastoma cells were used in place of glioblastoma cells.
[b]Standard error, $n = 3$.

fetal calf serum. The growth medium was removed and replaced by Earle's balanced salt solution containing various radiolabeled compounds, incubated for 30 min, and filtered. As shown in Table IX, norepinephrine had no effect on the incorporation of label from radioactive glucose in these cells.

The question examined in these experiments was whether norepinephrine affects the uptake of radioactive glucose, the release of radioactive compounds derived from radiolabeled glucose, or the metabolism of radioactive glucose in glioblastoma and neuroblastoma cells in culture. From the results presented, it appears that the addition of norepinephrine does have an effect on these processes in glioblastoma cells and not in neuroblastoma cells in cell culture.

It is of interest to speculate that what is occurring in glioblastoma cells can be explained as shown in Fig. 10. The breakdown of glycogen is activated by norepinephrine as a result of an increase in cyclic AMP, which activates the protein kinase for conversion of phosphorylase b to phosphorylase a. This then results in an increase of glucose within the cell. If radioactive glucose is added to the medium, less will be taken into the cell because of an increase in an intracellular pool of glucose or compounds derived from glucose. This is the result that was obtained (Tables V and VI). If the cells are prelabeled with glucose and the radioactive medium is removed, then it might be expected that radioactivity would be lost from the cell in the presence of norepinephrine. This was found to occur (Table VII). In addition, it might be expected that if norepinephrine causes an increased conversion of glycogen to glucose, increased oxidation of the glucose might also occur. The results shown in Table VIII are consistent with this postulate.

Fig. 10. Diagram of a glioblastoma cell, showing that its glucose metabolism is affected by norepinephrine by activating glycogenolysis and subsequently inducing CO_2 production by glycolysis. (From Newburgh and Rosenberg, 1972. Reproduced with the permission of *Proc. Natl. Acad. Sci.*)

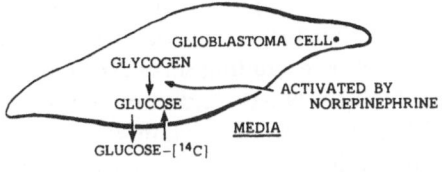

Although it is interesting to speculate that the effect of norepinephrine is on the breakdown of glycogen, the nature of the experiments does not permit an unequivocal conclusion in this regard. This would require determination of the products derived from the radioactive glucose and the nature of the compounds lost from the cell in the presence of norepinephrine.

Nevertheless, it is of interest to propose that *in vivo* these products from glial cells are made available to neurons and used for metabolic processes in the latter cells, assuming the present experiments might have relevance to the intact brain. Thus one can envision the relation of neurons and glial cells to be one whereby a neurotransmitter from neurons triggers a reaction in glial cells that results in the latter providing metabolites to the neurons for various synthetic reactions or to generate energy for cellular processes.

V. SPECULATION

A. *In Vivo* Neuronal Differentiation

A program of neuronal differentiation emerges from these mixed brain and neuroblastoma experiments which may have an important analogy to the development of the mammalian central nervous system. Rapidly dividing neuroblasts in fresh cultures or during *in vivo* embryogenesis appear morphologically dedifferentiated, rounded-up with little or no neurite formation. This type of immature neuroblast is seen in early embryos when these cells are migrating from the periependymal region adjacent to the primitive neurotube to the distant mantle and marginal zones of the developing telencephalon (Rakic and Sidman, 1968). A high serum concentration in brain extracellular fluid, as in a culture dish, might promote rapid cellular division. Cell–cell contact in the petri dish restricts cellular division, as it may also do in the developing brain. Cellular division can be rapidly stopped in culture, however, by the removal of serum from the growth medium followed by intense neurite outgrowth and enzyme induction for neurotransmission. A similar phenomenon of controlling the serum concentration in brain extracellular fluid may affect the onset of neuronal differentiation during embryogenesis.

The development and maturation of the blood–brain barrier in the mammalian brain may be one signal which initiates neuronal differentiated function by excluding serum from brain extracellular space and cerebrospinal fluid (CSF). Normal adult man has less than 1 % of the protein content in his CSF (50 mg %) that he has in serum (8 g %). Inhibition of transport of serum into brain by the blood–brain barrier may be one signal responsible for the activation of the program of (1) axon and dendrite formation, (2) synaptogenesis, (3) neurotransmitter synthesis, and (4) generation of propagated action potentials.

Regulation of the events of neuronal differentiation which have been described with mixed brain cultures and neuroblastoma cells may have a great deal to tell us about these events occurring in brain. The unraveling of the molecular biology of neuronal differentiation is just beginning, and the approaches taken to initiate this inquiry described in this chapter are based on the use of "simple systems" which can be manipulated in cell culture. In this way, the immense complexity of the mammalian brain can be broken down into more elementary components such as glia and neurons, which can be combined in culture systems under a variety of conditions in order to elucidate these mechanisms of regulation.

B. The Brain Code

The ultimate differentiated function of nervous system tissue is to encode, store, and retrieve information. The neurophysiological and biochemical principles and mechanisms which have evolved from simple metazoans to the formation of the mammalian brain remain quite far from our comprehension. The systems for handling the vast amounts of motor, sensory, language, perceptual, and cognitive functions which are inherently present in the brain of man are indeed complex ones, but perhaps decipherable if reduced to elementary units. A precedent for decoding enormous amounts of biological information in a short time has already been provided in Marshall Nirenberg's (1963, 1966) deciphering of the entire genetic code in terms of nucleotide triplets which code for a single amino acid. The code which the brain utilizes to fix experience and recall it, although foreboding and seemingly inaccessible at present, might be approachable by studying simple systems capable of learning.

The cell culture of neurons and glia under controlled conditions as described in the experiments cited previously might offer such a simple system. Neurons and glia might function as a "unit," as suggested by Galambos (1961). Several such neuronal–glial units could be grown in culture, become differentiated with synapse formation, and generate patterns of neuronal depolarizations characteristic for specific afferent stimuli. A cell culture neuron–glia system capable of learning would be an ideal one for studying

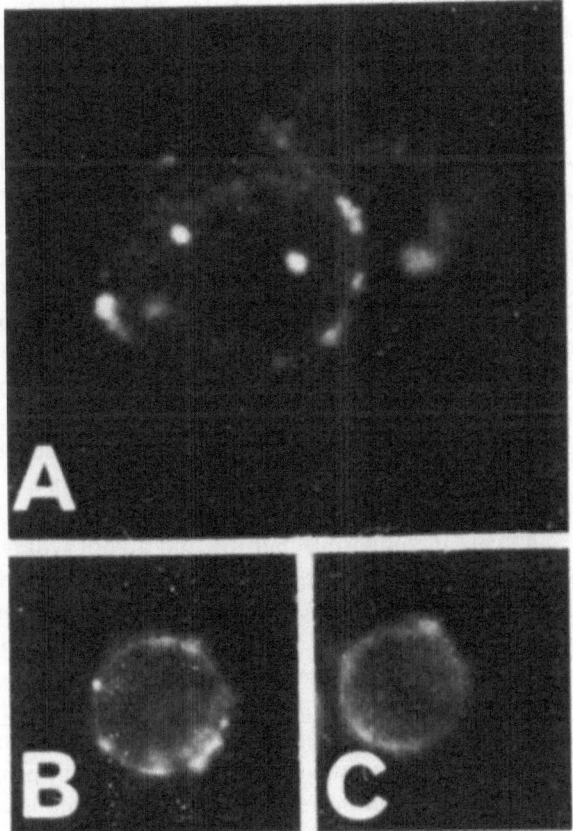

Fig. 11. Three neuroblastoma cells from the C1300 cell line stained by the fluorescent antibody technique for the θ-antigen. The cells show intense fluorescence on their surfaces, indicating that they contain an antigen which reacts with antibody from a thymus-derived lymphocyte. (From Oldstone and Rosenberg, 1971, unpublished observations.)

the "code," for it would utilize small numbers of the two important brain cell types, allow study of the biochemical interrelationships between glia and neurons, and permit a direct correlation between electrical events and the synthesis and turnover of specific macromolecules.

It is curious that although neuroblastoma cells in culture retain the abilities to metabolize cholinergic and adrenergic transmitters, produce action potentials, and form long neurites, they seem to lose the ability to form a synapse. Is the lack of synapse formation because they are tumor cells, or do the cultures perhaps represent incompatible classes of neurons? An important point in approaching the "brain code" is how many functional classes of neurons exist in brain. An analogous question was how many types of nucleotide bases exist in DNA or RNA. The knowledge of the number of types of bases in DNA and RNA, and how they are base paired or complementary, provided crucial data for our eventual understanding of the molecular structure of DNA, transcription of DNA, and RNA translation. There may be only a very small number of classes of neurons, as is the case with nucleotides, and these classes of neurons may have selective complementarity as determined by their cell-surface histocompatibility antigens: a class A neuron aggregates with or forms a synapse with a class C neuron but is incompatible with a class B neuron. Neurons in this way might segregate out and form multisynaptic circuits from relatively few subtypes. Cloned neuroblastoma cells in culture might represent only one histocompatibility class, as they are cloned from a single cell and thus are unable to form a synapse. It would require the recombination of two complementary clones to form a synapse by neuroblastoma cells in culture if this hypothesis is correct.

Selective circuit formation in brain involving four classes of neurons might look like this: -A-C-B-D-D-D-A-C-, etc. Thus A and C, B and D, D and A, D and D are complementary neuronal pairs and form a synapse, but A and B, and C and D are incompatible pairings and do not synapse. In this way, specific linkages of neurons in series would be produced, and the resulting circuit would be programmed to behave in an individual manner uniquely different from that of other linkages. Further, synapse formation may require the presence of a complementary class of glial cells.

Such a hypothesis of neuronal and glial classes can be tested in cell culture by defining cell-surface histocompatibility antigens of neurons and glia in mixed brain cultures and neuroblastoma clones. This approach has been taken by M. A. B. Oldstone and myself, and Fig. 11 demonstrates the presence of the θ-antigen on the surface of neuroblastoma cells from clones N18 and C46. In this manner, it might be found that synapse formation is a selective process of cell recognition, sorting out, and differentiated attachment.

The description of the molecular biology of certain aspects of neuronal differentiation in cell culture as outlined in this chapter was acquired in a very short period of time and allows speculation that this *in vitro* approach may have brought us closer to appreciating the "brain code" than we currently realize.

VI. REFERENCES

Amano, T., Richelson, E., and Nirenberg, M. 1972. Neurotransmitter synthesis by neuroblastoma clones. *Proc. Natl. Acad. Sci.* **69**:258–263.

Augusti-Tocco, G., and Sato, G. 1969. Establishment of functional clonal lines of neurons from mouse neuroblastoma. *Proc. Natl. Acad. Sci.* **64**:311–315.

Blume, A., Gilbert, F., Wilson, S., Farber, J., Rosenberg, R., and Nirenberg, M. 1970. Regulation of acetylcholinesterase in neuroblastoma cells. *Proc. Natl. Acad. Sci.* **67**: 786–792.

Clark, R., and Perkins, J. 1971. Regulation of adenosine 3':5'-cyclic monophosphate concentration in cultured human Astrocytoma cells by catecholamines and histamine. *Proc. Natl. Acad. Sci.* **68**:2757–2760.

Galambos, R. 1961. A glia–neural theory of brain function. *Proc. Natl. Acad. Sci.* **47**: 129–136.

Gilman, A., and Nirenberg, M. 1971. Effect of catecholamines on the adenosine 3':5'-cyclic monophosphate concentrations of clonal satellite cells of neurons. *Proc. Natl. Acad. Sci.* **68**:2165–2168.

Harrison, R. G. 1907. Observations on the living developing nerve fiber. *Anat. Rec.* **1**: 116–124.

Henn, F., and Hamberger, A. 1971. Glial cell function: Uptake of transmitter substances. *Proc. Natl. Acad. Sci.* **68**:2686–2690.

Lowry, O. H., Rosebrough, N., Farr, A., and Randall, R. 1951. Protein measurement with the Folin phenol reagent. *J. Biol. Chem.* **193**:265–275.

Murray, M. R. 1965. Nervous tissues *in vitro*. pp. 373–455. *In* E. N. Willmer (ed.). The Biology of Cells and Tissues in Culture, Vol. II. Academic Press, New York.

Nelson, P., Ruffner, W., and Nirenberg, M. 1969. Neuronal tumor cells with excitable membranes grown *in vitro*. *Proc. Natl. Acad. Sci.* **64**:1004–1010.

Newburgh, R. W., and Rosenberg, R. N. 1972. Effect of norepinephrine on glucose metabolism in glioblastoma and neuroblastoma cells in cell culture. *Proc. Natl. Acad. Sci.* **69**:1677–1680.

Nirenberg, M., Jones, O. W., Leder, P., Clark, B. F. C., Sly, W. S., and Pestka, S. 1963. On the coding of genetic information. *Cold Spring Harbor Symp. Quant Biol.* **28**: 549–557.

Nirenberg, M., Caskey, T., Marshall, R., Brimacombe, R., Kellogg, D., Doctor, B., Hatfield, D., Levin, J., Rottman, F., Pestka, S., Wilcox, M., and Anderson, F. 1966. The RNA code and protein synthesis. *Cold Spring Harbor Symp. Quant. Biol.* **31**:11–24.

Rakic, P., and Sidman, R. 1968. Supravital DNA synthesis in the developing human and mouse brain. *J. Neuropathol. Exptl. Neurol.* **27**:246–276.

Rosenberg, R. N., Vandeventer, L., DeFrancesco, L., and Friedkin, M. 1971. Regulation of the synthesis of choline-*O*-acetyltransferase and thymidylate synthetase in mouse neuroblastoma in cell culture. *Proc. Natl. Acad. Sci.* **68**:1436–1440.

Schrier, B. W., Rosenberg, R. N., Thompson, E., and Farber, J. 1970. Enzyme markers in mouse brain cell culture. *Fed. Proc.* **29**:480.

Schrier, B. K., Wilson, S. H., and Nirenberg, M. Assay of enzymes of transmitter metabolism of neuroblastoma and other cultured cells from the nervous system. *Meth. Enzymol.* (in press).

Schubert, O., Humphreys, S., Baroni, C., and Cohn, M. 1969. *In vitro* differentiation of a mouse neuroblastoma. *Proc. Natl. Acad. Sci.* **64**:316–323.

Seeds, N. W. 1971. Biochemical differentiation in reaggregating brain cell culture. *Proc. Natl. Acad. Sci.* **68**:1858–1861.

Seeds, N. W., and Gilman, A. 1971. Norepinephrine stimulated increase of cyclic-AMP levels in developing mouse brain cell cultures. *Science* **174**:292.

Seeds, N. W., and Vatter, A. E. 1971. Synaptogenesis in reaggregating brain cell culture. *Proc. Natl. Acad. Sci.* **68**:3219–3222.

Seeds, N. W., Gilman, A., Amano, T., and Nirenberg, M. 1970. Regulation of axon formation by clonal lines of a neural tumor. *Proc. Natl. Acad. Sci.* **66**:160–167.

Wilson, S. H., Schrier, B. K., Farber, J. L., Thompson, E. J., Rosenberg, R. N., Blume, A. J., and Nirenberg, M. W. 1972. Markers for gene expression in cultured cells from the nervous system. *J. Biol. Chem.* **247**:3159–3169

Chapter 6

Electrophysiological Studies of Normal and Neoplastic Cells in Tissue Culture

P. G. Nelson

Behavioral Biology Branch, National Institute of Child Health and Human Development
National Institutes of Health
Bethesda, Maryland

I. INTRODUCTION

A number of tissue culture preparations have been extensively studied electrophysiologically, and this chapter will seek to summarize some of the observations which have been made on a number of continuous cell lines and on long-term cultures of normal, dissociated nerve and muscle cells. No attempt will be made to cover the valuable studies of nerve and muscle explants which have appeared over the past several years (Corner and Crain, 1972; Crain *et al.*, 1970; Peterson and Crain, 1970).

It has been demonstrated that various cultured cell systems actively accumulate or exclude different ions and metabolites (Lamb and Mac Kinnon, 1971; Lamb and McCall, 1972), that various resting ionic conductance mechanisms develop in these preparations, that voltage-dependent conductances specific for both Na and Ca ions occur (Fischbach and Dichter, in preparation), that chemosensitivity to different neurohormones is coupled to excitatory and inhibitory membrane conductance mechanisms (Harris and Dennis, 1970; Nelson *et al.*, 1971a; Peacock and Nelson, 1972b), and that well-differentiated and specific synaptic connections may be established between the cellular elements (Fischbach, 1970, 1972). These neurobiologically important phenomena are thus accessible for study by a number of cell biological approaches. At present, electrical and chemical excitability are the electrophysiological phenomena which are most clearly expressed in continuous lines of neuronal cells, and these properties will be discussed first.

II. THE MOUSE C1300 NEUROBLASTOMA

The origin and many of the properties of the mouse C1300 neuroblastoma discussed in detail elsewhere in this volume. Carried for many years as a transplantable tumor in mice, it was adapted to tissue culture (Augusti-Tocco and Sato, 1969; Klebe and Ruddle, 1969) and has proven an extremely versatile neurobiological preparation.

A. Electrical Excitability

The question to be addressed is whether the property of electrical excitability is under any degree of regulation in the neuroblastoma cell lines. Two different positions have been advanced in this regard. One is that the excitable mechanism in neuroblastoma cells is not under any form of regulation and is fully expressed in all clones and in all states of growth (Schubert et al., this volume). The basis for this conclusion is twofold: (1) It is extremely difficult to be certain that a negative finding with regard to electrical excitability is meaningful. Technical limitations of electrophysiological intracellular stimulation and recording methods and of tissue culture may well account for a finding of reduced or absent electrical excitability. (2) Schubert and coworkers have seen a high degree of electrical excitability in cells grown in suspension soon after the cells have attached to the plastic surface of tissue culture plates.

Nelson et al. (1969, 1971b) and Peacock et al. (1972) have come to the conclusion that the property of electrical excitability is under a high degree of regulation and is differentially expressed in different clones of neuroblastoma cells and under different growth conditions in the same clone. The evidence for this latter position will be presented here.

Quantitative measures of the passive and active electrical properties of the neuroblastoma cells were required to approach the problem. Intracellular transmembrane potential recordings were made with conventional 3 M KCl–filled micropipette electrodes. A single microelectrode was usually used in a bridge circuit which allowed simultaneous passage of stimulating current and recording of transmembrane potential. Recordings were also obtained with two independent electrodes inserted within the same cell, for independent current passage and potential measurement. This method confirmed the validity of the single electrode bridge method as used in the studies to be described. When a single electrode is used, however, it is crucial to prepare and select the electrodes so that the required amount of stimulating current can be passed through them without altering their electrical resistance. The electrical properties of the neuroblastoma membrane are such that unambiguous distinction can, in general, be made between the time constant associated with the electrode characteristics (less than 1 msec) and that of the cell mem-

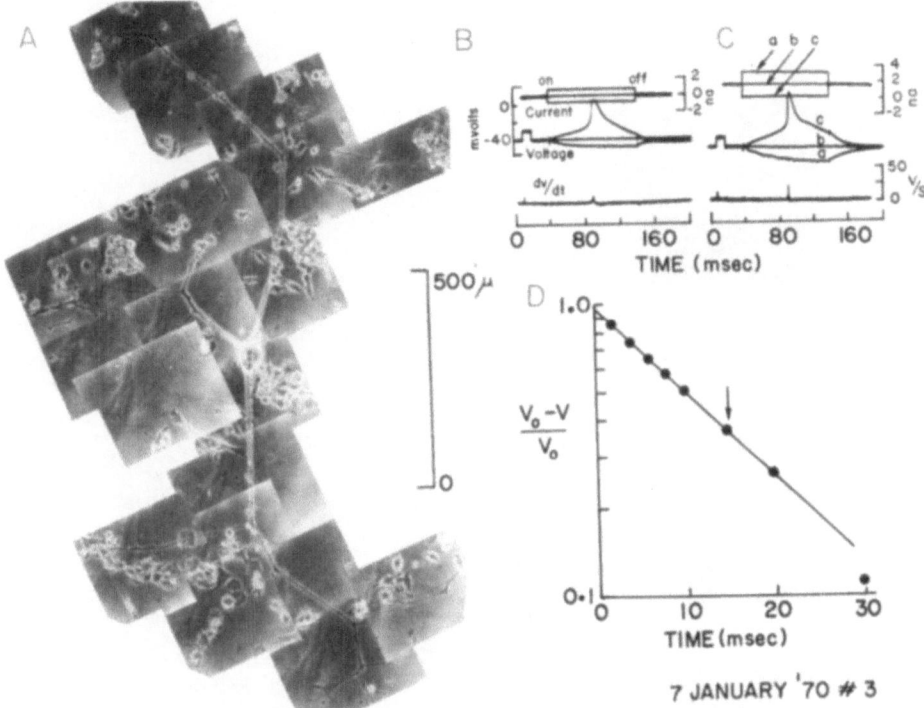

Fig. 1.   Clone N32, cells plated 8 days prior to experiment. (A) Phase-contrast photo-micrograph of cell; scale as indicated. (B and C) Oscilloscope recordings obtained with an intracellular microelectrode from the cell shown in A. Upper traces represent the currents passed across the cell membrane. Middle traces show the membrane potential changes produced by the current pulses. Lowest traces show the derivative of membrane potential with respect to time, dv/dt. The electronic system which generated the time derivative of membrane potential was approximately linear from 10 V/sec to 100 V/sec, but rates of change of membrane potential much below 10 V/sec were probably non-linear. Three sweeps of the oscilloscope are shown in B and C. On one sweep, a hyper-polarizing current pulse was delivered (trace a in C). On another sweep a depolarizing pulse was delivered (trace c in C), and on one sweep no current was passed (trace b in C). In C, a steady hyperpolarizing current of 1.7 namp was applied through the micropipette. (D) A plot on semilogarithmic axis of the hyperpolarizing voltage transient (trace a in C above). V_0 represents the voltage change at the end of the current pulse (the difference between traces b and a), V is the voltage change at various instants after the onset of the current pulse, and time is the elapsed time after the onset of the current pulse. The membrane time constant is the time required for $(V_0-V)/V_0$ to fall to a value $1/e$ of its initial value. (From Nelson *et al.*, 1971*b*.)

brane (approximately 15 msec; see below), so that the method allows the valid determination of cell membrane electrical properties.

The general format of the experimental derivations of the neuroblastoma membrane properties are shown in Fig. 1. The large cell shown in A generated

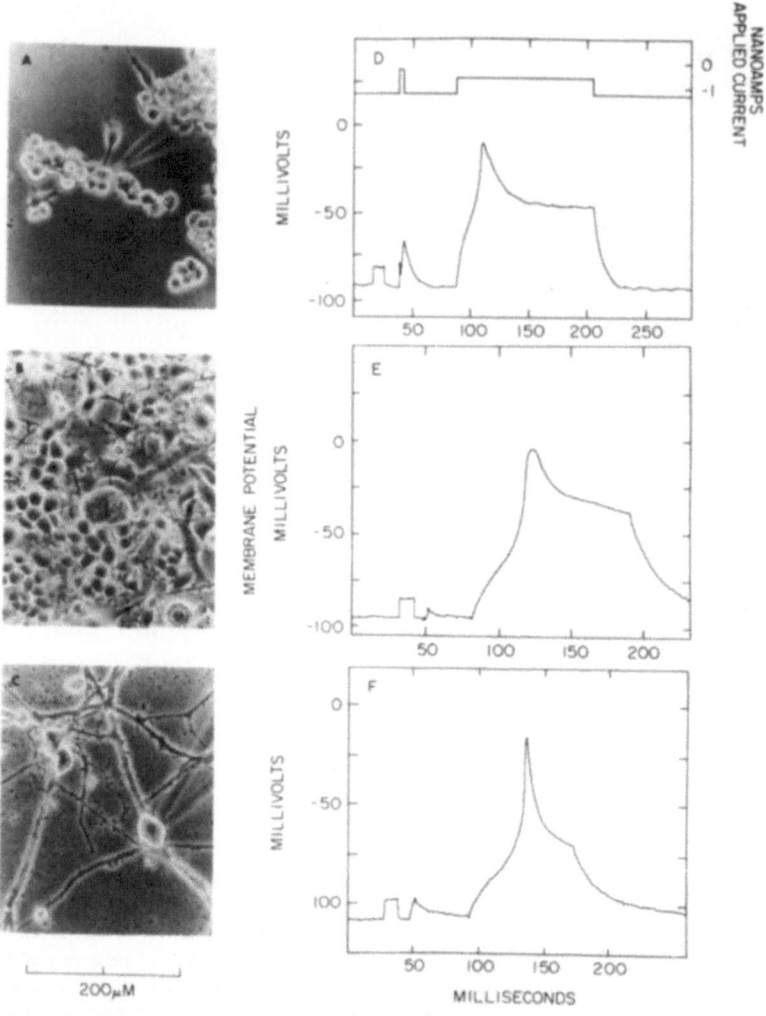

Fig. 2. Appearance of N18 cells under three culture conditions (phase-contrast photomicrographs on left side) and corresponding maximum action potentials (right side) obtained from the cell designated by microelectrode *in situ*. (A) Log phase culture 1 day after plating. (B) Minus serum culture plated 5 days earlier in solution A (see footnote Table I) and changed to solution A minus serum the day following plating. Commonly, the larger cells were tested. (C) Aminopterin-selected culture 14 days after plating. (D) Tracing of action potential (lower trace) elicited from cell in A in response to stimulating current pulse of about 100 msec as shown in the upper trace. At the beginning of the voltage record is a calibration pulse (10 mV and 10 msec) followed by a brief voltage deflection in response to the current calibration pulse (1 namp and 3 msec) on the upper trace. (E and F) Action potentials from cell in B and C, respectively, obtained by stimulating current pulse similar to that shown in D. Electrical recordings in D, E, F, and subsequent figures were obtained by computer-controlled X–Y plotter printout. (From Peacock *et al.*, 1972.)

action potentials when stimulated electrically (B and C). The action potential in C is slightly larger than that in B because in C the membrane potential had been increased by steady hyperpolarizing current prior to the depolarizing pulse of stimulating current which elicited the action potential. The peak rate of change of membrane potential with respect to time (dv/dt) was measured with a differentiating circuit and is displayed on the bottom traces of B and C. This peak dV/dT can be seen to be substantially greater in C than in B. This maximum action potential rate of rise is an index of membrane current during the action potential, and we have taken this as a quantitative measure of the degree of electrical excitability in the cells under study. We determined this for a wide range of steady membrane potentials in the cells studied and have taken the electrical excitability to be a function of the greatest peak dV/dT that a cell exhibited at any of the steady membrane potentials we examined. Passive membrane electrical properties (resistance and capacity) can be measured with hyperpolarizing current pulses. The negative slope of the plot shown in Fig. 1D gives the membrane time constant (equal to $R_m \cdot C_m$ or the total input resistance of the cell membrane times the total cell membrane capacity). The total input resistance of the cell is obtained as the quotient of the steady membrane potential change produced by a given pulse of current divided by the magnitude of that current.

Are any or all of these electrical parameters different when different clones of neuroblastoma cells are studied or when a given clone is studied under different culture conditions? Figures 2 and 3 and Table I (and data with regard to hybrid lines of cells; see below) indicate that the property of electrical excitability is differentially expressed in these different situations. The

TABLE I

Variation of Neuroblastoma Electrical Properties with Different Growth
Conditions and in Different Clones[a]

Clone	Culture medium	Growth phase	Membrane potential ($-mV$)	Membrane resistivity (ohm-cm²)	Action potential (μamp/cm²)
N18	Low serum	Stationary	41	2300	59
N18	Full medium +aminopterin	Stationary	43	2900	160
N18	Full medium	Logarithmic	14	680	1
N1A103	Full medium +aminopterin	Stationary	28	2000	10

Modified from Peacock *et al.* (1972).
[a]Full medium (solution A) is the Dulbecco–Vogt modification of Eagle's medium plus 10% fetal calf serum plus 50 units/ml of penicillin and 10 αg/ml of streptomycin sulfate. Aminopterin was used in concentrations of 10^{-5} or 10^{-6} M.

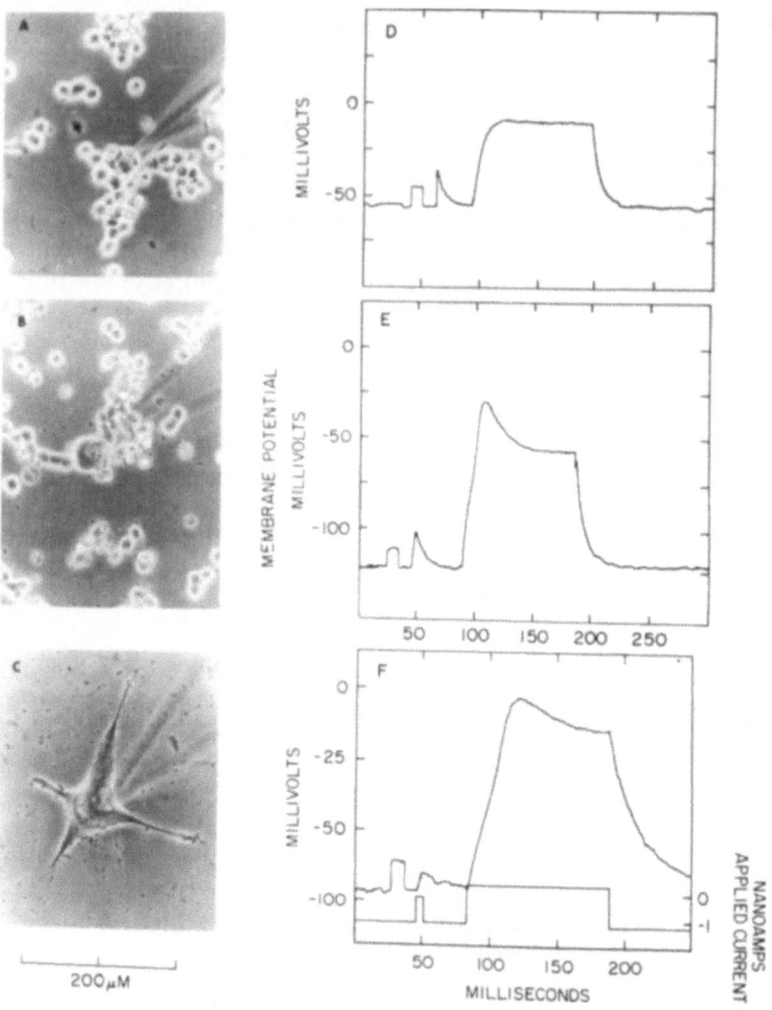

Fig. 3. N1A103 cultures studied electrically under three different conditions. (A) Log phase culture 3 days after plating. (B) Another culture, 3 days older than A but plated from same parent flask. N18 cells of comparable age have started to grow processes. (C) N1A103 cell after 9 days in aminopterin. Most cells were still round, but in some there was meager process formation. (From Peacock *et al.*, 1972.)

differences are quantitative ones, and individual cells under essentially all culture conditions in all clones may exhibit some degree of electrical excitability. However, a fifteenfold or greater range of action-potential generation capability is seen in the neuroblastoma, depending on the clone and conditions of examination. We will consider in detail the question of the validity of this conclusion, that the action-potential mechanism is under some degree of regulation in the neuroblastoma, after presenting further data with regard to electrical excitability in somatic cell hybrids (see below).

The N18 (Fig. 2) and N1A103 (Fig. 3) clones constitute two cell populations which are substantially different in a number of regards in addition to electrical excitability. For instance, unlike many other neuroblastoma clones including N18, N1A103 does not extend processes under any of the culture conditions we have used, and the percentage of cells killed by the aminopterin selection method is much higher in the N1A103 than in the N18 clone.

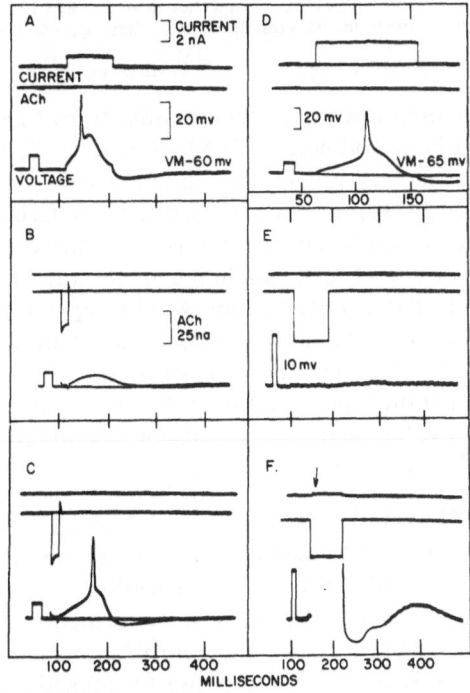

Fig. 4. Intracellular recordings of membrane potential to show electrical and chemical excitability of two neuroblastoma cells from the N18 clone selected in aminopterin. In all portions of this figure, the current passed through the intracellular pipette to electrically stimulate the cell is shown on the upper trace, the current passed through an acetylcholine-filled pipette whose tip is located immediately adjacent to the cell being recorded from is shown in the middle trace, and the intracellular recorded membrane potential is shown on the bottom trace. (A) Response to direct stimulating current pulse to show action potential. (B and C) Responses of cell illustrated to iontophoretically applied acetylcholine (ACh). ACh pulse is larger in C than in B, and higher depolarization evokes an action potential. Voltage calibration bar in A applies also to B and C. An acetylcholine calibration in B applies to C, E, and F as well. (D) Electrically induced action potential from second cell on same plate as that of A–C. (E) Lack of response to large long pulse of ACh. (F) Pulse of ACh elicits a direct electrical response when ACh electrode is pushed too far against cell. The 10-mV calibration in E applies also to F. (From Peacock and Nelson, 1972*b*.)

TABLE II

Acetylcholine Responses in N18 Cultures[a]

Medium	Depolarizing (%)	Hyperpolarizing[b] (%)	Mixed (%)	Cells tested
DMEM	7	14	4	83
F12	9	28	4	105

From Peacock and Nelson (1972b).
[a] F12 cells were initially grown in DMEM and then switched to F12 3–15 days prior to physiological study. Both media contained 10% fetal calf serum and 4×10^{-7} M aminopterin.
[b] P of difference in hyperpolarizing incidence in DMEM vs. F12 is < 0.025.

The action potential mechanism in neuroblastoma cells is largely but not completely blocked by tetrodotoxin (TTX) (Nelson et al., 1971b). The action potential waveform is very different in different cells (Harris and Dennis, 1970; Nelson et al., 1971b), and a delay on the repolarization phase of the action potential seen in some cells represents a similarity to the action-potential characteristics of dorsal root ganglion cells in normal dissociated preparations (see below). These observations would suggest that Ca ions may participate in the neuroblastoma action potential. It would be of interest to determine whether the TTX-resistant component of the neuroblastoma action potential is dependent on external Ca ions. If it is, the important question of Ca-Na specificity in voltage-sensitive membrane ionophores could be studied in detail in neuroblastoma cells.

B. Chemosensitivity

Harris and Dennis (1970) demonstrated that iontophoretically applied acetylcholine (ACh) could produce depolarization and initiation of action potentials in neuroblastoma cells. We have confirmed their findings (Fig. 4) and have shown in addition that some neuroblastoma cells develop hyperpolarizing, inhibitory potentials in response to applied ACh (Nelson et al., Peacock and Nelson, 1972b). Both types of responses may be elicited in the same cell, and Fig. 5 is an example of such a cell in which the different receptors were distributed over the surface of the cell in an organized topographic manner. Depolarizing responses were elicited by ACh applied to the cell body, while hyperpolarizing responses were elicited by ACh applied to any of the three major cell processes. Depolarizing ACh responses were blocked by d-tubocurarine (Fig. 6), while the hyperpolarizing responses were preferentially blocked by atropine. The latency and time course of the hyperpolarizing responses are substantially longer than is the case for the depolarizing responses. Hence different receptors and different ionic permeability channels associated with the receptors are synthesized and differentially distributed over the cell surface in these neuronal tumor cells.

We have examined the question of regulation of this differentiated function of chemosensitivity by studying a large population of cells from the N18 clone in two different culture media, DMEM plus 10% fetal calf serum (FCS) and F12 plus 10% FCS (Peacock and Nelson, 1972b). The cells were initially selected in DMEM plus 10% FCS plus 4×10^{-7} M aminopterin so that a stable population of cells, well differentiated from the standpoint of morphology and electrical excitability, were available (Peacock et al., 1972). A group of cultures were switched from DMEM plus 10% FCS plus 4×10^{-7} M aminopterin to F12 plus 10% FCS plus 4×10^{-7} M aminopterin, and these were studied 3–10 days after the switch along with cultures maintained in DMEM plus 10% FCS plus 4×10^{-7} M aminopterin. The incidence of depolarizing (D) responses, hyperpolarizing (H) responses, and combined D-H responses found in cells in the two cultures are shown in Table II. The incidence of H responses is doubled, while the D and D-H responses are not significantly changed. The

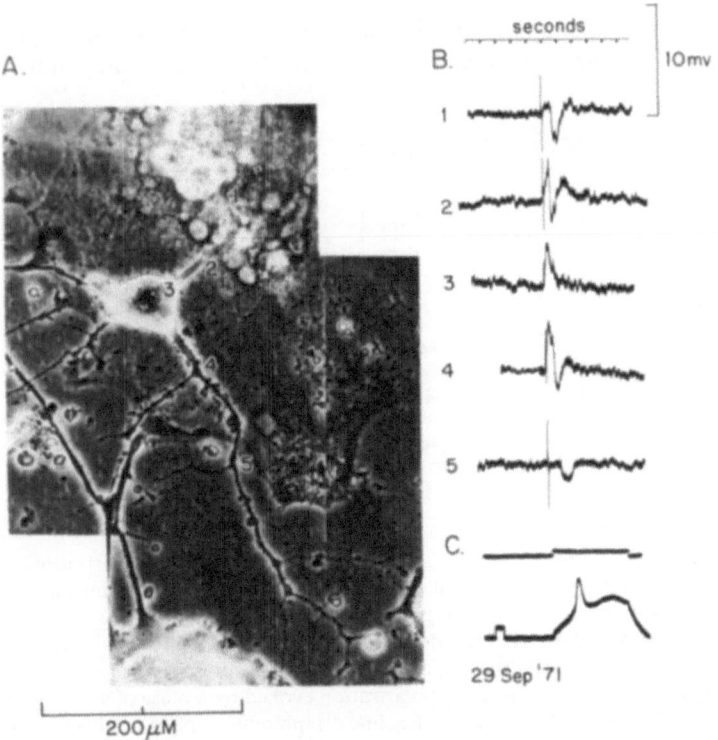

Fig. 5. NA neuroblastoma cell, X-irradiated. (B_{1-5}) Intracellularly recorded responses to short pulses of acetylcholine delivered to the cell surface at the locations indicated on A. (C) Action potential (lower trace) elicited by intracellularly applied current pulse (upper trace). (From Peacock et al., 1973.)

F12 medium contains sufficient hypoxanthine and thymidine to circumvent the aminopterin block of nucleic acid synthesis and cell division, and within 2 weeks after switching from the DMEM to F12 the cells in F12 were dividing rapidly. A large number of metabolic alterations therefore no doubt result from change in culture media. The results indicate, however, that the different ACh receptor mechanisms are under differential control and can be affected to different degrees by such factors as culture conditions.

A less extensive survey of the N18 clone was made with regard to possible chemosensitivity of the cells to other neurohormones (Peacock and Nelson, 1972*b*). Dopamine, norepinephrine, and serotonin were tested. Dopamine produced hyperpolarizing responses in 30% of cells, while of 18 cells tested with norepinephrine and 18 tested with serotonin, none showed any responsiveness. It is of interest that dopamine has been identified as being present in sympathetic ganglia and that it has been implicated in the production of slow hyperpolarizing responses in intact sympathetic ganglion (Libet and Tosaka, 1970).

In the many pairs of neuroblastoma cells we have tested in an attempt to demonstrate synaptic connections between these cells, no short-latency,

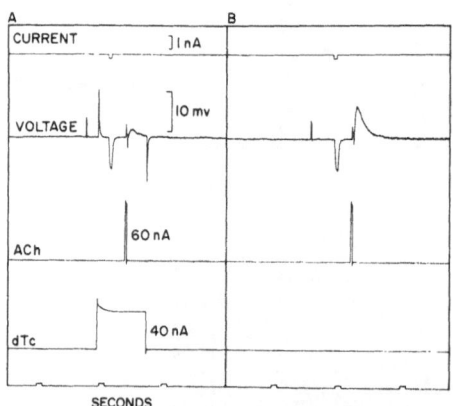

Fig. 6. Effect of iontophoretically applied *d*-tubocurarine on depolarization produced by a pulse of acetylcholine. In A and B, line 1 represents the current being passed through the intracellular electrode to measure cell membrane resistance, line 2 represents the transmembrane potential. The first deflection is a 10-mV, 10-msec calibration pulse, the first downward deflection is the response to the current pulse shown on line 1, and the following upward deflection is the depolarization evoked by a pulse of acetylcholine. Line 3 records the applied acetylcholine pulse, line 4 represents applied *d*-tubocurarine (dTC), and line 5 is a 1-sec calibration. Series A shows the ACh response elicited during an application of dTC, and B shows the large response elicited in the absence of applied *d*-tubocurarine. Artifacts occur on voltage trace on A at onset and termination of dTC pulse. (From Peacock *et al.*, 1973.)

depolarizing, excitatory connections have been seen. Long-latency, hyperpo-larizing potentials have been evoked on several occasions in one cell of a pair by strong depolarization of a connecting, second cell. These interactions are quite uncommon, are not always reproducible, and do not resemble typical synapses in their behavior. Harris *et al.* (1971) have shown that when neuro-blastoma cells are cocultured with a continuous line of muscle cells, contacts established between neuroblastoma and muscle are associated with a marked alteration of ACh sensitivity in the muscle cells. This is suggestive of a tropic interaction between these lines of cells.

Electrical coupling between neuroblastoma cells was described by Harris and Dennis (1970), and while it is quite uncommon we too have seen this type of interaction. Electrical coupling between various sorts of normal and neoplastic cell lines has been described and will be discussed below.

III. HYBRID CELL LINES

The technique of somatic cell hybridization has been widely used in cell biology as a means of studying such problems as the mechanism of control of differentiated characteristics and the establishment of linkage groups between different enzyme markers (Davidson, 1971; Ruddle, 1972). Minna (Minna *et al.*, 1971, 1972) and McMorris (Peacock *et al.*, 1973) have succeeded in producing a number of lines of hybrid cells by fusing mouse neuroblastoma cells and mouse L cells (a continuous line of fibroblasts) and cloning the heterokaryons. These hybrid lines have been studied electrophysiologically (Minna *et al.*, 1971; Peacock *et al.*, 1973).

L cells lack the capacity to generate action potentials, but they do exhibit an active electrical response, the hyperpolarizing activation or H.A. response (Nelson *et al.*, 1972). This can be elicited by electrical, mechanical, or chemical stimuli (Nelson and Peacock, 1972) and consists of a large increase in mem-brane permeability to potassium ions with consequent hyperpolarization of the membrane. The main features of this response and morphological charac-teristics of the L cells selected by X-irradiation are shown in Figs. 7 and 8. The steady resting potential is relatively low approximately ($-$ 20 mV) and the membrane resistivity and time constant are large, probably reflecting a low resting membrane potassium conductance. The neuroblastoma $\times$ L-cell hybrid clones exhibit a range of morphologies, resting membrane con-ductances, electrical excitability, chemosensitivity, and incidence of H.A. responses. The electrical characteristics of a given clone were quite homogene-ous under controlled culture conditions, but the various clones were markedly different in this regard. Examples of this are shown in Fig. 9, and data are summarized in Table III. The cells in these hybrid clones were large, and

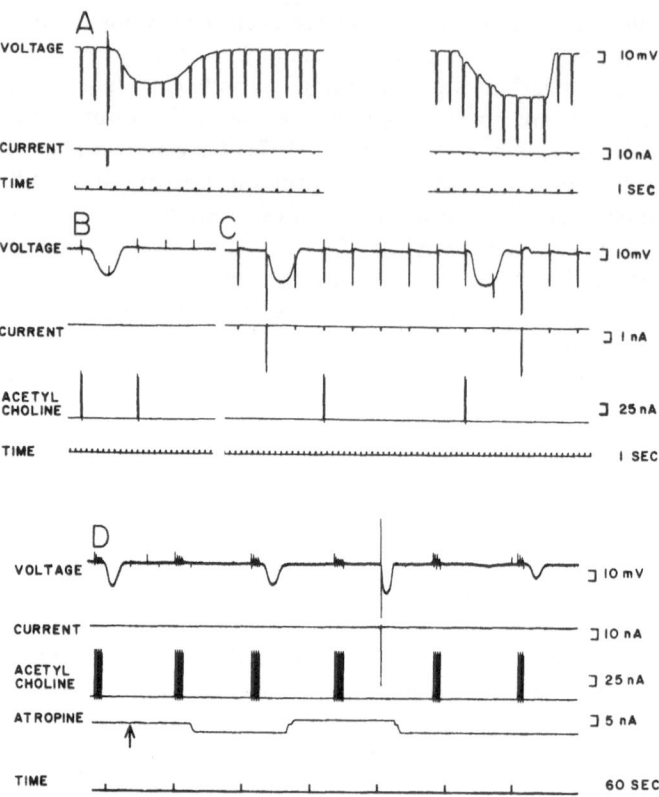

Fig. 7.   Records from three different cells shown in A, in B and C, and in D. Trace labeled VOLTAGE represent transmembrane voltage (negative downward) measured with an intracellular pipette. Traces labeled CURRENT represent current passed across the membrane (inward current down) by the intracellular pipette arranged in a bridge circuit. Traces labeled ACETYLCHOLINE represent total current passed through an acetylcholine-containing micropipette (outward current up). Steady levels of negative holding current of about 5 namp were passed from the ACh pipette between pulses. Trace-labeled ATROPINE represents total current passed through an atropine sulfate electrode (outward current up). All calibrations as marked. (A) Left portion: Hyperpolarizing activation response (H.A. response). Small pulses of current are used to test membrane resistance, and the larger pulse (third pulse on current trace) elicits the H.A. response. Note decrease in voltage response to small test current pulse during the H.A. Right portion: Membrane potential is increased by small steady current while testing with small pulses to show that voltage responses to these test pulses are essentially unchanged as a result of the increase in membrane potential as contrasted to the result during the H.A. response. Resting potential in this cell was −25 mV. (B)Response to ACh. Second pulse fails to elicit a change in membrane potential. Upward deflection on voltage traces are calibration pulses. (C) Interaction between directly elicited H.A. and the ACh responses. ACh pulse following H.A. response by some 10 sec fails to elicit a response even though membrane potential and resistance have returned to

stable recordings were readily obtained from them. It seems clear in these hybrid lines that the action-potential mechanism is differentially expressed.

The observation with regard to the electrical excitability of neuroblastoma and hybrid cells must be interpreted with caution, because of the technical limitations of the methods employed. We conclude that the data are incompatible with the position that electrical excitability is uniformly expressed in the various cell lines and with the corresponding inference that the measured differences between lines are due to inadequacies of the culturing or electrophysiological methods. Our conclusion is based on two considerations: (1) Considerable attention was given to treating the various lines of cells uniformly with respect to temperature, pH, and osmolarity of the cultures during the physiological experiments. Differences in electrophysiological properties should not have been caused by artifacts of the culturing conditions. (2) If differential cell injury resulting from the penetration of the cells by the recording microelectrodes were responsible for the different electrical excitabilities measured in the various populations, this should have been reflected in some of the measures of passive membrane properties. In particular, lower resting potentials and lower membrane resistivity (or membrane time constant) should correlate with lower electrical excitability. Probably the most sensitive passive membrane indicator of cell injury is the time constant, since any leakage resistance occurring at the site of microelectrode penetration will necessarily reduce the overall electrical resistance between the inside and outside of the cell and hence shorten the measured cell time constant. The time constant measurement has the advantage that it, unlike the cell resistance, is independent of cell surface area. In fact, within a given population of cells, no

---

normal. Similarly, a previously adequate direct stimulus does not elicit H.A. response when preceded by an ACh-elicited response. Resting membrane potential in B and C was −30 mV. (D) ACh but not H.A. responses blocked by atropine in consecutive trials of continuous recording. First series of ACh pulses elicited a response. At the arrow below the atropine trace, the atropine electrode was positioned with its tip close to the tip of the acetylcholine electrode with no negative steady current flowing so that some leakage of atropine would occur. The subsequent ACh pulses (second application of ACh) did not elicit a response (the refractory period of the ACh response was shown in other trials to be much shorter than the 70-sec period between these two ACh applications). Atropine flow was turned off when a negative current was passed through the atropine pipette, and the ACh response was recovered (third application of ACh). Positive atropine current released more atropine than before and again resulted in abolition of the ACh response (fourth application of ACh), but the H.A. response could still be elicited (note large stimulus pulse on current trace). After negative current was passed through the atropine electrode for about 1.5 min, the ACh response recovered (sixth application of ACh). Resting membrane potential was −20 mV. (From Nelson and Peacock, 1972.)

TABLE III

Electrical Properties of Neuroblastoma × L-Cell Hybrids

	Clone	Membrane potential (−mV)	Membrane time constant (msec)	Maximum action potential dv/dt (V/sec)
Series	NL1	27	11.5	5.1
A	NL2	34	15.5	1.0
Series	NLI8	37	16	32
B	NLI3	23	15	2

Series A from Minna *et al.* (1971); series B from Peacock *et al.* (1973).

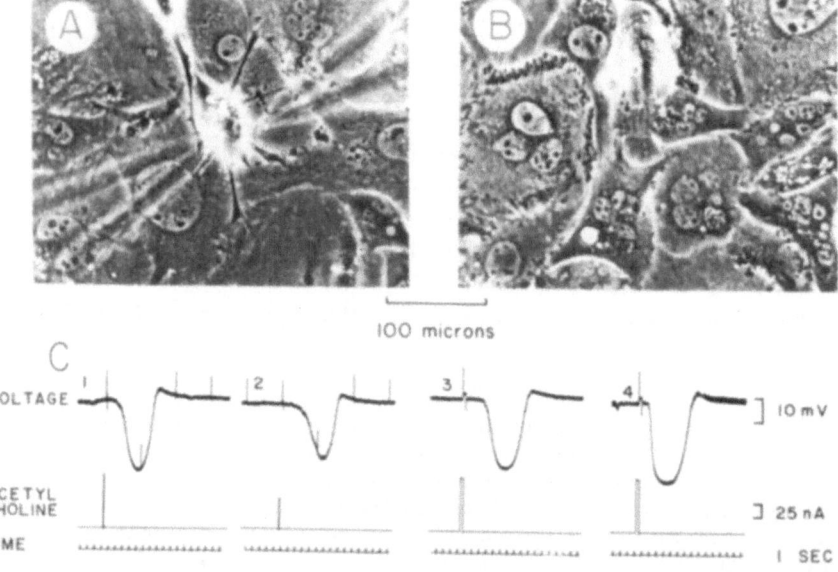

Fig. 8. (A) Cell from which the records shown in C were obtained is the phase-bright cell in the center of the field. Electrode shadow coming from lower left is from the intracellular microelectrode, that from upper right from the ACh electrode. (B) Phase-bright cell in middle top portion of the field exhibited hyperpolarizing responses when three out of five of the cells adjacent to it were stimulated with acetylcholine. (C₁). Membrane potential response of cell when ACh was applied to the cell body as shown in A. (C₂). Slower similar response obtained with smaller ACh pulse. (C₃). Response from same cell when ACh was applied to the cell body of the phase-bright cell at upper edge of field. (C₄). Faster, larger response when ACh was applied to the process of the upper cell. Response was abolished by withdrawing the electrode several microns up into the culture medium. Resting membrane potential of this cell was −30 mV. (From Nelson and Peacock, 1972.)

correlation between electrical excitability and passive properties was found (Fig. 6, Peacock *et al.*, 1972). In the two pairs of hybrid clones of Table III the membrane resistivity (or time constant) of the less excitable clones was either the same or actually larger than that of the more excitable clone. We are thus led to the interpretation that, as with other electrophysiological, enzymatic, and morphological properties of neuroblastoma and hybrid cells, the property of electrical excitability is indeed under a high degree of regulation.

Two possibilities may be suggested to explain the differences between the results presented above and the contrary interpretations arising from the experiments of Schubert *et al.* (this volume). First, different culture conditions were used in the two sets of experiments; Schubert and coworkers grew cells in suspension cultures to obtain cells in a dedifferentiated state and then studied these cells shortly after they had attached to plastic culture dishes. This method produces a morphologically undifferentiated population of cells, but it is possible that electrical excitability is more fully expressed in these cells than in, for instance, the logarithmically growing cells in surface cultures which were studied by Peacock *et al.* (1972). Second, a sampling

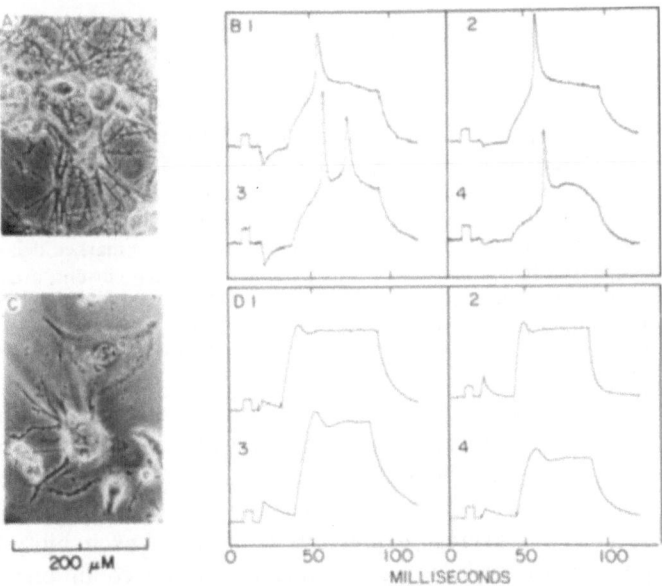

Fig. 9. Morphological and electrical characteristics of two different strains of NA × LM (TK⁻) hybrids. (A) Examples of a neuron-like hybrid line NLI8 after incubation in aminopterin (10^{-5} M) containing DMEM plus 10% FCS for 10 days. (B_{1-4}) For examples of action potentials generated by different cells of the NLI8 clone in response to stimulating current pulses. (C) Examples of more fibroblastic hybrid line NLI3 under culture conditions similar to those in A. (D_{1-4}) Four examples of nearly passive behavior of four different cells from clone NLI3 when stimulated by depolarizing pulses of current. Note great similarity of examples in B and in D and substantial difference between B and D. (From Peacock *et al.*, 1973.)

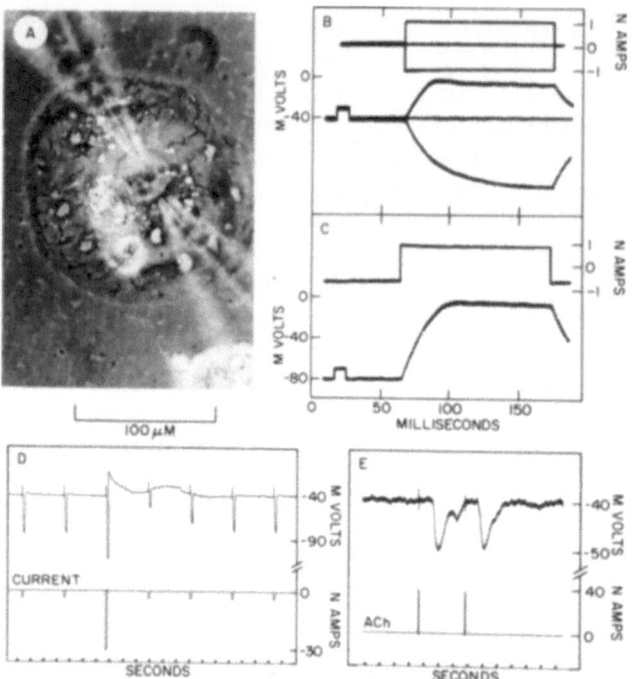

Fig. 10.   Morphology and electrical responses of N × M hybrid, NMVII10. (A) Photomicrograph of cell, recordings from which are shown in B–D. (B) Upper traces are currents passed through impaling microelectrode to hyperpolarize and depolarize the cell. Lower traces show membrane potential elicited by those currents. No action potential occurs, but marked asymmetry of voltage response demonstrates marked delayed rectification in this cell. (C) In the presence of steady hyperpolarizing current, a depolarizing current pulse still does not elicit an action potential. (D) Strong electrical stimulation (lower trace) does not elicit a H.A. response (upper trace). (E) Acetylcholine pulses (lower trace) elicit hyperpolarizing responses (upper trace). (From Peacock *et al.*, 1973.)

problem may be involved. A small population of cells in any culture conditions may well undergo some degree of differentiation, and Schubert and coworkers were concerned with the maximum degree of excitability that could be demonstrated in their cultures. Peacock and coworkers dealt with quantitative measures of the average expression of electrical excitability in a substantial sample of the cells under the various culture conditions explored.

The incidence of cells exhibiting ACh sensitivity was also different in the various neuroblastoma × L-cell hybrids. In general, a pattern of coordinate expression of neuronal and L-cell characteristics was seen: clones with prominent cell processes had a high degree of electrical excitability and a relatively high incidence of depolarizing responses to ACh. Process-poor clones had a high incidence of the L-cell H.A. response, a low degree of electrical excitability, and no depolarizing responses to ACh.

Hybrid clones were established by McMorris between neuroblastoma cells and a human diploid fibroblast, the MRC5 line (Peacock *et al.*, 1973). A considerable degree of morphological and electrophysiological heterogeneity characterized these clones despite a low degree of heteroploidy. Some of the cells exhibited a high degree of neuronal differentiation, and in others some dissection of neuronal characteristics occurred. Thus in Fig. 10 an example is shown of a cell with fibroblastic morphology and low electrical excitability along with the neuroblastoma type of chemosensitivity. The time course of the hyperpolarizing response in this cell was typical of that occurring in neuroblastoma cells and substantially faster than that of L cells.

IV. OTHER CONTINUOUS CELL LINES: ELECTRICAL COUPLING

Electrical transmission between nerve cells was demonstrated several years ago (Furshpan and Potter, 1959), and low-resistance intercellular coupling has been studied extensively since that time (Bennett, 1966; Bennett and Trinkhaus, 1970; Furshpan and Potter, 1968). Electrophysiological methods have shown that this form of close communication between cells is a very widespread phenomenon. Loewenstein and Kanno (1964) initially studied electrical coupling between gland cells, but this work has been extended to a number of other tissues and has dealt in particular with differences between normal and neoplastic cells, *in vivo* and *in vitro* (Azarnia and Loewenstein, 1971). Normal cells exhibited extensive electrical intercellular coupling, while cancerous cells did not. This has raised the question of whether electrical coupling reflects a mechanism which might account for control of cell division and tissue growth. Furshpan and Potter (1968) found evidence for electrical coupling in some lines of transformed cells, however, so that a causal relationship between electrical intercellular coupling and growth control does not seem to be entirely general.

Direct biochemical evidence has been obtained that interchange of metabolically important molecules occurs between cultured cells. By an ingenious technique allowing separation of different populations of cultured cells, Kolodny (1971) has shown that RNA can be transferred from one population of cells to another. The properties of the transferred material indicated that more or less intact ribosomes are probably transferred, so that relatively large particles are involved. DNA is not transferred from one cell population to the other, however, so that some mechanism other than cell disintegration and subsequent phagocytosis must be involved. Transfer takes place between transformed, non-contact-inhibited lines as well as between nontransformed lines, so that the exchange of material does not seem to be causally related to growth control (Kolodny, 1972).

Intercellular transfer of enzyme products has been shown with a number of cell lines (Subak-Sharp et al., 1969). Mutant lines of fibroblasts have been obtained which are deficient in the enzyme hypoxanthine-guanine phosphoribosyltransferase (HGPRT⁻). These cells cannot incorporate hypoxanthine into nucleic acid, and when the cells were incubated with radioactive hypoxanthine, subsequent autoradiography failed to show any labeling of the cells. If these deficient cells were cocultured with HGPRT-containing cells, however, the deficient cells did incorporate radioactive hypoxanthine. This could be shown to be due to uptake of hypoxanthine which had been metabolized by the HGPRT in the nondeficient cells, so that transfer of the enzyme product from competent to deficient cells must have taken place.

Morphological and electrophysiological studies of the mechanism that may underlie this phenomenon have been carried out (Gilula et al., 1972). Direct electrical coupling has been demonstrated between cells of the lines which do exhibit transfer of metabolites, and gap junctions between these same cell types have been shown electron microscopically. Conversely, cell lines which do not exchange metabolites exhibit neither electrical nor morphological evidence of low-resistance pathways between the cells of the different lines.

Electrical coupling has been demonstrated between cells in developing embryos (Bennett and Trinkhaus, 1970; Potter et al., 1966) and in embryonic cells which have reaggregated after an initial dissociation (Sheridan, 1971). Movement of dye molecules such as fluorescein correlates with the occurrence of electrical coupling in some cases, so that transcellular movement of molecules larger than inorganic ions is possible. The role that these widespread channels of intercellular communication play in normal development is of great interest but at present is far from clear. Furshpan and Potter (1968) have argued that movement of molecules of 200–300 mol wt. either could serve a regulatory role or could serve to effectively dilute the effects of focal metabolic activity that would otherwise deplete nutrients or lead to the accumulation of waste metabolites.

V. NORMAL DISSOCIATED CULTURES

A marked disadvantage of many of the continuous cell lines and in particular the neuroblastoma system is its substantial degree of aneuploidy and karyotypic instability. Clones of single-cell origin exhibit a considerable range in the number of chromosomes per cell. Considerable chromosomal and gene duplication characterizes these lines so that genetic studies are made complex. The neuroblastoma model system shows some crucial shortcomings in the range of neurobiological properties which it expresses, notably in the

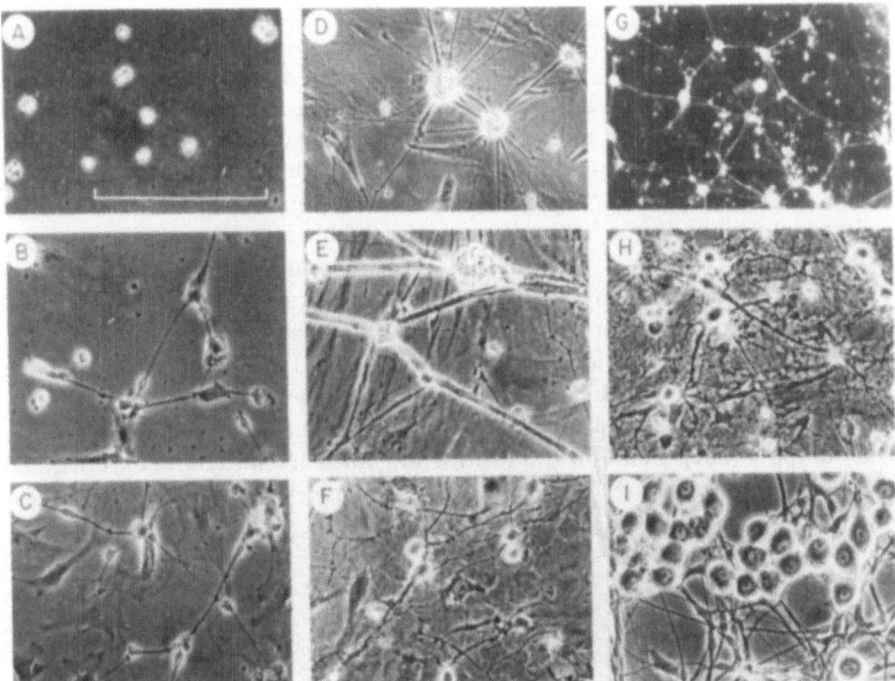

Fig. 11. Composite of phase-contrast photomicrographs (except for G, which is not phase) of various culture stages. Calibration bar in A is 200 μ for A, B, C, E, F, and H. For D, it is 275 μ; for G, 1.3mm; and for I, 225 μ. (A) Dissociated cord and ganglion cells from 11-day-old fetus; cells were attached to collagen-covered surface of dish about 6 hr after plating. Similar microscopic fields were seen at each fetal age used. (B) Cells with long processes 24 hr after plating. Surface was collagen covered. Fetal gestational age was 14 days. (C) Same culture as B, 72 hr after plating and after 48 hr of incubation in medium containing aminopterin. Note flat background cells. (D and G) High- and low-power microscopic fields from 1-week-old culture growing on collagen-covered surface. Fetal gestational age was 11 days. (E and F) Same dish as in C after 4 weeks in culture. (H) Field of SC cells after 4 weeks in culture on plastic surface. Fetal gestational age was 12–13 days. (I) Field of DRG cells after 6 weeks in culture on plastic surface. Fetal gestational age was 11–12 days. (From Peacock and Nelson, 1972*a*.)

capacity of these cells to form synapses. Several workers have diligently sought to demonstrate synaptic connections between the neuroblastoma and a number of potential target-cell types, so far without success. Interactions between neuroblastoma cells and a continuous line of muscle cells have been described (Harris *et al.*, 1971), but this system lacks the full range of phenomena characteristic of synaptic connections.

These considerations add to the great intrinsic interest of normal nervous system and muscle cells in culture.

A. Muscle Cultures

Normal chick embryonic muscle has been studied extensively by a variety of techniques, as it develops in culture from single myoblasts to multinucleated, striated, twitching muscle fibers (Hirakow and DeHaan, 1970; Konigsberg, 1963; Stockdale and Holzer, 1961; Yaffe, 1969). Membrane resistivity stays relatively constant, but membrane potential gradually increases as does electrical excitability as myotubes mature (Fishbach *et al.*, 1971). The synthesis of acetylcholine receptors has been measured electrophysiologically and autoradiographically by Fambrough and Rasch (1971). Nonuniform distribution of acetylcholine receptors along developing myotubes even in the absence of innervation has been demonstrated by Fischbach and Cohen (1973), with as much as a fortyfold range of sensitivity occurring along the surface of the same myotube. Single heart myocytes exhibit rhythmic action-potential generation and contraction, and the time course of functional coupling between these cells in culture has been elegantly shown by Hirakow

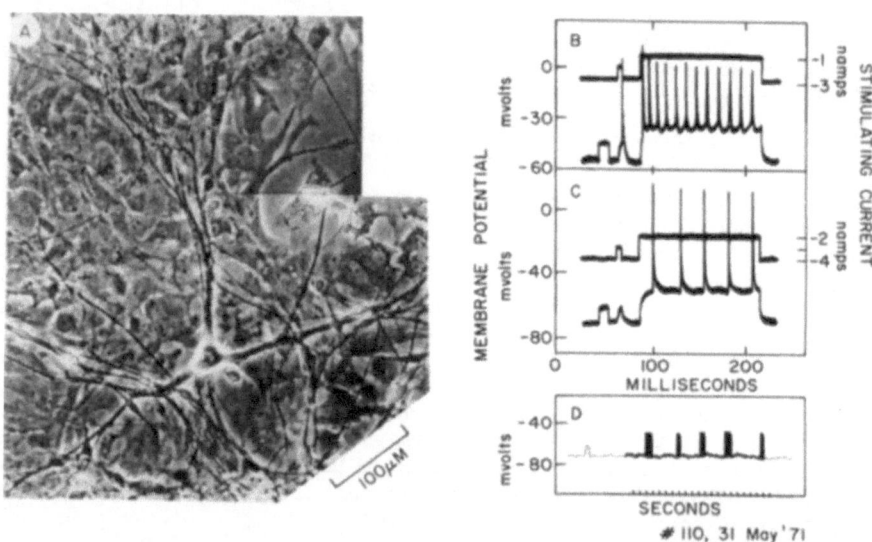

Fig. 12. (A) Phase-contrast photomicrograph of SC neuron in 17-day-old culture grown on plastic. Fetal gestational age was 11 days. (B and C) The lower or voltage trace of each shows action potential firing from cell in A during a long stimulation current pulse, upper trace of each. The first event on the voltage trace is a calibration pulse of 10 mV by 10 msec followed by a response to the current calibration of 1 namp immediately above on upper trace. Note that membrane potential is higher in C than in B. (D) Bursts of spontaneous action-potential firing from cell in A recorded on a penwriter at slower time base, seconds, and beginning as noted on abscissa after a faster recording period marked by a similar calibration pulse as above. Actual amplitudes of action potentials are higher than could be recorded on a penwriter, because of its limited frequency response. (From Peacock and Nelson, 1972*a*.)

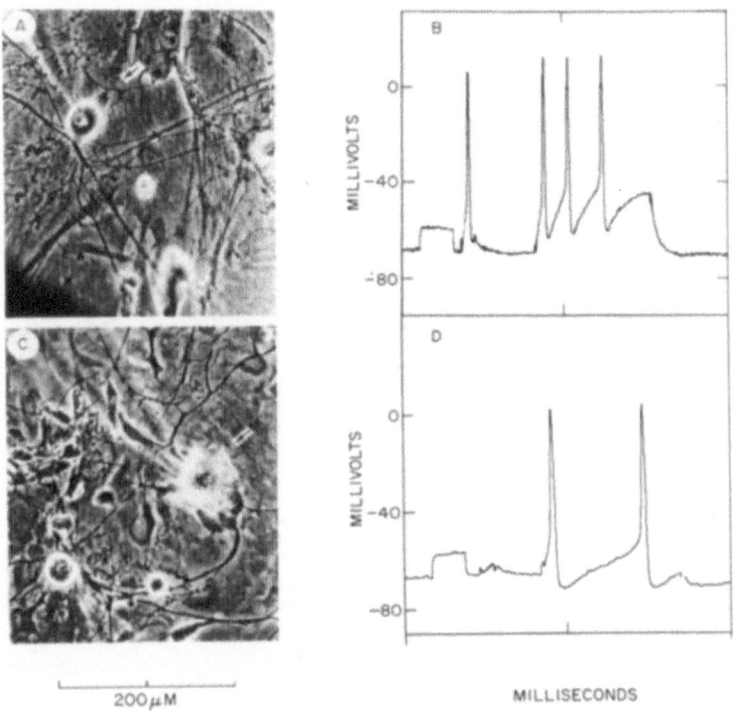

Fig. 13. In A and C are illustrated examples of DRG cells and action potentials recorded from each, respectively, in B and D. The action-potential traces were drawn by an $X-Y$ plotter from data stored on magnetic computer tape. Indicated cell in A was in 24-day-old culture grown on plastic and obtained from fetuses of 11 days gestational age. The cells shown in C were in a 20-day-old culture grown on plastic and were initially dissociated from a fetus of 17 days gestational age. (From Peacock and Nelson, 1972a.)

and DeHaan (1970). Within as little as 2 min after physical contact was made between independently contracting myocytes, synchronization of their contractions occurred. The morphological counterpart of this synchronization at the electron microscopic level was the formation of a specialized membrance structure, the nexus, between the coupled cells.

B. Nervous System Cultures

1. Spinal Cord and Dorsal Root Ganglia

Dissociated chick embryonic spinal cord and dorsal root ganglion (DRG) cells in low-density cultures survive and develop into large multiprocess neuronal networks in culture (Fischbach, 1970, 1972; Scott, 1971; Scott et al., 1969). This is true for mouse embryonic spinal cord and DRG preparations as well (Peacock and Nelson, 1972a), and typical chemical synaptic

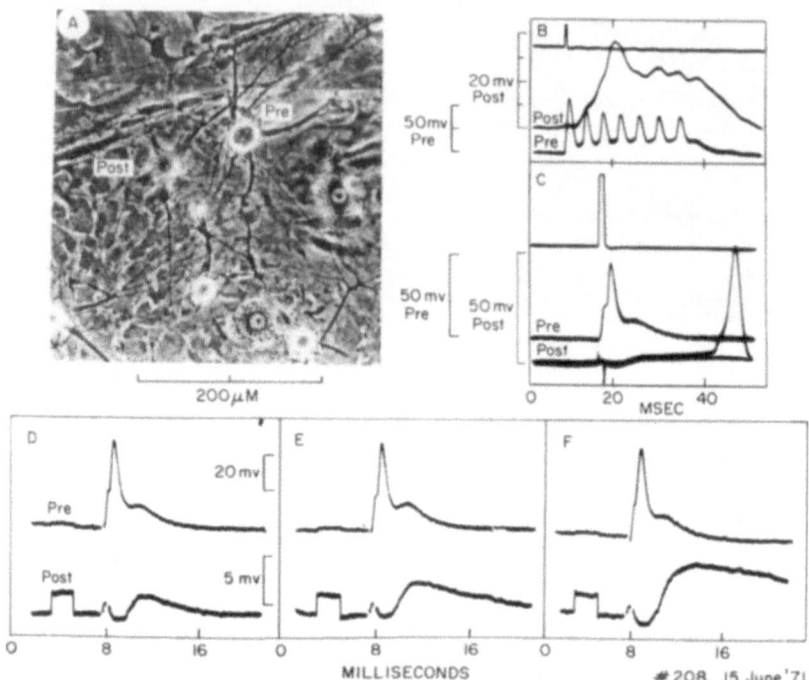

Fig. 14. (A) Synaptically coupled cells identified as "Pre" and "Post" in a 34-day-old culture grown on plastic. Fetal gestational age was 11 days. (B) Summated EPSP (middle trace) in Post to a burst of action potentials (lower trace) elicited in Pre by short current pulse (upper trace). (C) A postsynaptic action potential in Post (lower trace) following a presynaptic action potential (middle trace) response to current stimulation (upper trace). Recording was obtained on second penetration of cell. (D, E, and F) EPSPs of varying amplitudes (lower traces) follow presynaptic action potentials (upper traces). Upper calibration marker holds for Pre and lower calibration marker for Post. (From Peacock and Nelson, 1972a.)

transmission between pairs of neurons and between neurons and muscle cells has been demonstrated in both chick and mouse preparations (Fischbach, 1972; Peacock and Nelson, 1972a, b). Fischbach (1972) has utilized methods for suppressing fibroblast growth and promoting the survival and development of neurons so that rich neuronal preparations are available which are relatively free of contaminating, nonneuronal elements. A high degree of synaptic activity characterizes these cultures.

Spinal cord neurons and DRG cells exhibit different, characteristic action-potential configurations, and these differences are maintained for prolonged periods *in vitro*. Fischbach and Dichter (in preparation) have shown that the action-potential currents are carried exclusively by a tetrodotoxin-sensitive sodium mechanism in spinal cord cells, while calcium ions carry a substantial fraction of the action currents in DRG cells. Mouse dissociated material exhibits some of these same features (Peacock and Nelson, 1972a), and Figs. 11–13 show characteristic morphological and electrophysiological properties of mouse spinal cord and DRG cells. Synaptic coupling between two mouse spinal cord cells is shown in Fig. 14. Analysis of the failure rate and variance of the evoked postsynaptic potentials in a small sample of mouse spinal cord cells indicated that the quantum content of these synapses was probably in the range of 5–20.

2. Cerebellum

Dissociated preparations of neonatal rat and mouse embryo cerebellum have been made, and long-term survival of neurons has been demonstrated (Lasher and Zagon, 1972). Although the percentage of surviving neurons is less than is the case with spinal cord and DRG cultures, small clusters of neurons survive and exhibit rich synaptic interactions. Rhythmic bursts of synaptically mediated action potentials have been seen and both excitatory and inhibitory synaptic potentials recorded (Peacock and Nelson, 1973c).

3. Glia

Glial cells have been studied in culture by several workers (Hild and Tasaki, 1962; Trachtenberg, et al., 1972; Wardell, 1966). As expected, these cells do not generate action potentials, and the membrane time constant is very short, indicating that the resistivity of the membrane is very low. Glial cells may be electrically coupled to neuronal cell types so that direct metabolic interaction between the cells could occur (Walker and Hild, 1969). The cells of neuronal appearance which were coupled to glial cells were not electrically excitable, and it was suggested that the formation of electrical contacts with glial cells may be a mechanism for turning off electrical activity in neurons. The analysis of neuron–glia relationships is an important area for study and one in which tissue culture methodology may prove very useful.

One major disadvantage of dissociated normal preparations is that the cells represent a heterogeneous mixture of different cell types. Various cell separation techniques have been used to minimize this difficulty, but only partial success in separating specific cell types has been attained (Okun 1972; Scott, 1971; Varon and Raiborn, 1969). Nonetheless, the development of techniques for identifying different classes of cells in the mixed culture (Lasher and Zagon, 1972) and for combining cell populations from different regions of the nervous system should allow the study of cell-specific interaction in some detail.

VI. REFERENCES

Augusti-Tocco, G., and Sato, G. 1969. Establishment of functional clonal lines of neurons from mouse neuroblastoma. *Proc. Natl. Acad. Sci.* **64**:311–315.

Azarnia, R., and Loewenstein, W. R. 1971. Intercellular communication and tissue growth. V. A. cancer strain that fails to make permeable membrane junctions with normal cells. *J. Membrane Biol.* **6**:368–385.

Bennett, M. V. L. 1966. Physiology of electrotonic junctions. *Ann. N.Y. Acad. Sci.* **137**:509.

Bennett, M. V. L., and Trinkaus, J. P. 1970. Electrical coupling between embryonic cells by way of extracellular space and specialized junctions. *J. Cell Biol.* **44**:592–610.

Corner, M. A., and Crain, S. M. 1972. Patterns of spontaneous bioelectric activity during maturation in culture of fetal rodent medulla and spinal cord tissues. *J. Neurobiol.* **3**:25–45.

Crain, S. M., Alfei, L., and Peterson, E. R. 1970. Neuromuscular transmission in cultures of adult human and rodent skeletal muscle after innervation *in vitro* by fetal rodent spinal cord. *J. Neurobiol.* **1**: 471–490.

Davidson, R. L. 1971. Regulation of gene expression in somatic cell hybrids: A review. *In Vitro* **6**:411–426.

Fambrough, D., and Rash, J. E. 1971. Development of acetylcholine sensitivity during myogenesis. *Develop. Biol.* **26**:55–68.

Fischbach, G. D. 1970. Synaptic potentials recorded in cell cultures of nerve and muscle. *Science* **169**:1331–1333.

Fischbach, G. D. 1972. Synapse formation between dissociated nerve and muscle cells in low density cultures. *Develop. Biol.* **28**:407–429.

Fischbach, G., and Cohen, S. A. The distribution of acetylcholine sensitivity over uninnervated and innervated muscle fibers grown in cell culture. *Develop. Biol.* **31**:147–162.

Fischbach, G. D., and Dichter, M. The action potential of chick dorsal root ganglion neurons in cell culture. (In preparation.)

Fischbach, G. D., Nameroff, M., and Nelson, P. G. 1971. Electrical properties of chick skeletal muscle fibers developing in cell culture. *J. Cell. Physiol.* **78**:289–300.

Furshpan, E. J., and Potter, D. 1959. Transmission at the giant motor synapse of the crayfish. *J. Physiol.* **145**:289–325.

Furshpan, E. J., and Potter, D. D. 1968. Low resistance junctions between cells in embryo and tissue culture, pp. 95–127. *In* A. A. Moscona and A. Monray (eds.). Current Topics in Developmental Biology, Vol. 3. Academic Press, New York.

Gilula, N. B., Reeves, O. R., and Steinbach, A. 1972. Metabolic coupling, ionic coupling and cell contacts. *Nature* **235**:262–265.

Harris, A. J., and Dennis, M. J. 1970. Acetylcholine sensitivity and distribution on mouse neuroblastoma. *Science* **167**:1253–1255.

Harris, A. J., Heinemann, S., Schubert, D., and Tarakis, H. 1971. Trophic interaction between cloned culture lines of nerve and muscle. *Nature* **231**:296–301.

Hild, W., and Tasaki, I. 1962. Morphological and physiological properties of neurons and glial cells in tissue culture. *J. Neurophysiol.* **25**:277–304.

Hirakow, R., and DeHaan, R. L. 1970. Synchronization and the formation of nexal junction between isolated chick embryonic heart myocytes beating in culture. *J. Cell Biol.* **47**:88a.

Klebe, R. J., and Ruddle, F. H. 1969. Neuroblastoma: Cell culture analysis of a differentiating stem cell system. *J. Cell Biol.* **43**:69a.

Kolodny, G. M. 1971. Evidence for transfer of macromolecular RNA between mammalian cells in culture. *Exptl. Cell Res.* **65**:313–324.

Kolodny, G. M. 1972. Cell to cell transfer of RNA into transformed cells. *J. Cell Physiol.* **79**:147–150.

Konigsberg, I. R. 1963. Clonal analysis of myogenesis. *Science* **140**:1273–1274.

Lamb, J. F., and MacKinnon, M. G. A. 1971. Effect of ouabain and metabolic inhibitors of the Na and K movements and nucleotide contents of L-cells. *J. Physiol. (Lond.)* **213**:665–682.

Lamb, J. F., and McCall, D. 1972. Effect of prolonged ouabain treatment on Na, K, Cl and Ca concentration and fluxes in cultured human cells. *J. Physiol.* **225**:599–618.

Lasher, R. S., and Zagon, I. S. 1972. The effect of potassium on neuronal differentiation in cultures of dissociated newborn rat cerebellum. *Brain Res.* **41**:482–488.

Libet, B., and Tosaka, T. 1970. Dopamine as a synaptic transmitter and modulator in sympathetic ganglion: A different mode of synaptic action. *Proc. Natl. Acad. Sci.* **67**:667–673.

Loewenstein, W. R., and Kanno, Y. 1964. Studies on an epithelial (gland) cell junction. I. Modifications of surface membrane permeability. *J. Cell Biol.* **22**:565–586.

Loewenstein, W. R., and Kanno, Y. 1967. Intercellular communication and tissue growth. I. Cancerous growth. *J. Cell Biol.* **33**:225–234.

Minna, J., Nelson, P. G., Peacock, J., Glazer, D., and Nirenberg, M. 1971. Genes for neuronal properties expressed in neuroblastoma × L-cell hybrids. *Proc. Natl. Acad. Sci.* **68**:234–239.

Minna, J., Glazer, D., and Nirenberg, M. 1972. Genetic dissection of neural properties using somatic cell hybrids. *Nature New Biol.* **235**:225–231.

Nelson, P. G., and Peacock, J. 1972. Acetylcholine responses in L-cells. *Science* **177**:1005–1007.

Nelson, P. G., Ruffner, B. W., and Nirenberg, M. 1969. Neuronal tumor cells with excitable membranes grown *in vitro*. *Proc. Natl. Acad. Sci.* **64**:1004–1010.

Nelson, P. G., Peacock, J., and Amano, T. 1971*a*. Responses of neuroblastoma cells to iontophoretically applied acetylcholine. *J. Cell. Physiol.* **77**:353–362.

Nelson, P. G., Peacock, J., Amano, T., and Minna, J. 1971*b*. Electrogenesis in mouse neuroblastoma cells *in vitro*. *J. Cell. Physiol.* **77**:337–352.

Nelson, P. G., Peacock, J., and Minna, J. 1972. An active electrical response in fibroblasts. *J. Gen. Physiol.* **60**:58–71.

Okun, L. M. 1972. Isolated dorsal root ganglion neurons in culture: Cytological maturation and extension of electrically active processes. *J. Neurobiol.* **3**:111–152.

Peacock, J., and Nelson, P. G. 1973*a*. Electrophysiologic study of cultured neurons dissociated from spinal cords and dorsal root ganglia of fetal mice. *Develop. Biol.* **30**:137–152.

Peacock, J., and Nelson, P. G. 1973*b*. Chemosensitivity of neuroblastoma cells. *J. Neurobiol.* (in press).

Peacock, J., and Nelson, P. G. 1973*c*. Electrical activity in dissociated cell cultures from fetal mouse cerebellum. *Brain Res.* (in press.)

Peacock, J., Minna, J., Nelson, P. G., and Nirenberg, M. 1972. Use of aminopterin in selecting electrically active neuroblastoma cells. *Exptl. Cell. Res.* **73**:367–377.

Peacock, J., McMorris, F. A., and Nelson, P. G. 1973. Electrical excitability and chemosensitivity of mouse neuroblastoma × mouse or human fibroblast hybrids. *Exptl. Cell Res.* (submitted for publication).

Peterson, E. R., and Crain, S. M. 1970. Innervation in cultures of fetal rodent skeletal muscle by organotypic explants of spinal cord from different animals. *Z. Zellforsch. Mikroskop. Anat.* **106**:1–21.

Potter, E. E., Furshpan, E. J., and Lennox, E. S. 1966. Connections between cells of the developing squid as revealed by electrophysiological methods. *Proc. Natl. Acad. Sci.* **55**:328–336.

Robbins, N., and Yonezawa, T. 1971. Physiological studies during formation and development of rat neuromuscular junctions in tissue culture. *J. Gen. Physiol.* **58**:467–481.

Ruddle, F. H. 1972. Linkage analysis using somatic cell hybrids. *Advan. Hum. Gent.* **3**: 173–235.

Scott, B. S. 1971. Effect of potassium on neuron survival in cultures of dissociated human nervous tissue. *Exptl. Neurol.* **30**:297–308.

Scott, B. S., Engelbert, V. E., and Fisher, K. C. 1969. Morphological and physiological characteristics of dissociated chick embryo spinal ganglion cells in cultures. *Exptl. Neurol.* **23**:230–248.

Sheridan, J. D. 1971. Dye movement and low-resistance junctions between reaggregated embryonic cells. *Develop. Biol.* **26**:627–636.

Stockdale, F., and Holzer, H. 1961. DNA synthesis and myogenesis. *Exptl. Cell Res.* **24**: 508–519.

Subak-Sharp, J. H., Burk, R. R., and Pitts, J. D. 1969. Metabolic cooperation between biochemically marked mammalian cells in tissue culture. *J. Cell Sci.* **4**:353–367.

Trachtenberg, M. G., Kornblith, P. L., and Hauptli, J. 1972. Biophysical properties of cultured human glial cells. *Brain Res.* **38**:279–298.

Varon, S., and Raiborn, C. W., Jr. 1969. Dissociation, fractionation and culture of embryonic brain cells. *Brain Res.* **12**:180–199.

Walker, F. D., and Hild, W. J. 1969. Neuroglia electrically coupled to neurons. *Science* **165**:602–603.

Wardell, W. M. 1966. Electrical and pharmacological properties of mammalian neuroglial cells in tissue culture. *Proc. Roy. Soc. Lond. Ser. B* **165**:326–361.

Yaffe, D. 1969. Cellular aspects of muscle differentiation *in vitro*. *Curr. Topics Develop. Biol.* **4**:37–77.

Chapter 7

Genetic Analysis of the Mammalian Nervous System Using Somatic Cell Culture Techniques

John D. Minna
Laboratory of Biochemical Genetics, National Heart and Lung Institute
National Institutes of Health
Bethesda, Maryland

I. GENERAL METHODS FOR GENETIC ANALYSIS OF THE NERVOUS SYSTEM

The success of genetic analysis of complex biochemical pathways, morphogenetic events, and their regulation in phage, bacteria, and yeast has suggested to many workers that such an analysis would be invaluable in the study of development and differentiation. The available information indicates that differentiation in higher organisms represents in part a mitotically inherited program of gene expression with commitment of different somatic cell lines to unique programs of gene expression (Gehring, 1969). Genetic analysis of developmental steps would seem to be both possible and necessary in order for us to understand differentiation.

Work with a variety of organisms indicates that the nervous system can be genetically probed (Hotta and Benzer, 1970; Ikeda and Kaplan, 1970; Kung and Eckert, 1972; Sidman *et al.,* 1965). At present, fruit flies, nematodes, mice, snails, and paramecia are being analyzed genetically for functions relating to the nervous system. Several analytical methods are possible: first, mutations that affect behavior can be produced (or detected) and the defective gene product determined. In this way, the number and types of gene

The author is a member of the United States Public Health Service and a Research Associate of the Laboratory of Biochemical Genetics, National Heart and Lung Institute.

TABLE I

Nervous System Functions Inherited Mitotically by Clonal Cell Lines in Tissue Culture[a]

Property	Representative	
	Cell line	Reference
Process formation		
Neurites	Neuroblastoma	Seeds et al. (1970)
Neurofibrils (silver staining)	Neuroblastoma	Schubert et al. (1969)
Glial fibrils	Glioblastoma	Benda et al. (1968)
Electrically excitable membranes		
A response (Na$^+$, ?Ca^{++}influx)	Neuroblastoma	Minna et al. (1971)
B response (K$^+$ efflux)	Neuroblastoma	Minna et al. (1971)
Hyperpolarizing activation		
(?K$^+$ efflux)	L cell	Nelson et al. (1972)
Neurohormone synthesis		
Acetylcholine (CAT)	Neuroblastoma	Amano et al. (1972)
Catecholamine (TH)	Neuroblastoma	Amano et al. (1972)
ACTH	Pituitary adenoma	Yasumura et al. (1966)
Growth hormone	Pituitary adenoma	Tashjian et al. (1968)
Neurohormone receptors		
Acetylcholine chemosensitivity	Neuroblastoma	Harris and Dennis (1970)
	Myogenic line	Patrick et al. (1972)
	L cell	Nelson and Peacock (1972)
Localization of ACh receptors	Neuroblastoma	Harris and Dennis (1970)
Catecholamine chemosensitivity	Glioblastoma	Gilmam and Nirenberg (1971a)
Histamine sensitivity	Glioblastoma	Clark and Perkins (1971)
PGE$_1$ chemosensitivity	Neuroblastoma	Gilman and Nirenberg (1971b)
Neurohormone degradation		
AChE	Neuroblastoma	Blume et al. (1970)
COMT	Neuroblastoma	Blume et al. (1970)
Contractile myotubes	Myogenic line	Yaffee (1968)
Miscellaneous		
S100 protein	Glioblastoma	Benda et al. (1968)
Myelin basic protein	Glioblastoma	Pfeiffer and Wechsler (1972)
Cortisol-inducible GPDH	Glioblastoma	Davidson and Benda (1970)
Complex glycoproteins,		
glycolipids	Glioblastoma	Stoolmiller et al.
	Neuroblastoma	Stoolmiller et al.

[a]Abbreviations are as follows: CAT, choline acetyltransferase (E.C. 2.3.1.6); TH, tyrosine hydroxylase (E.C. 1.14.3a); GPDH, glycerol-3-phosphate dehydrogenase (E.C. 1.1.1.8); COMT, catechol-O-methyltransferase (E.C. 2.1.1.1); AChE, acetylcholinesterase (E.C. 3.1.1.7); ACTH, adrenocorticotropic hormone; PGE$_1$, prostaglandin E$_1$; A response, inflection on upswing of voltage trace of action potential (active response); B response, inflection on late part of action potential (delayed rectification).

products involved in a specific function can be elucidated. The second approach is to produce mutations that will affect similar functions, but in specific parts of the nervous system. Thus mutation is used as a scalpel to cleave the nervous system along anatomical rather than biological lines (Hotta and Benzer, 1970). The third approach is to induce mutations that affect the development of the nervous system rather than any specific final function. A fourth type of analysis makes use of mosaicism (resulting from allopheny, gynandromorphs or induced by somatic mutation/recombination) to follow cell lineage within individual animals.

Another form of genetic analysis is also possible. Clonal lines of cells derived from the nervous system and maintained *in vitro* allow genetic manipulation and provide large quantities of material for elucidating the biochemical mechanisms underlying neural function. Clones can be used to assign functions to specific cell types, to study the stability and inheritance of a differentiated phenotype, and be perturbed with mutagens or environmental manipulation (Augusti-Tocco and Sato, 1969; Benda *et al.,* 1968; Seeds *et al.,* 1970; Amano *et al.,* 1972; Schubert *et al.,* 1969, 1971; Klebe and Ruddle, 1969; Pfeiffer and Wechsler, 1972; Lightbody *et al.,* 1970; Yasumura *et al.,* 1966). By fusing cells which differ in the expression of specific genes, the mechanisms controlling gene expression can be explored while chromosomal alterations occur at various rates to generate genetically different cell lines (Ephrussi, 1972; Harris *et al.,* 1966; Davidson, 1971; Weiss and Green, 1967; Minna *et al.,* 1971, 1972). This chapter will deal with the use of somatic cell hybridization as a tool for genetic analysis of neural properties.

II. MITOTIC INHERITANCE OF DIFFERENTIATED FUNCTIONS

In order to study the inheritance of a trait using sexual genetics, a polymorphism within the species is needed. In contrast, clonal lines of cells that express tissue-specific functions *in vitro* provide the built-in polymorphism that exists between different tissue types by virtue of differentiation. For many genetic studies, then, one does not have to induce mutation but simply selects lines of cells expressing different tissue-specific functions.

Perhaps the most striking piece of genetic information that clonal lines have yielded is that information controlling expression of nervous system functions can be transmitted from one cell generation to the next. This inheritance can occur *in vitro* under defined environmental conditions (Table I). Thus mysterious *in vivo* clues, three-dimensional architectonics, or other cell types are not necessary for the expression of at least part of the neural, glial, or muscle phenotypes. Such factors may of course be necessary for determination of primordial cells or the fullest differentiation *in vivo* (Seeds,

1971). Two interesting examples of mitotic inheritance in clonal lines of neuro-blastoma cells are the ability to actively synthesize the neurotransmitter acetylcholine (ACh) (high specific activities of choline acetyltransferase, CAT, E.C. 2.3.1.6) (Amano *et al.*, 1972) and a degree of cellular localization of ACh receptors (Harris and Dennis, 1970). Thus fundamental parts of synaptic specificity (neurotransmitter production and reception) are genetically programmed before neuroblasts stop dividing.

III. HYBRIDIZATION EXPERIMENTS

A. General Considerations

Analysis by somatic cell hybridization begins with the fusion of two cells which differ in the expression of specific genes (Ephrussi, 1972; Harris *et al.*, 1966). This fusion can occur spontaneously or be increased with the addition of inactivated virus (most commonly β-propiolactone-inactivated Sendai virus) (Coon and Weiss, 1969).

Two fusion products are of interest. The first is the multinucleated heter-okaryon (two or more different parental nuclei are present in a common cytoplasm). The influence of cytoplasmic mixing and internuclear relations on one another can be studied. However, heterokaryons require single-cell assays, for the culture population becomes heterogeneous after fusion because both parental cells and heterokaryons are present. Also, the half-lives of preexisting products introduced into the mating must be known. Little has been done with heterokaryons related to neural function. Jacobson (1968) observed reactivation of DNA synthesis in neurons fused to fibroblasts. Process for-mation dependent on nerve growth factor was found in heterokaryons between HeLa and superior cervical ganglion neurons of rat (DiZerega and Morrow, 1970). However, it is not entirely clear that the multinucleated cells under study were indeed heterokaryons, that a neuron was involved in the fusion, or that the properties studied were definitely related to a neuron. Hetero-karyons should provide a fruitful area for future study using electrophysio-logical and autoradiographic methods.

The second type of fusion product is the replicating, uninuclear hybrid cell with the genes of both parents residing in a common nucleus. These prop-agating hybrid cell lines can be cloned and in a very few divisions (by the time a colony of 1000 cells is formed) will have diluted out the original components present at the time of fusion. This chapter will concentrate on the analysis of replicating hybrid cell lines. The parental cells introduced into such matings are mouse neuroblastoma and rat glioma cell lines discussed at length in other chapters.

B. Neuroblastoma × L-Cell Matings

The phenotypes of the parental clones used in hybridization experiments are summarized in Table II. These lines are deficient in the incorporation of exogenous purines and pyrimidines, and thus hybrid cells between various parental lines survive in Littlefield's HAT medium by intergenic complementation while parental cells cannot replicate (Littlefield, 1964).

Neuroblastoma cells (process positive, silver impregnation positive, AChE positive, AChE regulation positive, bearing electrically excitable membranes with ACh receptors) were fused to mouse fibroblasts not expressing these characters, using inactivated Sendai virus, and then hybrid cells were selected in HAT medium. Neuroblastoma cells fuse easily, and large numbers of independently derived hybrid clones can be generated (approximately one hybrid colony arising per 10^3 input neuroblastoma cells.) Initially, it was preferable to select for independent mating events rather than to obtain many subclones from the same mixed-cell population. Using the latter technique, cell lines with a higher plating efficiency or more rapid growth rate would be repeatedly selected. Analysis of independent mating events represents an attempt to ascertain if variation exists among the fusion products.

The formal proof that the clones selected in HAT medium are indeed hybrid resides in the case of neuroblastoma × L-cell hybrids (N × L hybrids) in chromosome and isozyme markers specific for each parental cell type and simultaneously present in the hybrid cells.

For purposes of clonal analysis, one must be sure that the progeny within a given hybrid cell population have arisen from one progenitor cell (and thus one mating event) and do not represent mixtures of hybrid cells derived from different mating events. To insure clonal purity, the N × L hybrids were all recloned in microwells. We then asked, are any neural properties expressed in hybrid cells, and, if so, are any nonparental phenotypes found? (Minna et al., 1971, 1972).

1. Phenotype Analysis

a. *Process Formation.* The large majority of hybrid clones had cells that extended long (greater than 100 µ) processes under growth conditions that selected for nondividing cells (medium minus serum, aminopterin without hypoxanthine and thymidine, or 10^{-3} M dibutyryl cyclic adenosine monophosphate; Seeds et al., 1970; Peacock et al., 1972; Prasad and Vernadakis, 1972 (Fig. 1). In addition, many hybrid clones extended processes even when the population was in the logarithmic phase of growth. This latter finding contrasts with work on the parental neuroblastoma clone N18 (Seeds et al., 1970) and may indicate a change in the regulation of process formation in hybrid cells.

NLIF　　　　　　　　　　　　　　　　NL7AC

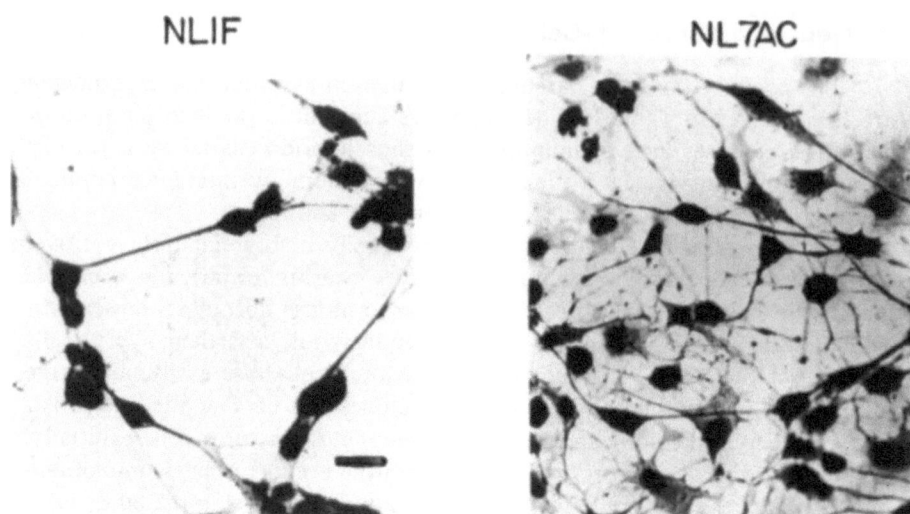

Fig. 1.　Silver stain (Bodian's) of neuroblastoma × L-cell (N4TG1 × B82) hybrid clones NL1F and NL7AC 100 generations after fusion. Bar in left frame is 50 μm.

TABLE II

Parental Clones with Drug-Resistance Markers Suitable for Hybridization Experiments and Phenotypes for Some Neuroectodermal Functions[a]

Cell line[b]	HGPRT	TK	CAT	AChE	AChEreg.	Processes	Bodian	A	B	D	H
Neuroblastoma											
N4TG1	−	+	−	+	+	+	+	+	+	rare	
N18TG2	−	+	−	++	++	+	+	++	++	+	
N18BU1G	+	−	−	low		rare	−				
S20TG	−	+	++	++	++	++	+	++	++		
Glioblastoma											
C6TG	−	+	low	low		++	−				
C6 (TK⁻)	+	−	−	low							
Fibroblast											
B82 (L cell)	+	−	−	−	−	rare	−	−	−	−	+
A9(L cell)	−	+	−	−		rare	−	−	−		+
3T34E,C	+	−	−	low		rare	−	−	−		+

(Header groups: "Electrical excitability" spans Bodian, A; "Ach receptors" spans B, D, H.)

[a]Abbreviations used: HGPRT, hypoxanthine-guanine phosphoribosyltransferase (E.C. 2.4.2.8); TK, thymidine kinase (E.C. 2.7.1.21); AChE, acetylcholinesterase; CAT, choline acetyltransferase; AChE reg., regulation of AChE specific activity. +, ++, Moderate to high activity; −, very low activity; blank, uncertain or not tested.

[b]Cell-line reference: N4TG1, N18TG2, B82, A9 (Minna *et al.*, 1971, 1972); N18BU1G, S20TG, C6TG, 3T34E, 3T34C (Minna, unpublished results); C6 (TK⁻) (B. Hamprecht, personal communication.)

Process formation occurred as early as ten and as late as 120 generations after fusion. In some cases, much longer, thicker, and more extensively branching processes were found in the hybrid compared to the parental neuroblastoma cells. The amount and type of process formation were stable characteristics of a clone over 20–40 generations of observation. However, process formation *per se* should be viewed with some degree of caution as regards its neuronal specificity. Many types of hybrids formed between fibroblasts (L cell or 3T3 cells) and a variety of tissue types can show marked degrees of process formation (Minna, unpublished observations). Some hybrid clones formed few or no processes, and at least one neuroblastoma clone exhibits this phenotype (Amano *et al.*, 1972). With silver stains (e.g., Bodian's), some hybrid clones had cells with extensive impregnation of processes, while other clones did not. Thus process-positive and process-negative clones were found, and within process-positive clones, Bodian-positive and Bodian-negative subgroups were detected.

b. Electrical Activity. The ability of a nerve to develop an action potential is at the heart of the reception, storage, and transmission of information within the nervous system. Using intracellular microelectrodes, the change in transmembrane potential as a function of time can be recorded when pulses of current or neurotransmitters are applied to individual cells in culture (Nelson *et al.*, 1971; Harris and Dennis, 1970). Three general types of responses were seen following depolarizing stimulation (Nelson *et al.*, 1969; Minna *et al.*, 1971). First, no inflections appeared on the curve of transmembrane potential as a function of time (a passive response, A^-B^-). Second, an inflection occurred on the downswing of the curve (delayed rectification, A^-B^+ response). The available evidence suggests that this response results from the facilitated diffusion of K^+ out of the cell (Hodgkin and Huxley, 1952). Third, an inflection occurred on the upswing of the curve (active response, $A^+B^{\pm}$). The available evidence suggests that this results from the facilitated diffusion of Na^+ and/or Ca^{2+} into the cell (Hodgkin and Huxley, 1952; Nelson *et al.*, 1971b). Quantitative differences in the steepness of the inflection can be determined by measuring the first derivative of $\Delta V/\Delta t$ (Nelson *et al.*, 1971b; Minna *et al.*, 1971). These quantitative differences in A^+ or B^+ response can be expressed as the amount of current (ion flow) per square centimeter of cell membrane.

The main disadvantages of the microelectrode assay are cell damage by the microelectrode impalement and selection of certain cell types due to easier microelectrode placement (e.g., large *vs.* small cells; thick *vs.* flat cells). Under appropriate culture conditions, neuroblastoma and hybrid cells are quite stable for electrophysiological study (minutes to hours of stimulation and recording). Likewise, there are certain membrane characteristics (resistance, capacitance, and time constant) which do not depend on active electrical responses and serve as a check on cell damage (Nelson *et al.*, 1971*b*; Minna *et al.*, 1971). A major advantage of microelectrode study is that comparison of cells within as well as between clones can be made.

Parental and N × L hybrid cells have been examined early (ten generations) and late (40–120 generations) after fusion for their electrical phenotype following depolarizing and hyperpolarizing stimulation. At all time points, hybrid cells with electrically excitable membranes were found (Minna *et al.*, 1971, 1972). The incidence of active hybrid cells equaled or surpassed the incidence of electrically active parental neuroblastoma cells tested under the same growth conditions (in the 1971 studies in medium minus serum). In cells expressing an A response, quantitative measurements were comparable between hybrid and parental cells.

Within a clone, both parental and hybrid cells exhibited several different states of excitability: some were passive (A$^-$B$^-$), some had delayed rectification (A$^-$B$^+$), and some had action potentials (A$^+$B$^+$). This was true if the cells were placed in medium minus serum, or in aminopterin-containing medium with serum. Similarly, when electrical excitability of cells within a neuroblastoma clone was tested during different stages of growth (logarithmic phase, stationary phase, in medium minus serum, or after aminopterin selection), changes in electrical excitability of the population were noted. Again, cells within a clone appeared able to regulate their state of electrical excitability (Peacock *et al.*, 1972; Nelson, this volume). The mechanism(s) by which this occurs is as yet obscure, and we could not relate it to cell damage or electrode artifact. Other investigators would debate this point (see Schubert *et al.*, in this volume). In order to resolve this issue, other laboratories will have to study neuroblastoma and hybrid cells electrophysiologically under various growth conditions and quantitatively present their data.

The maximal electrical excitability that a cell could exhibit has been the main focus of our attention. To achieve this, cells must be tested over a range of stimulating currents (0–5 namp) and a range of membrane potentials (resting to −80 mV) (Nelson *et al.*, 1971*b*). In addition, a variety of culture conditions have been tried to optimize electrical activity. Rigid control of temperature, *p*H, and nutrition are routinely used before and during the time of recording (Nelson *et al.*, 1971*b*). So far, the culture conditions that have yielded the optimal results with hybrid cells are aminopterin selection (Peacock *et al.*, 1972), irradiation (P. G. Nelson, personal communication), and growth in dibutyryl cyclic adenosine monophosphate (B. Hamprecht, personal communication). Removal of serum from the medium, while enhancing neurite outgrowth (Seeds *et al.*, 1970), does not yield optimal electrical activity (Peacock *et al.*, 1972).

The aminopterin selection method has been used in the most recent studies (Minna *et al.*, 1972; P. G. Nelson, personal communication). After hybrid cells have been grown in aminopterin (4×10^{-7} M) without exogenous purines or pyrimidines for 1 week, the dividing cells are killed and a population (10–20% of the starting cell number) of nondividing, electrically mature cells remains (Peacock *et al.*, 1972). The cells can be maintained for weeks to months in this medium, and neuroblastoma cells so selected have extensive neurite formation (in length, thickness, and branching), a high frequency (greater than 90%) of silver-staining cells, and very high specific activities of AChE (500 nmoles/mg protein/min for clone N 18). If hypoxanthine and thymidine are added to the culture medium, wild-type neuroblastoma and hybrid cells (HGPRT+, TK+) resume growth and become less differentiated (Peacock *et al.*, 1972; Minna, unpublished observations).

Clonal analysis revealed several different N × L phenotypes. On the basis of maximal electrical excitability found within a clone, clones could be scored as A+B,+A−B+, or A−B−. The second category (A−B+) is especially important since it represents a nonparental phenotype (nonneuroblastoma or non–L cell). It should be noted that A−B− and A−B+ clone phenotypes were found when resting membrane potentials were adequate for testing so that no steady hyperpolarizing current had to be passed. This makes recording electrode artifacts unlikely. In addition, the clone phenotype was stable over 20 generations of growth, was stable to freezing and thawing, and was exhibited by the majority of cells within such a clone. A correlation of clone phenotype with cell phenotype within a clone yields highly significant differences when A−B+ and A+B+ clones are compared (Table III). Thus parental neuroblastoma clones of phenotype A+B+ after fusion yielded hybrid clones, some of which expressed only part of the action-potential mechanism (Minna *et al.*, 1972).

L cells have an active electrical response not expressed by parental neuroblastoma cells that is termed "hyperpolarizing activation" (H.A. or C+ response) (Minna *et al.*, 1971; Nelson *et al.*, 1972). This response is elicited by mechanical stimulation or large pulses of hyperpolarizing current (50 namp) or occurs spontaneously. It is manifested by a long (1–5 sec) increase in membrane hyperpolarization which is accompanied by a decrease in membrane resistance and an increase in permeability to K+ ions (Nelson *et al.*, 1972). It was detected in N × L hybrid clones, but at a lower incidence and with less amplitude than in parental L cells (Minna *et al.*, 1972). Detailed studies on clonal variation of the H.A. response in hybrid cells have yet to be reported (Minna *et al.*, 1971; see also Nelson, this volume).

c. Acetylcholine (ACH) Chemosensitivity. Neuroblastoma cells can exhibit chemosensitivity to applied ACh (Harris and Dennis, 1970; Nelson *et al.*, 1971*a*). Both depolarizing (D) and hyperpolarizing (H) responses have been noted (Nelson *et al.*, 1971*a*). However, the vast majority of clones tested exhibit chemosensitivity in only a fraction of the cells despite culture conditions designed to select for maximally differentiated cells by other criteria. This problem may be related to clonal differences or in part to the reported localized areas of chemosensitivity (Harris and Dennis, 1970). This localization may represent a more differentiated state than generalized sensitivity if the analogy is made to the progressive localization of ACh chemosensitivity seen with muscle differentiation (Katz and Miledi, 1964). Quantitative comparison of reponse incidence between clones is difficult, and large numbers of cells and multiple sites on each cell must be tested in order to classify cell lines. An additional problem is the existence of ACh chemosensitivity in fibroblasts (Peacock and Nelson, 1972). Many fibroblast lines will exhibit a hyperpolarizing response to applied ACh (H_{slow}) which appears muscarinic in nature. This response may be different from the H response seen in neuroblastoma cells by its prolonged time course (seconds as opposed to milliseconds). In some $N \times L$ hybrid clones, D and H responses have been found (P. G. Nelson, personal communication; Chalazonitis, Minna, and Nirenberg, unpublished observations).

The ACh chemosensitivity inherited in $N \times L$ hybrids from the L-cell parent could be an extremely useful tool. By varying membrane potential on either side of the reversal potential for the H response, both excitatory (depolarizing) and inhibitory (hyperpolarizing) responses to ACh can be achieved. Thus new cell lines with some physiological relationship to classes of neurons found *in vivo* can be created.

d. Acetycholinesterase (ACHE, E.C. 3.1.1.7) Activity. The specific activity of AChE in neuroblastoma cells is relatively low in the logarithmic phase of growth but rises as the cells enter the stationary phase (Blume *et al.,* 1970; see Rosenberg, this volume). The maximal specific activity of AChE was either 40 (parental clone N4TG1) or 330 times (N18TG2) that found with

TABLE III

Correlation of Clone Phenotype for Electrical Excitability with Phenotype
of Cells Within the Clone

	Cell phenotype[a] (% of cells)	
	A^-B^+	A^+B^+
Clone phenotype		
A^-B^+	57	0
A^+B^+	34	40

[a]$N = 240$ cells tested in 15 independently derived $N \times L$ hybrid clones. A^+, Inflection on upswing of action potential; B^+, inflection on downswing of action potential (delayed rectification).

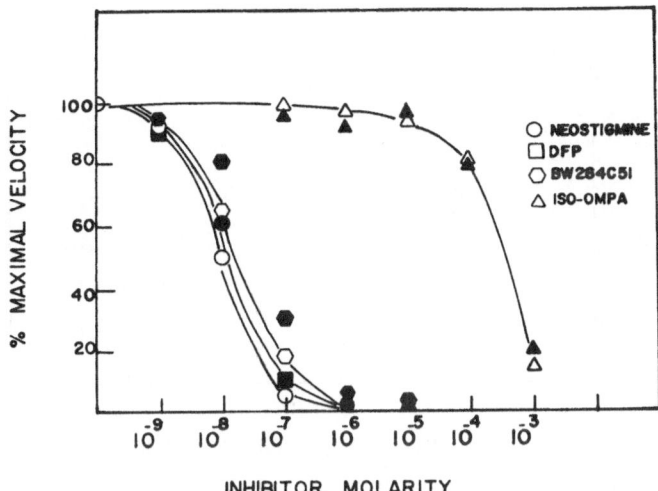

Fig. 2. Inhibition of acetylcholinesterase activity in parental (N18TG2, open symbols) and hybrid cell homogenates (clone NL308, filled symbols) by various inhibitors. Note inhibition of enzyme activity at low concentrations of inhibitors by neostigmine, DFP (diisopropylfluorophosphate), and BW284C51 [1, 5-bis (4-allyldimethylammoniumphenyl) pentane-1, 3-dibromide] but only at high concentrations by Iso-Ompa (tetrammonoisopropyl pyrophosphortetramide).

L (B82, A9) cells. While the parental neuroblastoma clones showed regulation (fourfold, to 22-fold rises) of AChE, L cells showed a slight fall in specific AChE activity as the cells became confluent in the culture vessels.

N × L hybrid clones fell into three general classes: clones with activities equal to or higher than those of the parental neuroblastoma clones, clones with activities intermediate between those of the parental lines, and clones with low AChE activity (Minna et al., 1972). In addition, the AChE specific activity in most hybrid clones was low during the logarithmic phase of growth and increased as the cells became confluent. Thus some hybrid clones inherited the ability to both synthesize AChE and regulate its specific activity, while other clones did not. Cell viability remained essentially constant during these experiments, ruling out any possible artifacts secondary to cell death.

The AChE activity in parental and N × L hybrid cells appears to be "true" AChE (E.C. 3.1.1.7). Thus the activity is inhibited by 2×10^{-7} M BW284C51, a selective inhibitor of AChE, but only by 3×10^{-4} M Iso-Ompa, a more potent inhibitor of cholinesterase (E.C. 3.1.1.8) (Austin and Berry, 1953). The activity is also very sensitive to neostigmine sulfate and diisopropylfluorophosphate (Minna et al., 1972) (Fig. 2) and can be demonstrated with acetyl-β-methylcholine, a substrate preferred by AChE.

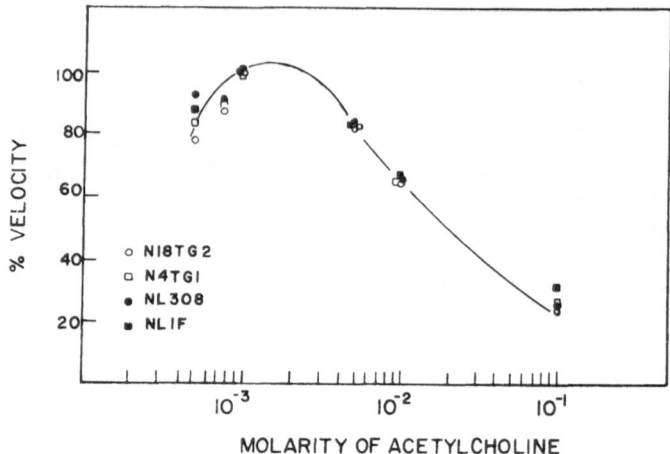

MOLARITY OF ACETYLCHOLINE

Fig. 3.   Effect of substrate concentration on acetylcholinesterase activity in homogenates of parental (N4TG1, N18TG2) and hybrid (NL308, NL1F) clones. Note fall in reaction velocity with increasing concentration of substrate, a phenomenon characteristic of acetylcholinesterase.

Last, parental and hybrid AChE activity exhibited substrate inhibition, a phenomenon found with AChE from other sources (Augustinsson, 1957) (Fig. 3). It would seem appropriate to carefully analyze all enzyme activities in biologically unique systems such as hybrid cells by using selective inhibitors, kinetic properties, substrate specificity, and product identification (Wilson et al., 1972).

One possible explanation for the different AChE phenotypes seen in N × L hybrid cells is that parental neuroblastoma clones are heterogeneous with respect to transmission of the phenotype to daughter cells. This is known to exist in immunoglobulin-producing plasmacytoma clones (Coffino et al., 1970). By histochemical staining of many subclones of parental neuroblastoma and L cells, the AChE phenotype was found to be remarkably stable (Minna et al., 1972). The data showed a reversion frequency for the AChE neuroblastoma marker of less than 1.5×10^{-4} per colony-forming unit. Likewise, the low activity of AChE in L-cell populations was not explained by a rare propagating L cell with high AChE activity (reversion frequency for L cells of AChE phenotype of less than 1.2×10^{-4}). By staining hybrid colonies approximately ten generations after fusion, one can ascertain when the various phenotypes arose and avoid any selection involved in growing and transferring cells from colonies to mass populations. The different AChE phenotypes (AChE+ and AChE−) were seen in the early generations after fusion. When the data from many crosses had been pooled, approximately 40% of the N × L colonies tested were AChE+ ten generations after fusion (Minna et al., 1972).

Thus the commitment of a hybrid clone to express this differentiated function occurs quite early in its life history.

e. Choline Acetyltransferase (CAT E.C.2.3.1.6) The CAT phenotype is currently being assayed in hybrid cells in which one of the parents is a neuroblastoma cell that is CAT⁺ (high specific activity of this enzyme). Preliminary evidence suggests that this property can be inherited in some hybrid clones. In addition, hybrids between CAT⁻ neuroblastoma and CAT⁻ fibroblast or glioblastoma cells may yield some CAT⁺ hybrid clones (T. Amano and B. Hamprecht, personal communication; F. A. McMorris, personal communication), indicating that some form of complementation exists.

2. Phenotypic Classes N × L Hybrid Clones

The pattern of neuronal markers expressed by various clones is summarized in Table IV. N × L hybrid clones expressing all parental neuroblastoma properties were found. Similar results have been obtained independently by McMorris, Gilbert, Nelson, Peacock, and Ruddle (personal communication). Five nonparental phenotypes were also found. This result indicates that it is possible to mate neuroblastoma cells expressing complex "black box" functions (such as neurite formation or synthesis of action-potential components) and recover some hybrid clones with a less complex phenotype. The new phenotypes are then mitotically inherited as the hybrid cells replicate.

Whatever the mechanism(s) by which such simplification occurs, it would appear to fulfill criteria for "genetic dissection": the generation of replicating cell lines which inherit a more elementary phenotype than that present in

TABLE IV

Phenotypic Classes of N × L Hybrid Clones

Process formation	B⁺	AChE	Silver stain	A⁺	ACh	Percent chromosomes[a]	Reference N × L clones
+	+	+	+	+	+	78–91	NLIF, NL308, NL3093
+	+	+	+	+		62	NL7AC
+	+	+	−	−		44, 70	NL2N, NL3H
+	+	−	−	−		64, 69	NL14J, NL304
+	−	−	−	−		73	NL305
−	−	−	−	−		40	NL303C
−	+	+	−	−		57	NL13C

Data rearranged from Minna *et al.* (1972).
[a]Percent of expected number of chromosomes from fusion of two modal cells, Karyology was performed 50–100 generations after fusion.

parental cells. In sexual genetics, this phenotypic simplification is usually achieved by mutation. A similar simplification of the action-potential mechanism analogous to the A^+B^+, A^-B^+, A^-B^- transition occurred in paramecia. In this unicellular organism, mutants defective in response to environmental cationic stimuli were defective in inflections on the upswing of the action potential (Kung and Eckert, 1972). In N × L hybrids, the simplification probably occurs by the introduction of non-neuroblastoma regulatory elements (genes?) or by subsequent changes in hybrid-cell gene content that occur with chromosome segregation. Heritable differences in expression of a differentiated phenotype appear to be more readily produced using hybridization rather than mutational methodology. The ease of generation of the variant phenotypes should be compared with the relative stability of this phenotype in parental neuroblastoma cells.

About 20 independently derived clones have been fully phenotyped, and some, but not all, possible "recombinant" (nonparental) phenotypes have been seen. This could represent a sampling problem since only a few clones have yet been analyzed. However, this finding could have functional and/or genetic implications for neuronal maturation. Various neural properties could be functionally related in such a way that a given property requires the presence of another property for assembly, maintenance, regulation, or expression. Conversely, certain properties appear to be functionally independent. Thus on the clonal level, action-potential step B can be expressed independently of step A and high AChE levels. Process formation can be expressed independently of neurofibril formation. The participation of AChE in the action-potential mechanism has long been debated (Nachmansohn, 1971). The facilitated diffusion of K^+ (delayed rectification, B^+ step) does not appear to require the high levels of AChE seen in neurons. A hybrid variant of great interest that has not been detected would retain action-potential step A but have low levels of AChE.

The clonally inherited variant phenotypes could represent differences in gene content and/or heritable differences in regulation of gene expression. The different phenotypic classes would then suggest linkage groups or heritable hierarchies of gene regulation taking place in neural maturation. The available data from N × L hybrids suggest the following as a possible sequence of steps in such maturation: neuroblast→step B, process formation → AChE → neurofibrils → step A.

With analysis of hybrids resulting from matings involving neuroblastoma clones with additional markers (e.g., choline acetyltransferase, tyrosine hydroxylase, or localization of ACh chemosensitivity), other steps could be fitted into the above scheme. Likewise, by mating neuroblastoma cells to cells expressing other tissue-specific characteristics e.g., glial cells, muscle cells, or liver cells), it may be possible to determine if there are common or unique genetic programs for differentiation. Hybrids of the above types have been made and are now being analyzed.

Chromosome analysis suggests that some N × L clonal differences may represent differences in gene content (Minna et al., 1972). At present, expression or regulation of a neural character (or set of characters) cannot be assigned to a specific chromosome.

Reduction in chromosome number occurs more rapidly in interspecific than in intraspecific hybrid cells (Weiss and Green, 1967; Engle et al., 1969). In order to achieve maximum stability in chromosome complement, intraspecific (mouse × mouse) hybrids were first generated. However, after 80–120 generations, intraspecific hybrids also can show significant reduction in chromosome number (Engle et al., 1969). At this time and in earlier generations, the variant N × L hybrids expressing only part of the neuroblastoma phenotype showed a reduction in expected total chromosome number (Minna et al., 1972) (Table IV).

When chromosome number is examined in hybrids expressing high vs. very low levels of AChE, a correlation with chromosome number is seen. Clones that were AChE− (very low levels of AChE) had lower modal numbers of total chromosomes than those that were AChE+ (very high levels of AChE) (Minna et al., 1972). The correlation of low chromosome number and lack of expression of high AChE levels was seen in some hybrids as early as 30–40 generations after fusion.

These data suggest, but do not prove, that the variant phenotypes arose by chromosome segregation. A formal proof would require that expression of a neural marker be constantly associated with a particular chromosome(s). By use of newer chromosome-staining techniques for generating banded chromosomes (Drets and Shaw, 1971; Caspersson et al., 1970), it should be possible to follow a large number of chromosomes in hybrids and assign expression of differentiated functions to individual chromosomes.

The expression of neural characters in some N × L hybrids stands in contrast to the generally reported extinction of differentiated functions in hybrid cells (Davidson, 1971). The mechanism(s) responsible for expression of neural characters has not been elucidated. This could occur because of gene dosage effects, (Fougere et al., 1972; Davidson, 1972), by loss of regulator genes (Klebe et al., 1970; Weiss and Chaplain, 1971), by changes in regulatory events, or by genetic variability within parental clones.

Neuroblastoma cells have more chromosomes than L cells, but as yet it is not possible to definitively relate chromosome number to amount of specific genetic information. Since some genes may be expressed at only certain times during the cell cycle or during differentiation, clonal but unphased populations may be heterogeneous with respect to gene expression. This difference in gene expression may be heritable in hybrid cells. By synchronizing parental cell populations, mating across species lines, and quantitating marker isozymes for each parental cell type, it should be possible to delineate the rules for expression of neuroblastoma characters in hybrid cells.

Some hybrid clones expressed quantitatively higher levels of neural characters than their parental neuroblastoma cells. Higher levels of AChE, more electrically active membranes, and more extensive process formation were found (Minna *et al.*, 1971, 1972). Possible mechanisms to explain these phenomena are gene dosage effects, complementation, activation of fibroblast genes (Peterson and Weiss, 1972), segregation of regulating genes, and parental heterogeneity. It will be worthwhile to look for neural characters qualitatively not present in certain parental neuroblastoma clones such as neurotransmitter synthesis, neurohormone receptors, and synapse formation.

In searching for complementation, neuroblastoma cells have been fused to normal neural tissue from a variety of sources and in various stages of development, including brain, retina, spinal cord, and sensory ganglia of several different species (e.g., mouse, rat, and hamster) (Minna and Coon, unpublished observation). In addition, fusion to a variety of clonal propagating cell lines of diverse origin has been made and is being analyzed. One attractive possibility is that neuroblastoma cells would be "permissive" for expression of some neural characters that they do not now express. Thus new neural lines may be generated by rescue of some necessary structural genes or exposure to the action of certain regulatory genes (or products) capable of

TABLE V

Regulation of cAMP Metabolism in Hybrid Cells

Parental phenotypes[a]	Hybrid phenotype	Mating[b]
$\beta^+ \times \beta^+$	β^+	C6 × BRL
$\beta^+ \times \beta^-$	β^-	C6 × L, C6 × 3T3, C6 × N
$\beta^- \times \beta^-$	β^-	N × L, L × L
$PGE_1^{+++} \times PGE_1^+$	PGE_1^{+++}	N × L
$PGE_1^{+++} \times PGE_1^-$	PGE_1^{+++}	3T3 × C6, L × C6
$Theo_p \times Theo_p^-$	$Theo_p^+$	N × L, 3T3 × C6
$Theo_p^- \times Theo_p^-$	$Theo_p^-$	L × L, C6 × L

[a]β^+, Response to β-adrenergic agonists (e.g., isoproterenol, norepinephrine); PGE_1^+, response to prostaglandin E_1; Theo, significant potentiation of peak PGE_1 hormone effect. β^+, PGE_1^+, Four- to hundred-fold rises in intracellular cAMP (adenosine-3',5'-cyclic monophosphate) following neurohormone exposure of clonal lines of cells *in vitro*; β^-, PGE_1^-, less than 1-fold rises in cAMP following hormone exposure.
[b]Cell-line abbreviations: C6, rat glia, clone C6TG; BRL, Buffalo rat liver clone BRL30E of H. Coon; 3T3, mouse fibroblast clones 3T34E, 3T34C2; N, mouse neuroblastoma clones N4TG1, N18TG2; L, mouse fibroblast clones B82, A9.

activating additional programs of neural differentiation. The introduction of L-cell ACh chemosensitivity mentioned above is an example of one such line. Obviously, the same tack could be taken with replicating glial cells in culture.

C. Regulation of Adenosine 3′, 5′-Cyclic Monophosphate (cAMP)

Good evidence exists that the response of a variety of cell types to specific hormones is mediated via changing the intracellular level of cyclic AMP (cAMP) (Sutherland *et al.*, 1968). The data pertinent to the nervous system have been reviewed (Rall and Gilman, 1970). In collaboration with Dr. Alfred Gilman of the Department of Pharmacology, University of Virginia, a variety of parental cell types and their resulting hybrids have been examined for their response in terms of intracellular cAMP accumulation to β-adrenergic agonists (β^+), to prostaglandins (PGE_1), and to the potentiation of peak hormone effect by the phosphodiesterase inhibitor theophylline ($Theo^+$) (Gilman and Minna, 1972). The data from a variety of crosses are summarized in Table V. The main conclusions that can be drawn at the present time are as follows: First, catecholamine responsiveness is extinguished in hybrid cells, while PGE_1 responsiveness is not. This would imply that different types of gene regulation obtain for these neurohormone receptors. The observation of Davidson and Benda (1970) that glia × fibroblast hybrids did not increase lactic dehydrogenase levels after β-agonist stimulation is probably a reflection of this. Benda is also exploring the expression of adenylcyclase following β-stimulation in glial hybrids (personal communication). Second, theophylline sensitivity is inherited in hybrid cells, and thus some component of the phosphodiesterase system is not under negative control. We hope to establish the rules of expression in hybrid cells for other known and potential neurohormones (and their related adenylcyclase systems) that act via regulating levels of cAMP and to generate variant lines with novel (nonparental) combinations of neurohormone receptors and adenylcyclase systems.

D. Evidence for Pleiotropic Negative Control of Neuroectodermal Properties

While some N × L hybrids have expressed a complete set of parental neuroblastoma characters, many hybrids in this mating and in other matings involving neuroectodermal tissues do not exhibit the full set of differentiated functions in hybrid cells (Table VI). As indicated from AChE histochemical staining and melanin production (both detectable on single cells or colonies of cells), this lack of expression can occur within the earliest generations of a hybrid cell's life (Davidson *et al.*, 1966; Minna *et al.*, 1972). The lack of expression of several glial and neuronal properties in some hybrids is highly suggestive of pleiotropic negative control of a set of neuroectodermal functions (Davidson and Benda, 1970); Minna et al., 1972).

Is there more than one mechanism or site for negative control of a particular program of tissue differentiation in hybrid cells? One approach is to perform complementation analysis of clones that are extinguished for the expression of a particular function. This could be accomplished by heterokaryon formation between different hybrid clones or by intercrossing hybrid clones to generate new hybrid clones that would be analogous to an *in vivo* F_2 generation. To this end, 15 different combinations of AChE⁻-N × L hybrid clones were fused to yield heterokaryons and then histochemically stained for AChE activity. All combinations were still AChE⁻. This suggests that only one AChE regulation group has been detected. This method is a potential source of new genetic information. For example, it would be of great interest if complementation could take place only in hybrid cells (genes located in the same nucleus) and not in heterokaryons (genes in different nuclei in a common cytoplasm).

IV. GENERATION OF PROPAGATING CELL LINES FROM NORMAL NEURONS AND GLIA

New sources of replicating neural and glial lines would allow rapid advances in neurobiology. The approaches include direct cloning from normal embryonic tissue, transformation either *in vivo* or *in vitro* of neuroblasts and glioblasts with oncogenic viruses or chemical carcinogens, as discussed in other chapters (see Pfeiffer, this volume; Schubert et al., this volume), and hybridization. The work of Gurdon (1966), Harris (1967), Rao and Johnson (1970) and Jacobson (1968) suggests that cells capable of replication can initiate DNA synthesis in fully differentiated nondiving cells. Work with N × L hybrids suggests that it should be possible to generate replicating hybrid cells that still express neural characters.

Thus it would seem reasonable to try to reawaken a neuron or glial cell to division by fusing it to a fibroblast capable of replication in culture. Hayden Coon of the National Cancer Institute and I have been actively following such a line of action. We have assumed that to express neural functions fully, as much genetic information as possible from the normal neuron parent should be retained in the hybrid cell and as little information as possible from the fibroblast parent. (This assumption, of course, will have to be tested.) If one considers the existing literature on chromosome segregation (Weiss and Green, 1967), an interspecific cross of the type human fibroblast × rodent neuron seems most logical. A replicating hybrid of human fibroblast × mouse neuron should tend to lose human chromosomes while retaining those of murine origin. We have succeeded in generating several hundred replicating hybrid cell lines between the human fibroblast VA2 (Weiss and Green, 1967) deficient in hypoxanthine-guanine phosphoribosyltransferase and normal nervous tissue of rat, mouse, and Chinese hamster (neural retina, brain, spinal cord, and dorsal root ganglia). The human fibroblast cannot replicate in HAT medium, and the normal nervous tissue has a very low plating efficiency and/or a limited life span in this medium so that hybrid clones are easily isolated. To date, no hybrids from these crosses have expressed high levels of AChE of the several hundred tested during early generations. It is possible that a large degree of chromosome segregation must take place for expression to occur.

One interesting sidelight is that the "normal" rules of chromosome segregation appear to be violated in a large proportion of hybrids generated by these crosses. That is, human chromosomes are often retained while rodent chromosomes are lost. This will undoubtedly be of biological interest. How-

TABLE VI

Neuroectodermal Functions Extinguished in Some Somatic Cell Hybrids

Function extinguished	Mating[a]	
Neural		
Acetylcholinesterase	Neuroblastoma × L cell (mouse × mouse)	
Neurites		
Process formation	//	//
Silver impregnation	//	//
Electrical excitability		
A+ response	//	//
B+ response	//	//
Acetylcholine receptors, depolarizing	//	//
Choline acetyltransferase	//	//
Glial		
S100 protein	Glioblastoma × fibroblast (rat × mouse)	
Glycerol-3-phosphate dehydrogenase		
cortisol induction	//	//
LDH induction with catecholamine	//	//
cAMP accumulation with catecholamine (β+)	//	//
Neuroendocrine		
Growth hormone production	Pituitary adenoma × fibroblast (rat × mouse)	
Miscellaneous		
Melanin production	Melanoma × fibroblast (hamster × mouse)	

[a]References for matings: Neuroblastoma × L, Minna *et al.* (1971, 1972, and unpublished data). Glioblastoma × fibroblast, Davidson and Benda (1970) and Gilman and Minna (1972). Pituitary adenoma × fibroblast, Sonnerschein *et al.* (1968). Melanoma × fibroblast, Davidson *et al.* (1966).

ever, a certain fraction of these hybrids are segregating chromosomes in the expected fashion, and these are now being extensively analyzed.

By working with nonneoplastic tissue, we hope for a better chance at elucidating pathways of genetic regulation in neuronal maturation closely related to those occurring *in vivo* and correlating these events with karyology. In addition, information on growth regulation occurring in normal neuronal and glial maturation should be gained from studying these hybrids.

V. CONCLUSIONS AND FUTURE FORECAST

The genetic analysis of nervous system functions in mammalian cells *in vitro* is in its infancy. Neuroblastoma hybrids suggest that a form of genetic dissection of complex properties can be carried out. The variant cell lines should be useful for biochemical analysis of the neural phenotype by providing large amounts of material with novel phenotypes. While the neural markers so far studied are not single-cistron products, their inheritance can be studied. The patterns of nonparental phenotypes yield new phenomenology which will have to be incorporated into any scheme of the genetic program for neural maturation.

An optimistic projection from this work would suggest that more complex neural functions such as synapse and network formation could also be attacked using somatic cell hybrids. At least part of the specificity for synapse formation is determined by the types of neurotransmitters synthesized by a neuron and the types of neurohormone receptors present on its surface. These sites would appear to be a logical first step for further investigation.

Two major advantages of sexual genetics are the establishment of Mendelian inheritance for the characteristic observed and the ability to "saturate" the genetic map for a particular phenomenon. The parasexual genetics of somatic cells in culture is sadly deficient in these characteristics. While a standard hybridization experiment allows for a form of F_1 dominance test, there is no way of knowing whether one or many cistrons are being studied. Likewise, while only a limited number of phenotypes of hybrid cells have been detected to date, it is reasonable to ask how many independent mating events or segregants have to be tested in order to be sure of detecting all possible phenotypes. This will have to be approached by statistical analysis and will require the laborious testing of many different clones. At present, even simple culture techniques are tedious and the assays for differentiated function complicated. In contrast, analysis of a whole animal requires only observation of some gross distortion of a normal physiological process (e.g., perception of light or maintenance of posture).

Potential advantages of somatic cell hybrids or mutants are the immediate availability of large quantities of clonally purified material for biochemical analysis and the generation of certain variant phenotypes which may be difficult to achieve in the whole animal. For example, while AChE⁻ hybrid clones can be readily generated, it may be lethal for the whole animal to be generally defective in the production of AChE. This would necessitate the generation of conditional lethals to study such characteristics. Mammalian cells in culture are well suited for electrophysiological studies, while fruit fly and nematode neurons are too small to study with present intracellular recording techniques. The genetics of snails with giant neurons should prove useful for such analysis. Finally, replicating cell lines in cultures can be dealt with as reagents with the clone as the unit of study. Thus the generation of lines capable of synapse formation immediately suggests clone-mixing experiments to ascertain if there are certain general synaptic classes (rules). While such mixing experiments cannot be done in germinal genetics, it should be possible to see if certain mutations in whole animals affect particular classes of synapses throughout the nervous system. The two approaches thus appear complementary.

There has been no mention of direct mutagenesis of neuroblast or glioblast lines to derive defective mutants, since this work is as yet in its infancy (Siman-Tov and Sachs, 1972). The development of selective techniques which rely on the expression of differentiated functions is eagerly awaited. Such techniques would greatly reduce the technical effort required to generate differentiated clones.

VI. ACKNOWLEDGMENTS

I thank Drs. Xandra Breakefield, Hayden Coon, Alfred Gilman, Marshall Nirenberg, Phillip Nelson, John Peacock, Ms. Alcmene Chalazonitis, and Ms. Devera Glazer for collaboration and discussions during this work, and Drs. B. Hamprecht and T. Amano for allowing me to discuss their unpublished work. I particularly note the encouragement and discussion with Marshall Nirenberg, in whose laboratory this work was performed.

VII. REFERENCES

Amano, T., Richelson, E., and Nirenberg, M. 1972. Neurotransmitter synthesis by neuroblastoma clones. *Proc. Natl. Acad. Sci.* **69**:258–263.

Augusti-Tocco, G., and Sato, G. 1969. Establishment of functional clonal lines of neurons from mouse neuroblastoma. *Proc. Natl. Acad. Sci.* **64**:311–315.

Augustinsson, K.–B. 1957. Assay methods for cholinesterases, pp. 1–63. *In* D. Glick (ed.). Methods in Biochemical Analysis. Interscience Publishers, New York.

Austin, L., and Berry, W. K. 1953. Two selective inhibitors of cholinesterase. *Biochem. J.* **54**:695–700.

Benda, P., Lightbody, J., Sato, G., Levine, L., and Sweet, W. 1968. Differentiated rat glial cell strain in tissue culture. *Science* **161**:370–371.

Blume, A., Gilbert, F., Wilson, S., Farber, J., Rosenberg, R., and Nirenberg, M. 1970. Regulation of acetylcholinesterase in neuroblastoma cells. *Proc. Natl. Acad. Sci.* **67**: 786–792.

Caspersson, T., Zech, L., and Johansson, C., 1970. Differential binding of alkylating fluorochromes in human chromosomes. *Exptl. Cell Res.* **60**:315–319.

Clark, R. B., and Perkins, J. P. 1971. Regulation of adenosine 3′,5′-cyclic monophosphate concentration in cultured human astrocytoma cells by catecholamines and histamine. *Proc. Natl. Acad. Sci.* **68**:2757–2760.

Coffino, P., Laskov, R., and Scharff, M. D. 1970. Immunoglobulin production: Method for quantitatively detecting variant myeloma cells. *Science* **167**:186–188.

Coon, H. G., and Weiss, M. C. 1969. A quantitative comparison of formation of spontaneous and virus-produced viable hybrids. *Proc. Natl. Acad. Sci.* **62**:852–859.

Davidson, R. L., 1971. Regulation of gene expression in somatic cell hybrids: A review. *In Vitro* **6**:411–426.

Davidson, R. L. 1972. Regulation of melanin synthesis in mammalian cells: Effect of gene dosage on the expression of differentiation. *Proc. Natl. Acad. Sci.* **69**:951–955.

Davidson, R. L., and Benda, P. 1970. Regulation of specific functions of glial cells in somatic hybrids. II. Control of inducibility of glycerol-3-phosphate dehydrogenase. *Proc. Natl. Acad. Sci.* **64**:1870–1877.

Davidson, R. L., and Yamamoto, K. 1968. Regulation of melanin synthesis in mammalian cells, as studied by somatic hybridization. II. The levels of regulation of 3,4-dihydroxyphenylalanine oxidase. *Proc. Natl. Acad. Sci.* **60**:894–901.

Davidson, R. L., Ephrussi, B., and Yamamoto, K. 1966. Regulation of pigment synthesis in mammalian cells, as studied by somatic hybridization. *Proc. Natl. Acad. Sci.* **56**: 1437–1440.

Dawson, G., Kemp, S. F., Stoolmiller, A. C., and Dorfman, A. 1971. Biosynthesis of glycosphingolipids by mouse neuroblastoma (NB41A), rat glia (RGC-6) and human glia (CHB-4) in cell culture. *Biochem. Biophys. Res. Commun.* **44**:687–694.

DiZerega, G., and Morrow, J. 1970. The effect of nerve growth factor on dispersed neuronal–HeLa heterokaryons. *Exptl. Neurol.* **28**:206–212.

Drets, M. E., and Shaw, M. W. 1971. Specific banding patterns of human chromosomes. *Proc. Natl. Acad. Sci.* **68**:2073–2077.

Engle, E., McGee, B. J., and Harris, H. 1969. Recombination and segregation in somatic cell hybrids. *Nature* **223**:152–155.

Ephrussi, B. 1972. Hybridization of Somatic Cells. Princeton University Press, Princeton, N.J. 175 pp.

Ephrussi, B., and Weiss, M. C. 1965. Interspecific hybridization of somatic cells. *Proc. Natl. Acad. Sci.* **53**:1040–1042.

Ephrussi, B., and Weiss, M. C. 1968. Regulation of the cell cycle in mammalian cells: Inferences and speculations based on observations of interspecific somatic hybrids. *In* Control Mechanisms in Developmental Processes. Proceedings of the 26th symposium of the Society for Developmental Biology (*Develop. Biol.,* Suppl. I). Academic Press, New York.

Finch, B. W., and Ephrussi, B. 1967. Retention of multiple developmental potentialities by cells of a mouse testicular teratocarcinoma during prolonged culture *in vitro* and their extinction upon hybridization with cells of permanent lines. *Proc. Natl. Acad. Sci.* **57**:615–621.

Fougere, C., Ruiz, F., and Ephrussi, B. 1972. Gene dosage dependence of pigment synthesis in melanoma × fibroblast hybrids. *Proc. Natl. Acad. Sci.* **69**:330–334.

Gehring, W. 1969. Problems of cell determination and differentiation in *Drosophila*, pp. 231–299. *In* E. W. Hanly (ed.). Problems in Biology: RNA in Development. University of Utah Press, Salt Lake City.

Gilman, A., and Minna, J., 1972. Adenosine 3′,5′-cyclic monophosphate (cAMP) regulation in somatic cell hybrids. *Am. Soc. Cell Biol. (St. Louis)*, abst.

Gilman, A. G., and Nirenberg, M. 1971a. Effect of catecholamines on the adenosine 3′,5′-cyclic monophosphate concentrations of clonal satellite cells of neurons. *Proc. Natl. Acad. Sci.* **68**:2165–2168.

Gilman, A. G., and Nirenberg, M. 1971b. Regulation of adenosine 3′,5′-cyclic monophosphate metabolism in cultured neuroblastoma cells. *Nature* **234**:356–357.

Gurdon, J. B. 1966. Nuclear transplantation in amphibia and the importance of stable nuclear changes in promoting cellular differentiation. *Quart. Rev. Biol.* **38**:54–78.

Harris, H. 1967. The reactivation of the red cell nucleus. *J. Cell Sci.* **2**:23–32.

Harris, A. J., and Dennis, M. J. 1970. Acetylcholine sensitivity and distribution on mouse neuroblastoma cells. *Science* **167**:1253–1255.

Harris, H., Watkins, J. F., Ford, C. E., and Scheefl, G. I. 1966. Artificial heterokaryons of animal cells from different species. *J. Cell Sci.* **1**:1–30.

Harris, A. J., Heinemann, S., Schubert, D., and Tarakis, H. 1971. Trophic interaction between cloned tissue culture lines of nerve and muscle. *Nature* **231**:296–301.

Hodgkin, A. L., and Huxley, A. F. 1952. Currents carried by sodium and potassium ions through the membrane of the giant axon of *Loligo*. *J.* Physiol. **116**:449–472.

Hotta, Y., and Benzer, S. 1970. Genetic dissection of the *Drosophila* nervous system by means of mosaics. *Proc. Natl. Acad. Sci.* **67**:1156–1163.

Ikeda, K., and Kaplan, W. D. 1970. Unilaterally patterned neural activity of gynandromorphs, mosaic for a neurological mutant of *Drosophila melanogaster*. *Proc. Natl. Acad. Sci.* **67**:1480–1487.

Jacobson, C. 1968. Reactivation of DNA synthesis in mammalian neuron nuclei after fusion with cells of an undifferentiated fibroblast line. *Exptl. Cell Res.* **53**:316–318.

Kao, F., Johnson, R. T., and Puck, T. T. 1969. Complementation analysis on virus fused Chinese hamster cells with nutritional markers. *Science* **164**:312–314.

Kates, J. R., Winterton, R., and Schlessinger, K. 1970. Induction of acetylcholinesterase activity in mouse neuroblastoma tissue culture cells. *Nature* **229**:345–346.

Katz, B., and Miledi, R. 1964. The development of acetylcholine sensitivity in nerve-free segments of skeletal muscle. *J. Physiol. (Lond.)* **170**:389–396.

Klebe, R. J., and Ruddle, F. 1969. Neuroblastoma: Cell culture analysis of a differentiating stem cell system. *J. Cell Biol.* **43**:69a.

Klebe, R. J., Chen, T., and Ruddle, F. R. 1970. Mapping of a human genetic regulator element by somatic cell genetic analysis. *Proc. Natl. Acad. Sci.* **66**:1220–1227.

Kung, C., and Eckert, R. 1972. Genetic modification of electric properties in an excitable membrane. *Proc. Natl. Acad. Sci.* **69**:93–97.

Lightbody, J., Pfeiffer, S. E., Kornblith, P. L., and Herschman, H. R. 1970. Biochemically differentiated clonal human glial cells in tissue culture. *J. Neurobiol.* **1**:411–417.

Littlefield, J. W. 1964. Selection of hybrids from matings of fibroblasts *in vitro* and their presumed recombinants. *Science* **145**:709–710.

Minna, J., Nelson, P., Peacock, J., Glazer, D., and Nirenberg, M. 1971. Genes for neuronal properties expressed in neuroblastoma × L cell hybrids. *Proc. Natl. Acad. Sci.* **68**: 234–239.

Minna, J., Glazer, D., and Nirenberg, M. 1972. Genetic dissection of neural properties using somatic cell hybrids. *Nature New Biol.* **235**:225–231.

Mohit, B. 1971. Immunoglobulin G and free kappa-chain synthesis in different clones of a hybrid cell line. *Proc. Natl. Acad. Sci.* **68**:3045–3048.

Nachmansohn, D. 1971. Chemical event in conducting and synaptic membranes during electrical activity. *Proc. Natl. Acad. Sci.* **68**:3107–3174.

Nelson, P. G., and Peacock, J. H. 1972. Acetylcholine responses in L cells. *Science* **177**: 1005–1007.

Nelson, P., Ruffner, W., and Nirenberg, M. 1969. Neuronal tumor cells with excitable membranes grown *in vitro*. *Proc. Natl. Acad. Sci.* **64**:1004–1010.

Nelson, P. G., Peacock, J., and Amano, T. 1971a. Reponses of neuroblastoma cells to iontophoretically applied acetylcholine. *J. Cell. Physiol.* **77**:353–362.

Nelson, P. G., Peacock, J. H., Amano, T., and Minna, J. 1971b. Electrogenesis in mouse neuroblastoma cells *in vitro*. *J. Cell. Physiol.* **77**:337–352.

Nelson, P., Peacock, J., and Minna, J. 1972. An active electrical response in L cells. *J. Gen. Physiol.* **60**:58–71.

Olmsted, J. B., Carlson, K., Klebe, R., Ruddle, F., and Rosenbaum, J. 1970. Isolation of microtubule protein from cultured mouse neuroblastoma cells. *Proc. Natl. Acad. Sci.* **65**:129–136.

Patrick, J., Heinemánn, S., Lindstrom, J., Schubert, D., and Stainbach, J. H. 1972. Appearance of acetylcholine receptors during differentiation of a myogenic cell line. *Proc. Natl. Acad. Sci.* **69**:2762–2766.

Peacock, J., Minna, J., Nelson, P., and Nirenberg, M. 1972. The use of aminopterin in selecting electrically active neuroblastoma cells. *Exptl. Cell Res.* **73**:367–377.

Peterson, J. A., and Weiss, M. C. 1972. Expression of differentiated functions in hepatoma cell hybrids: Induction of mouse albumin production in rat hepatoma–mouse fibroblast hybrids. *Proc. Natl. Acad. Sci.* **69**:571–575.

Pfeiffer, S. E., and Wechsler, W. 1972. Biochemically differentiated neoplastic clone of Schwann cells. *Proc. Natl. Acad. Sci.* **69**:2885–2889.

Prasad, K. N., and Vernadakis, A. 1972. Morphological and biochemical study in x-ray and dibutyryl cyclic AMP–induced differentiated neuroblastoma cells. *Exptl. Cell Res.* **70**:27–32.

Rall, T. W., and Gilman, A. G. 1970. The role of cyclic AMP in the nervous system. *Neurosic. Res. Bull.* **8(3)**.

Rao, P. N., and Johnson, R. T. 1970. Mammalian cell fusion. I. Studies on the regulation of DNA synthesis and mitosis. *Nature* **225**:159–164.

Schneider, J. A., and Weiss, M. C. 1971. Expression of differentiated functions in hepatoma cell hybrids. I. Tyrosine aminotransferase in hepatoma–fibroblast hybrids. *Proc. Natl. Acad. Sci.* **68**:127–131.

Schubert, D., Humphreys, S., Baroni, C., and Cohn, M. 1969. *In vitro* differentiation of a mouse neuroblastoma. *Proc. Natl. Acad. Sci.* **64**:316–323.

Schubert, D., Humphreys, S., De Vitry, F., and Jacob, F. 1971. Induced differentiation of a neuroblastoma. *Develop. Biol.* **25**:514–546.

Seecof, R. L., Teplitz, R. L., Gerson, I., Ikeda, K., and Donady, J. 1972. Differentiation of neuromuscular junctions in cultures of embryonic *Drosophila* cells. *Proc. Natl. Acad. Sci.* **69**:566–570.

Seeds, N. W. 1971. Biochemical differentiation in reaggregating brain cell culture. *Pro. Natl. Acad. Sci.* **68**:1859–1861.

Seeds, N. W., Gilman, A. G., Amano, T., and Nirenberg, M. W. 1970. Regulation of axon formation by clonal lines of a neural tumor. *Proc. Natl. Acad. Sci.* **66**:160–167.

Sidman, R. L., Green, M. C., and Appel, S. H. 1965. Catalog of the Neurological Mutants of the Mouse. Harvard University Press, Cambridge, Mass.

Siman-Tov, R., and Sachs, L. 1972. Enzyme regulation in neuroblastoma cells. *Europ. J. Biochem.* **30**:123–129.

Sonnerschein, C., Tashjian, A. H., Jr., and Richardson, U. I. 1968. Somatic cell hybridiza-tion: Mouse–rat hybrid cell line involving a growth-hormone producing parent. *Genetics* **60**:227–228.

Sutherland, E. W., Robison, G. A., and Butcher, R. W. 1968. Some aspects of the biologic role of adenosine 3′,5′-monophosphate (cyclic AMP). *Circulation* **3**:279–306.

Tashjian, A., Yasumura, Y., Levine, L., Sato, G., and Parker, M. 1968. Establishment of clonal strains of rat pituitary tumor cells that secrete growth hormone. *Endocrinology* **82**:342–352.

Vogel, Z., Sytkowski, A. J., and Nirenberg, M. W. 1972. Acetylcholine receptors of muscle grown *in vitro*. *Proc. Natl. Acad. Sci.* (in press).

Weiss, M. C., and Chaplain, M. 1971. Expression of differentiated functions in hepatoma cell hybrids: Reappearance of tyrosine aminotransferase inducibility after loss of chromosomes. *Proc. Natl. Acad. Sci.* **68**:3026–3030.

Weiss, M. C., and Ephrussi, B. 1966. Studies of interspecific (rat × mouse) somatic hybrids, I: Isolation, growth and evolution of the karyotype. *Genetics* **54**:1095–1109.

Weiss, M. C., and Green, H. 1967. Human–mouse hybrid cell lines containing partial complements of human chromosomes and functioning human genes. *Proc. Natl. Acad. Sci.* **58**:1104–1111.

Wilson, S. H., Schrier, B. K., Farber, J. L., Thompson, E. J., Rosenberg, R. N., Blume, A. J., and Nirenberg, M. W. 1972. Markers for gene expression in cultured cells from the nervous system. *J. Biol. Chem.* **247**:3159–3169.

Yaffee, D. 1968. Retention of differentiation potentialities during prolonged cultivation of myogenic cells. *Proc. Natl. Acad. Sci.* **61**:477–483.

Yasumura, Y., Tashjian, A. H., and Sato, G. H. 1966. Establishment of four functional, clonal strains of animal cells in culture. *Science* **154**:1186–1189.

Zanetta, J. P., Benda, P., Gombos, G., and Morgan, I. G. 1972. The presence of 2′ 3′-cyclic AMP 3′-phosphohydrolase in glial cells in tissue culture. *J. Neurochem.* **19**: 881–883.

Chapter 8

Nervous System–Specific Proteins in Cultured Neural Cells

Harvey R. Herschman, Barbara P. Grauling, and Michael P. Lerner

The Departments of Biological Chemistry and Neurosciences
and
Laboratory of Nuclear Medicine and Radiation Biology
School of Medicine
University of California
Los Angeles, California

I. INTRODUCTION

The earliest reports of differentiated functions in serially cultured cell strains and lines are difficult to trace completely and depend to some degree on an acceptable definition of the term "differentiated." Should we, for example, consider the species and strain-specific antigens of cells as "functional" or "differentiated" markers? Several early references describe serially cultured cells which maintained such antigenic distinctions (Brand and Syverton, 1960; Stulberg, *et al.*, 1961; Coombs, 1962). The consensus arising from an analysis of much of the cell culture studies of the 1950s and early 1960s, however, suggested that serially cultured cells generally lose the ability to carry out differentiated functions characteristic of their tissue of origin. Occasional reports to the contrary, the loss of differentiated function was thought to be a relatively general feature of dispersed cell culture. In the early 1960s loss of function in cultured cells was ascribed to two different mechanisms. The first

This work was supported by Contract AT(04)-GEN-12 between the Atomic Energy Commission and the Regents of the University of California and by Grant No. P598 from the American Cancer Society to H.R.H. B.P.G. is a predoctoral fellow supported by Mental Health Training Program MH06415 of the N. I. M. H.

of these phenomena was termed "dedifferentiation," a process inherent in cells propagated in dispersed culture. Alternatively, selective overgrowth by un-differentiated cells in the mixed cultures was postulated as the factor respon-sible for loss of function. The review of Levintow and Eagle (1961) describes the debate over these two phenomena as it existed at that time, while Yasu-mura (1968) provides a retrospective discussion of the controversy. Sato and his associates were able to resolve at least some aspects of this debate when they isolated from neoplasms of various endocrine organs a variety of clonal cell strains which were capable of producing organ-specific products in culture (Buonassisi *et al.,* 1962; Yasumura *et al.,* 1966). These results clearly demonstrated that selective overgrowth was responsible for the observed "dedifferentiation" in some cases; growth in culture did not *ipso facto* mean loss of function for the progeny of a functional cell. The clonal isolation of functional cell strains from neoplastic tissue has since become a major tool in a number of areas, including cell biology, endocrinology, and, most re-cently, neurobiology.

Several potential functional markers for neuronal tumors can be sug-gested, the bulk of which are related to biosynthetic or degradative pathways for neurotransmitters. With the exception of myelin and its components, no comparable markers for glial-specific function are obvious, due to our lack of knowledge of the functional role of glia. Several laboratories have described the existence of nervous system–specific antigens (Moore and McGregor, 1965; Kosinski and Grabar, 1967; Warecka and Baur, 1967) which have been detected by serological techniques. Several of these nervous system-specific antigens have been purified and extensively characterized (Moore, 1965; Moore and Perez, 1968; Bennett and Edelman, 1968). One approach our laboratory has taken to this question of the establishment of differentiated lines of neural origin has been the characterization of the production of ner-vous system–specific antigens in serially propagated cells from tumors of neural origin.

II. EXPERIMENTAL NEURAL TUMORS

Druckrey and his associates have described several carcinogens which are "organotropic" for the nervous system (Druckrey *et al.,* 1965). A variety of neural tumors including astrocytomas, oligodendrogliomas, ependymomas, and spongeoblastomas could be induced when adult rats were injected with weekly intravenous injections of the carcinogen *N*-nitrosomethylurea (NMU) at a dose of 5–10 mg/kg. Benda and his associates (Benda *et al.,* 1968) were able to successfully induce tumors of this type and adapt them to cell culture. Several of these lines were subsequently cloned, in collaboration with Dr. Sato. In this case, histological characterization of the original tumors suggested an astrocytic origin. Several other tumors induced by NMU administration (or the closely related carcinogen N-nitrosoethylurea) have recently been adapted to cell culture, as described in other chapters of this book.

The clonal cell lines derived by Benda et al. (1968) came from tumors which produced the nervous system–specific antigen S100 protein. This protein is a highly acidic macromolecule of molecular weight 20,000 (Moore, 1965) which has been shown by serologic techniques to be specific to neural tissue. One rat glial cell strain, termed C6, produced easily detectable amounts of S100 protein in culture.

III.   S100 PROTEIN PRODUCTION BY C6 RAT GLIAL CELLS

The relationship between cell division and expression of differentiated function is a controversial and active area of cell biology. Expression of differentiated function is limited to nondividing cells in a number of culture systems, such as fibroblastic collagen synthesis (Green and Goldberg, 1964) and proline hydroxylase activity (Gribble et al., 1969). In contrast, synthesis of specialized cell products concurrent with cellular proliferation has been observed in other cultured cells (Cahn and Lasher, 1967; Richardson et al., 1969). Many other examples from the literature can be cited which either support or refute the popular contention that cellular proliferation and expression of differentiated function are mutually exclusive conditions.

The appearance of the nervous system–specific S100 protein in developing rat brain is a relatively late ontogenic event (Herschman et al., 1971b). Its presence therefore suggests a relatively mature neural cell. We decided to investigate the relationship between cell growth and S100 protein levels in the C6 cell strain in order to see whether any indication of specific neural maturation as a function of culture state or condition might occur in these cells.

Monolayer C6 cells grow rapidly in horse and fetal calf serum supplemented Nutrient Mixture F10 (Ham, 1972). Doubling time for this cell strain in exponential growth is about 18 hr until a density of 2.5–3×10^5 cells/cm^2 is reached, when cell division is significantly reduced (Fig. 1). Analysis of S100 protein levels by quantitative microcomplement fixation (Levine, 1967) at various points in the growth curve reveals that significant accumulation of S100 protein occurs only after the cessation of rapid-cell proliferation. While cell number increases some twentyfold during the first 120 hr (Fig. 1), the S100 per bottle is less than doubled. As a result of continued cell division, S100 protein per cell is continuously reduced during the exponential phase and reaches a minimum when the cells enter stationary phase. At this point, accumu-

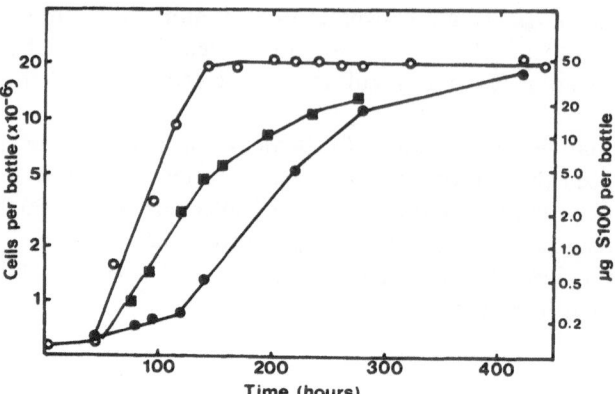

Fig. 1.   Growth and S100 protein production in C6 cells. Stationary-phase monolayers of C6 cells were harvested by trypsinization and subcultured at zero time in 75-cm² Falcon tissue culture flasks at an initial density of 5 × 10⁵ cells per flask. At the points indicated, flasks were either harvested by trypsinization for determination of cell number per bottle by hemocytometer (open circles) counting or washed twice with 0.01 M tris–HCl pH 7.3 buffer containing 0.15 M NaCl, harvested in this buffer, and frozen for S100 protein analysis. After all flasks were harvested, the cell suspensions were thawed, homogenized in Dounce homogenizers, and centrifuged at 35,000 × g for 10 min. The amount of S100 protein per bottle (filled circles) was determined by comparison of the complement fixation curve for each extract with that of a standard S100 protein preparation (Zuckerman *et al.*, 1970). The calculated levels of S100 protein, assuming that exponential- and stationary-phase cells accumulate this protein at the same rate, are shown by the filled squares. A description of the assumptions made and the nature of this calculation is in the text. (Redrawn from Pfeiffer *et al.*, 1970.)

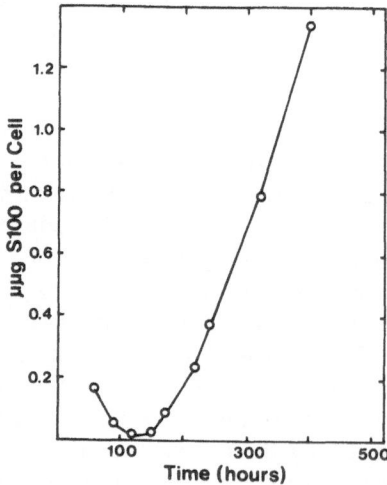

Fig. 2.   S100 protein per cell as a function of cell growth. Data are calculated from the values given in Fig. 1 for cell number per bottle and S100 protein per bottle.

lation begins and the level of S100 protein increases (Fig. 2). To assure ourselves that the accumulation data illustrated in Fig. 1 were not an artifact of the limitations of the sensitivity of the complement fixation assay, we generated an accumulation curve for S100 protein during the growth curve. We assumed that accumulation per cell in exponential phase was equivalent to that in stationary phase and used the expression $S_1 - S_0 = \frac{1}{c} N_0 K (e^{ct} - 1)$, where S_0 and S_1 are amounts of S100 protein per culture at times t_0 and t_1, respectively, $t = t_0 - t_1$, $c = \ln 2 / T_d$ (T_d is the doubling time), and K is the rate of S100 protein accumulation per cell in stationary phase. In the experiment shown in Fig. 1, K has a value of 0.0065 μμg/cell/hr.

The calculated accumulation curve is also shown in Fig. 1. Our assay method clearly would be sensitive enough to detect such accumulation. C6 cells are obliged to enter stationary phase before accumulation of S100 protein will occur.

Two potentially separable phenomena, cessation of cell division and initial cellular contact, occur at the point in the growth curve where S100 accumulation begins. Several experiments suggested that cell–cell contact is required for this accumulation. Cultures in which division of exponentially growing nonconfluent C6 cells was arrested by (1) hydroxyurea inhibition of DNA synthesis, (2) fluorodeoxyuridine inhibition of DNA synthesis, or (3) withdrawal of serum from the culture medium failed to initiate S100 protein accumulation. These procedures did not prevent either the onset or the continuation of S100 protein accumulation in confluent stationary-phase cultures. C6 cells in suspension culture grow to a cell density at which further cell division is suppressed, i.e., a stationary phase. S100 protein accumulation does not occur in stationary-phase C6 suspension cultures. These data suggest that cessation of cell division in C6 cultures is not a sufficient condition to initiate S100 protein accumulation. Mixed culture experiments with a cell line which does not produce S100 protein suggested that this accumulation requires homologous C6 cell–cell contact (Pfeiffer et al., 1970).

Several alternative explanations are available to account for the regulated initiation of accumulation of S100 protein in monolayer cultures. Probably the most parsimonious one suggests that cell contact induces the synthesis of this protein in cells which do not produce this differentiated gene product while growing in sparse culture. Alternatively, the pool of S100 protein could be continuously turned over, i.e., synthesized and degraded, at a balanced rate in exponential cultures but not in stationary cultures. Finally, a serologically inactive precursor might be made during growth and subsequently converted to the detectable form. The data presented above describe only the net increase in this protein. Analyses of rates of synthesis and degradation, rather than the balance between the two, are needed to distinguish among these alternative explanations.

IV. SYNTHESIS AND DEGRADATION OF S100 PROTEIN IN C6 CELLS

Several isotopic–electrophoretic and isotopic–serological techniques for the analysis of S100 protein synthesis and/or degradation have been described previously (Rubin and Stenzel, 1965; McEwen and Hyden, 1966). We have demonstrated that the application of such techniques to control cell lines which do not synthesize this protein yields unacceptably high background values (Herschman and Pfeiffer, unpublished). In order to devise a sufficiently specific assay for radiolabeled S100 protein in cultured cells, we exploited (Herschman, 1971) three unique features of S100 protein: (1) its heat stability in the presence of mercaptoethanol (Kessler *et al.,* 1968), (2) its reaction with anti-S100 antisera (Levine and Moore, 1966), and (3) its rapid migration on SDS–acrylamide gels (Herschman, unpublished; Dannies and Levine, 1969). When an immune precipitate between S100 protein and its antiserum is dis-

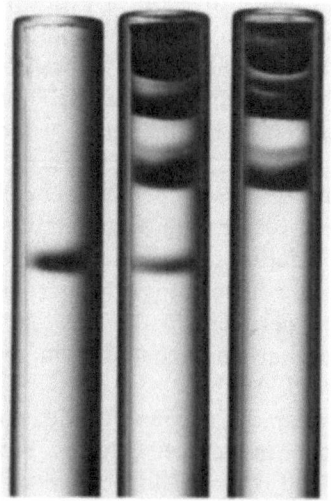

Fig. 3. SDS–acrylamide gel electrophoresis of solubilized S100 protein and rat serum albumin immune precipitates. Immune precipitation of S100 protein (23 µg S100 protein and 0.1 ml antiserum to S100 protein) and rabbit serum albumin (25 µg RSA and 0.2 ml antiserum to RSA) was carried out in 3 ml of 0.01 M pH 7.3 potassium phosphate buffer, containing 0.15 M NaCl. The reactions were incubated 1 hr at 37°C, then overnight at 4°C. Precipitates were removed by centrifugation in the cold at 2300 rpm for 10 min. The precipitates were washed three times in the potassium phosphate–NaCl buffer by resuspension and centrifugation. The final pellets were solubilized in 0.075 ml of a dissolving buffer containing 0.01 M sodium phosphate, 1% SDS, 10% sucrose, 1.0% β-mercaptoethanol, and a trace of tracking dye. These samples, as well as a 23-µg sample of S100 protein in 0.075 ml of dissolving buffer, were incubated at 37°C for 3 hr. A 50-µl portion of each sample was subjected to electrophoresis for 3 hr at 5 ma per gel in the SDS–acrylamide gel system described by Weber and Osborn (1969). Gels were stained with 1% Amido Schwartz for 20 min, then destained in 7% acetic acid. The gel on the left contains only S100 protein; the center gel contains the dissolved S100 protein immune precipitate; the gel on the right contains the dissolved RSA immune precipitate.

solved in an SDS buffer and electrophoresed in SDS-containing polyacrylamide gels, the S100 protein migrates quite rapidly and separates cleanly from the rest of the polypeptide chains involved in the immune precipitate (Fig. 3). A peak of labeled material coelectrophoresing with S100 protein may be demonstrated in extracts of L-leucine-H^3-labeled stationary-phase C6 cells after heating, immune precipitation, and electrophoresis of the dissolved pellet (Fig. 4). Control cells which do not produce S100 protein have no appreciable label in the S100 region and thus demonstrate the specificity of the method. Quantitative isolation of S100 protein from labeled extracts of S100-synthesizing cells has been demonstrated by analyzing a second immune precipitate from the supernatant of the first precipitation. All labeled S100 protein is present in the initial precipitation reaction. The technique described here provides the specificity and quantitative recovery of S100 protein necessary for the study of its synthesis and degradation. Details of the procedure are provided in the caption of Fig. 4.

A. Synthesis of S100 Protein by C6 Cells

The data illustrated in Fig. 4 are taken from an experiment in which stationary-phase C6 cells were labeled for 6hr with L-leucine-H^3. Incorporation of the radioactive precursor into TCA-precipitable protein is linear for this entire period under the conditions in which this experiment was performed. The relative rate of S100 protein synthesis, defined as cpm in S100 protein/ total TCA-precipitable cpm, in stationary-phase C6 cells is 0.026% in this experiment. When a correction is made for the nonspecific counts found in the S100 region of the gel (by subtracting the value found for L6 cells, a non-S100 protein producing rat muscle cell line), the relative rate of S100 protein synthesis in C6 stationary-phase cells is 0.020%.

Exponentially growing C6 cells do not incorporate radioactive leucine into S100 protein at a relative rate as great as that of stationary-phase cells. The radioactive profiles of S100 anti-S100 precipitates prepared from exponentially growing C6 cells and rat muscle cells are shown in Fig. 5. The S100 region of the gel prepared from an exponential C6 culture does not show extensive labeling. Background radioactivity (i.e., radioactive material which precipitates with the S100 protein immune precipitate but separates from S100 protein during electrophoresis) is always greater in exponentially growing cultures than in stationary cultures. The reasons for this are not clear. The relatively high background counts and the occasional presence of other peaks of radioactivity (e.g., the peak at fraction 10 in Fig. 5 for L6 cells) emphasize the lack of complete specificity of the immune precipitate alone and underscore the requirement for subsequent electrophoresis of the dissolved pellet. When a

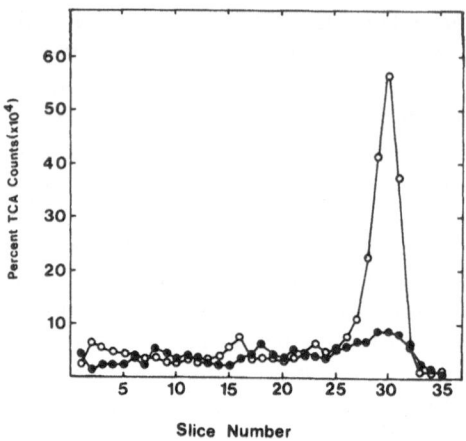

Fig. 4. Specificity of immune SDS–acrylamide gel isolation of labeled S100 protein from stationary-phase C6 cells. Confluent stationary-phase C6 cells (3.4×10^7 cells per plate) and L6 rat muscle cells (2.0×10^7 cells per plate) in 100-mm Falcon plates were labeled for 6 hr with 100 µc L-leucine-H^3 (specific activity 51 c/m M) in 10 ml of Nutrient Mixture F10, supplemented with 10% fetal calf serum. Cells were washed on the plate three times with cold 0.01 M potassium phosphate buffer, pH 7.3, containing 0.15 M NaCl and 1 mg/ml L-leucine (PBSL). The cells were scraped with a rubber policeman into 2.0 ml of PBSL. Samples were frozen until analysis. The thawed cell suspensions were made 0.05 M in β-mercaptoethanol, then sonicated in the cold (three 10-sec sonications at an intensity setting of 30 with a Bronwill Biosonic III Sonifier, using a microprobe). Samples were removed for TCA precipitation as described by Mans and Novelli (1961). There were 9.2×10^6 TCA-precipitable cpm in the C6 sample, 6.6×10^6 TCA-precipitable cpm in the L6 suspension. The sonicated samples were centrifuged at $40,000 \times g$ for 10 min. After the addition of 50 µl of 2 M mercaptoethanol, the supernatants were heated to 70°C for 10 min and again centrifuged. About 85% of the soluble protein is removed by heating in the presence of β-mercaptoethanol, but no S100 protein is lost. A drop of concentrated sheep red cell lysate was added to each supernatant. The samples were passed over Sephadex G25 columns prepared in disposable 10-ml pipettes and equilibrated with PBSL. The entire excluded volume of the column was collected, as judged by hemoglobin elution. Carrier S100 protein (23 µg) and antiserum to S100 protein (0.1 ml) were added to each tube. Immune precipitation, washing, solubilization, and electrophoresis were performed as described in the caption of Fig. 3. The stained gels were cut into 1-mm segments with a commercial gel slicer (Diversified Scientific Instruments). Each segment was dissolved in 0.5 ml of hydrogen peroxide for 3 hr at 75°C and counted in a scintillation mixture containing Liquifluor, toluene, and Triton X100 in a ratio of 1:9:5. Data are given as the percentage in each gel segment of the total TCA-precipitable counts in the sonicated cell suspension. Open circles, C6 cells; filled circles, L6 cells.

correction is made for nonspecific labeling by subtracting the counts found in the L6 S100 region from that of the C6 values, the relative rate of S100 protein synthesis in exponentially growing C6 cells is calculated to be 0.002%. We regard this value as an upper limit for S100 protein synthesis in C6 cells during exponential growth. The relative rate of synthesis of this protein in stationary cells is thus tenfold greater than in exponential phase.

Since we have not measured free leucine pool sizes, we cannot calculate the absolute rate of incorporation of labeled leucine into S100 protein in stationary and exponential cultures of C6 cells. Accurate knowledge of precursor pool specific activity is not required for a comparison of *relative* rates of synthesis, since the specific activities of the pool for total protein and that for S100 protein are operationally considered to be the same and cancel in the calculation. The rate of incorporation of label into protein in stationary-phase cells drops 40–50% from that observed in exponentially growing C6 cells. If we assume that pool sizes are the same for stationary-phase and exponentially growing cells, the absolute rate of synthesis of S100 protein, i.e., counts per minute of radioactive leucine entering S100 per microgram of protein, *increases* by a factor of at least 5–6 when C6 cells enter stationary phase. We plan to measure amino acid pool sizes in stationary and exponential cultures to determine absolute rates of synthesis of this protein in the two phases of growth.

B. Degradation of S100 Protein in C6 Cells

A study published shortly after the initial discovery of S100 protein concluded that in rat brain this protein has a half-life of several hours, while total protein has a half-life of several days (McEwen and Hyden, 1966). The pro-

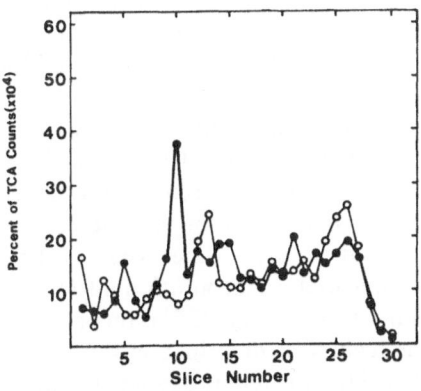

Fig. 5. SDS–acrylamide gel electrophoresis of S100 protein immune precipitates of exponentially growing C6 and L6 cells. Two 100-mm plates of C6 cells (5.35 × 10⁶ cells per plate) and three plates of L6 cells (5.8 × 10⁶ cells per plate) were labeled for 6 hr with L-leucine-H³ (specific activity 51 c/m M). Cells were washed, harvested in a total of 2.0 ml of PBSL, and sonicated as described in the caption of Fig. 4. There were 1.45 × 10⁷ TCA-precipitable cpm in the C6 cell suspension, 1.79 × 10⁷ TCA-precipitable cpm in the L6 cell suspension. A 1.2-ml portion of the C6 supernatant and a 0.9-ml portion of the L6 supernatant were each diluted to 2.0 ml with PBSL. Both samples were heated, centrifuged, chromatographed, and subjected to immune precipitation, solubilization, and electrophoresis as described previously. Data are expressed as the percentage in each gel segment of the total TCA-precipitable cpm present in the sonicated cell suspensions for C6 cells (open circles) and for L6 cells (filled circles).

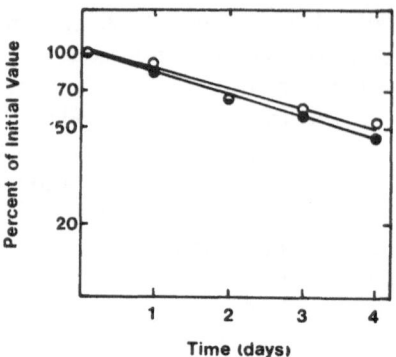

Fig. 6. Degradation of S100 protein and total protein in C6 cells. Confluent 100–mm plates of C6 cells were labeled for 24 hr with 100 μc of L-leucine-H³ (51 c/mM) in 10 ml of Nutrient Mixture F10 supplemented with 10% fetal calf serum. At zero time, one plate was washed with PBSL, scraped into 2.0 ml of PBSL, and frozen. The remaining plates were washed two times with nonradioactive medium and fed with 10 ml of fresh medium. At 24-hr intervals thereafter, one plate was harvested and frozen; the remaining plates were washed and refed. The cell suspensions were thawed and sonicated after all samples were harvested. Incorporation into total TCA-precipitable protein and S100 protein was determined as described previously. Data are presented as the percentage of the zero-time value for incorporation into total protein (filled circles) and S100 protein (open circles). Total amounts of protein per plate (Lowry *et al.*, 1951) and S100 protein per plate (determined by microcomplement fixation) increase throughout the experiment.

cedures used for this analysis, which included a Triton X100 extraction rather than a buffered aqueous extraction and the use of acrylamide gel electrophoresis as the sole isolation method and criterion of purity for the S100 fraction, suggested that other labeled components might be contaminating the fractions characterized as uniquely containing S100 protein. We decided to reinvestigate this problem with cultured C6 cells. The degradation of S100 protein in stationary-phase cells is illustrated in Fig. 6. Parallel culture plates were labeled with L-leucine-H³ for 24 hr, washed, and fed with fresh medium. At 24-hr intervals, a plate was removed and the cells were harvested in phosphate-buffered saline containing nonradioactive leucine (1 mg/ml). Remaining plates were fed at the same time. After all the samples had been harvested, the cells were sonicated. Incorporation into total protein was measured by the method of Mans and Novelli (1961). Incorporation into S100 protein was determined by the technique described in the caption of Fig. 4. It is clear that in the C6 cell line S100 protein is degraded at approximately the same rate that one observes for total protein. This cell culture result agrees completely with the *in vivo* degradation data obtained by Cicero and Moore (1970) and suggests that the observation of McEwen and Hyden is an artifact of the analytical methods employed. We are currently attempting to measure the rate of degradation of S100 protein in exponentially growing C6 cells to determine whether a change in this rate contributes to the observed kinetics of accumulation.

V. PRODUCTION OF 14-3-2 PROTEIN BY HUMAN NEUROBLASTOMA CELLS IN CULTURE

Moore and Perez (1968) reported the isolation from bovine brain of a second nervous system–specific protein, which they called "14-3-2 protein." This protein is serologically identical (Moore, personal communication) to the α-protein of Bennett and Edelman (1968). Moore and his coworkers feel that the 14-3-2 protein is primarily neuronal in origin.

The physiological and biochemical exploitation of clonal lines derived from the mouse neuroblastoma C1300 tumor has been extensive during their brief history. Electrophysiological and biochemical properties unique to neurons have been demonsrated in clonal C1300 lines by a number of laboratories. Much of this work is summarized and reviewed in other chapters of this book. We decided to analyze C1300 clones for the presence of 14-3-2 protein, to see if this presumptive neuronal marker is produced by functional neuroblastoma cells in culture.

Rabbit antisera to purified bovine 14-3-2 protein (the generous gift of Dr. Blake Moore) were prepared by our standard immunization procedures. Three toepad and intradermal injections of 5 mg of bovine 14-3-2 protein and 5 mg of methylated bovine serum albumin in Freund's adjuvant were given at weekly intervals to female New Zealand albino rabbits. The animals were boosted with an ear-vein injection of 5 mg of 14-3-2 protein in phosphate-buffered saline 3 weeks after the final adjuvant-containing immunization. The animals were bled from the ear vein on the sixth and seventh days after the boost. Microcomplement fixation titers of the two antisera with the homologous beef-brain 14-3-2 antigen were 1:1000 and 1:1200, respectively. Immunodiffusion studies (Ouchterlony, 1958) with extracts of various mouse organs suggested the restriction of this antigen to the nervous system. Microcomplement fixation analysis confirmed this result. Cross-reacting material could be detected in mouse brain extracts at concentrations of protein as low as 1–2 µg/ml, with antiserum used at a dilution of 1:350 (homologous titer 1:1000). No cross-reacting material was observed with extracts of mouse liver, kidney, spleen, or heart at protein concentrations up to 1000 µg/ml, the highest tested. The serologic cross-reaction between mouse-brain and beef-brain 14-3-2 protein is not nearly so extensive as that observed for S100 protein from the corresponding species. It is for this reason that a threefold increase in antibody concentration is required in the complement fixation reaction when analyzing for a heterologous reaction with extracts of mouse organs.

We have analyzed extracts of mouse neuroblastoma C1300 clones C1a (Schubert et al., 1971), NB41A (Augusti-Tocco and Sato, 1969), and N18 (Seeds et al., 1970) for 14-3-2 protein by complement fixation, using antisera dilutions appropriate for the detection of mouse-brain 14-3-2 protein. No

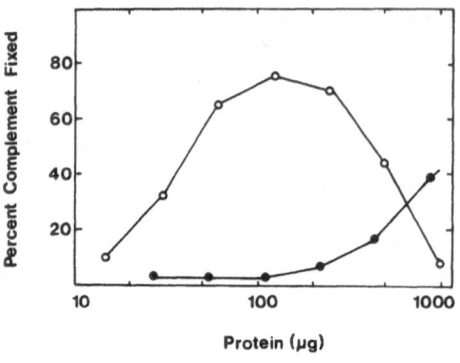

Fig. 7. Complement fixation reaction between extracts of human neuroblastoma IMR-32 cells, HeLa cells, and antiserum to bovine 14-3-2 protein. Stationary monolayer cultures of IMR-32 cells and HeLa cells in 100-mm plates were washed twice with 0.01 M tris–HCl buffer containing 0.15 M NaCl. Cells from a single plate were scraped with a rubber policeman into 1.0 ml of this buffer and frozen. Samples were thawed, sonicated (two 5-sec sonications), and centrifuged as described previously. Complement fixation analysis of these supernatants was performed in a final volume of 1.2 ml, using a dilution of 1:300 of antiserum to bovine 14-3-2 protein (homologous titer 1:1000). Protein was determined by the method of Lowry et al., (1951). Open circles, IMR-32 cells; filled circles, HeLa cells. (From Herschman and Lerner, 1973.)

14-3-2 protein was found in any of these clones. We have not as yet analyzed the parent tumor from which the various clones have been derived, however.

There have been several reports of the establishment of long-term serially cultured human neuroblastoma strains (Goldstein *et al.*, 1964; Tumilowicz *et al.*, 1970; Lyon, 1970). These strains of human neuroblastomas have not been nearly so intensively studied as the mouse C1300 clones. We obtained the human neuroblastoma strain IMR-32 (Tumilowicz *et. al,* 1970) from the American Type Culture Collection (Rockville, Md.) and adapted it to Nutrient Mixture F10 supplemented with 10% fetal calf serum. The results of a microcomplement fixation analysis of extracts of IMR-32 and HeLa cells (a clone derived from a human cervical cancer) with antisera to bovine 14-3-2 protein are presented in Fig. 7. Extracts of IMR-32 cells react extensively with antisera to bovine 14-3-2 protein. HeLa cell extracts react with antisera to 14-3-2 protein only at protein concentrations thirtyfold greater than those required with IMR-32 extracts. Complement fixation reactions occurring at such high protein concentrations are difficult to interpret. Such reactions may be due to nonspecific effects. However, the alternative proposition, i.e., the production of small amounts of 14-3-2 protein by a nonneural cell line in culture, cannot be eliminated. We are currently analyzing other human cell lines and preparing a radioimmunoprecipitation assay similar to that presented for S100 protein to pursue this question. Cells from the human neuroblastoma tumor contain easily detectable amounts of this protein, however, while cells of a nonneuronal origin have only marginal amounts at best.

The production of 14-3-2 protein by IMR-32 cells provided us with another opportunity to investigate the relationship between cell division and the expression of a differentiated function in cultured neural cells. This protein appears relatively late in development, at a time similar to the appearance of the S100 protein (Moore *et al.,* 1971). Its presence is characteristic, therefore, of a *relatively* mature neural cell. Levels of the 14-3-2 protein might reflect a cyclic maturation and dedifferentiation in stationary- and exponential-phase IMR-32 cells, respectively. Parallel plates of IMR-32 cells were analyzed for total protein, cell number, and amount of 14-3-2 protein throughout the growth curve. The amount of 14-3-2 protein could not be determined in microgram values by comparison to a standard curve, as had been done for S100 protein, since the serologic cross-reactivity of the human protein with antisera to bovine 14–3–2 protein is not sufficiently extensive. An arbitrary unit, termed a "14-3-2 C′ unit," was defined as the amount of extract required to give 40% complement fixation in the antibody-excess region of the curve with an antiserum dilution of 1:280 (with purified bovine 14-3-2 protein this value is

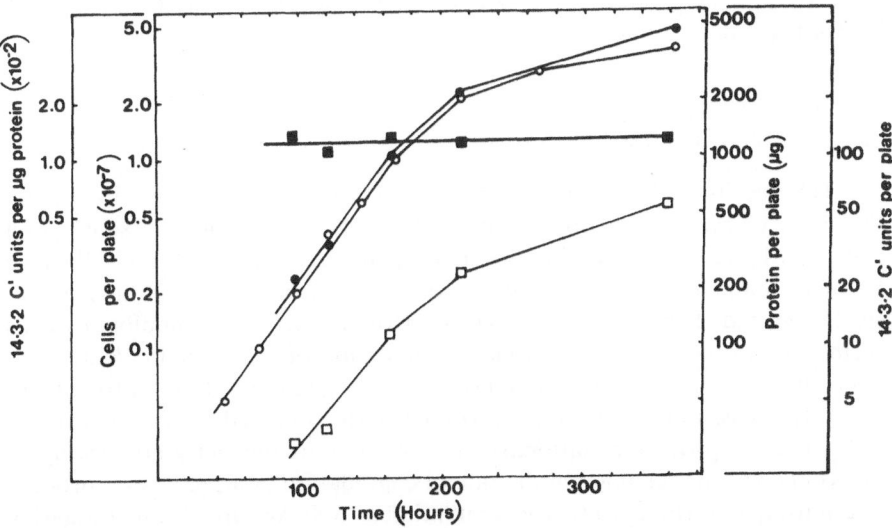

Fig. 8.   Growth and 14-3-2 protein production in IMR-32 cells. Stationary-phase mono-layers of IMR-32 cells were harvested by trypsinization and subcultured in 100-mm culture plates in Nutrient Mixture F10 supplemented with 10% fetal calf serum. Cells were fed at 48-hr intervals. Cell number per plate (open circles) was determined by hemocytometer count of trypsinized cell suspensions. At the points indicated, appropriate numbers of plates were washed, harvested in 1.0 ml of tris–HCl buffered saline, and frozen for total protein and 14-3-2 protein analysis. Total protein per plate (filled circles) and 14-3-2 C′ units per plate (open squares) were determined after all plates had been harvested. (See text for definition of 14-3-2 C′ unit.) 14-3-2 C′ units per microgram of total protein values are given by the filled squares. (From Herschman and Lerner, 1973.)

38 mµg). The total number of 14-3-2 C′ units is calculated as [the reciprocal of the dilution of IMR-32 cell extract required to give 40% complement fixation] × [volume of the extract]. IMR-32 cells had a doubling time of about 25 hr in Nutrient Mixture F10 supplemented with 10% fetal calf serum (Fig. 8). This is somewhat faster than the doubling time originally reported for IMR-32 cells grown on Medium 199 supplemented with 20% fetal calf serum (Tumilowicz et al., 1970). The amounts of 14-3-2 protein per plate and total protein per plate both increase as division of IMR cells proceeds, in contrast to the results obtained with C6 cells for S100 protein. The relative amounts of 14-3-2 protein (i.e., 14-3-2 C′ units per microgram of protein) are similar for exponentially growing and stationary-phase cells. This protein is apparently constitutive in IMR-32 cells. It is clear that cell division and production of 14-3-2 protein are not mutually exclusive. During the course of these experiments with IMR-32 cells, Drs. Milton Goldstein and Blake Moore informed us of their similar results with IMR-32 cells, as well as with NJB cells, a strain isolated by Dr. Goldstein. We have also demonstrated that extracts of NJB cells (sent to us by Dr. Goldstein) react with antiserum to bovine 14-3-2 protein.

VI. CONCLUSIONS

Our results to date on the production of S100 protein by C6 cells suggest that little or no synthesis of this protein occurs in growing, sparsely plated cells. Synthesis of this protein appears to be initiated only after the cells have become confluent, are in intimate contact with one another, and have extensively reduced their rate of cell division. Contact between homologous cells seems to be necessary for maximal accumulation of this protein. A density-dependent contact-mediated induction of the synthesis of this protein apparently occurs in C6 cells and contributes to the observed increase in accumulation of this protein in stationary cultures. We are currently attempting to determine whether changes in the rate of degradation or a precursor– product relationship contribute to this accumulation as well. We are also investigating the effects on S100 protein synthesis of a variety of treatments known to affect cell division and/or cell-surface mediated phenomena in other culture systems.

The induced "differentiation" of mouse C1300 neuroblastoma clones by a variety of agents including X-rays (Prasad, 1971), prostaglandins (Prasad, 1972), cyclic AMP derivatives (Prasad and Hsie, 1971; Furmanski et al., 1971), and serum withdrawal (Seeds et al., 1970) has been the subject of a number of reports. Whether the morphological, electrophysiological, and biochemical correlates of these treatments truly reflect a developmental program leading from a less differentiated neuronal precursor type of cell to a more differentiated cell is a topic of considerable controversy and is discussed in some detail in other chapters of this volume. We are currently initiating a program to determine whether these or other agents known to affect growth and/or differentiation of cells in culture will have any effect on the levels of 14-3-2 protein in cultured human neuroblastomas (IMR-32 and NJB) which produce this nervous system–specific marker.

VII. ACKNOWLEDGMENTS

We thank Mrs. Bella Konya and Ms. Jilla Wolsy for technical assistance.

VIII. REFERENCES

Augusti-Tocco, G., and Sato, G. 1969. *Proc. Natl. Acad. Sci.* **64**:311.
Benda, P. J., Lightbody, J., Sato, G. H., Levine, L., and Sweet, W. 1968. *Science* **161**:370.
Bennett, G. S., and Edelman, G. M. 1968. *J. Biol. Chem.* **243**:6234.
Brand, K. G., and Syverton, J. T. 1960. *J. Natl. Cancer Inst.* **24**:1007.
Buonassisi, V., Sato, G. H., and Cohen, A. I. 1962. *Proc. Natl. Acad. Sci.* **48**:1184.
Cahn, R. D., and Lasher, R. 1967. *Proc. Natl. Acad. Sci.* **58**:1131.
Cicero, T. J., and Moore, B. W. 1970. *Science* **169**:1333.
Coombs, R. R. A. 1962. *Natl. Cancer Inst. Monogr.* **7**:91.
Dannies, P. S., and Levine, L. 1969. *Biochem. Biophys. Res. Commun.* **37**:587.
Druckrey, H., Ivankovic, S., and Preussmann, R. 1965. *Z. Krebsforsch.* **66**:389.
Furmanski, P., Silverman, D. J., and Lubin, M. 1971. *Nature* **233**:413.
Goldstein, M. N., Burdman, J. A., and Journey, L. J. 1964. *J. Natl. Cancer Inst.* **32**:165.
Green, H., and Goldberg, B. 1964. *Nature* **200**:1097.
Gribble, T. J., Comstock, J. P., and Udenfriend, S., 1969. *Arch. Biochem. Biophys.* **129**:308.
Ham, R. G., 1972. *In* D. Prescott (ed.). Methods in Cell Physiology, Vol. 5, p. 37. Academic Press, New York.
Herschman, H. R. 1971. *J. Biol. Chem.* **246**:7569.
Herschman, H. R., Breeding, J., and Nedrud, J. 1971a. *J. Cell. Physiol.* **79**:249.
Herschman, H. R., Levine, L., and de Vellis, J. 1971b. *J. Neurochem.* **18**:629.
Herschman, H. R., and Lerner, M. P., 1973. *Nature New Biology* **241**:242.
Kessler, D., Levine, L., and Fasman, G. D. 1968. *Biochemistry* **7**:758.
Kosinski, E., and Grabar, P. 1967. *J. Neurochem.* **14**:273.
Levine, L. 1967. *In* D. M. Weir (ed.). Handbook of Experimental Immunochemistry, p. 707. Blackwell Scientific Publications, Oxford.
Levine, L., and Moore, B. W. 1966. *In* F. O. Schmitt and T. Melnechuk (eds.). Neurosciences Research Symposium Summaries, p. 454. MIT Press, Cambridge, Mass.
Levintow, L., and Eagle, H. 1961. *Ann. Rev. Biochem.* **30**:605.
Lowry, O. H., Rosebrough, N. J., Farr, A. L., and Randall, R. J. 1951. *J. Biol. Chem.* **193**:265.
Lyon, G. M., Jr. 1970. *Cancer Res.* **30**:2521.
Mans, R. J., and Novelli, G. D. 1961. *Arch. Biochem. Biophys.* **94**:48.
McEwen, B. S., and Hyden. H. 1966. *J. Neurochem.* **13**:823.

Moore, B. W. 1965. *Biochem. Biophys. Res. Commun.* **19**:739.

Moore, B. W., and McGregor, D. J. 1965. *J. Biol. Chem.* **240**:1647.

Moore, B. W., and Perez, V. J. 1968. *In* F. D. Carlson (ed.). Physiological and Biochemical Aspects of Nervous Integration, p. 43. Prentice-Hall, Englewood Cliffs, N. J.

Moore, B. W., Cicaro, T. J., Perez, V. J., and Cowan, W. M. 1971. *In* D. E. Pease (ed.). Cellular Aspects of Neural Growth and Differentiation, p. 481. University of California Press, Berkeley and Los Angeles.

Ouchterlony, O. 1958. *In* P. Kallos (ed.). Progress in Allergy, Vol. 5, p. 1. Karger, Basel.

Pfeiffer, S. E., Herschman, H. R., Lightbody, J., and Sato, G. 1970. *J. Cell Physiol.* **75**: 329.

Pfeiffer, S. E., Herschman, H. R., Lightbody, J., Sato, G., and Levine, L. 1971. *J. Cell. Physiol.* **78**:145.

Prasad, K. N. 1971. *Nature* **234**:471.

Prasad, K. N. 1972. *Nature New Biol.* **236**:49.

Prasad, K. N., and Hsie, A. W. 1971. *Nature New Biol.* **233**:141.

Richardson, U. I., Tashjian, A. H., Jr., and Levine, L. 1969. *J. Cell Biol.* **40**:236.

Rubin, A. L., and Stenzel, K. H. 1965. *Proc. Natl. Acad. Sci.* **53**:963.

Schubert, D., Humphreys, S., DeVitry, F., and Jacob, F. 1971. *Develop. Biol.* **25**:514.

Seeds, N. W., Gilman, A. G., Amano, T., and Nirenberg, M. W. 1970. *Proc. Natl. Acad. Sci.* **66**:160.

Stulberg, C. S., Simonson, W. F., and Berman, L. 1961. *Proc. Soc. Exptl. Biol. Med.* **108**: 434.

Tumilowicz, J. J., Nichols, W. W., Cholon, J. J., and Greene, A. E. 1970. *Cancer Res.* **30**: 2110.

Warecka, K., and Baur, H. J. 1967. *J. Neurochem.* **14**:783.

Weber, K., and Osborn, M. 1969. *J. Biol. Chem.* **244**:4406.

Yasumura, Y. 1968. *Am. Zoologist* **8**:285.

Yasumura, Y., Tashjian, A. H., Jr., and Sato, G. 1966. *Science* **154**:1186.

Zuckerman, J. E., Herschman, H. R., and Levine, L. 1970. *J. Neurochem.* **17**:247.

Chapter 9

Clonal Lines of Glial Cells

S. E. Pfeiffer

Department of Microbiology
University of Connecticut Health Center
Farmington, Connecticut

I. INTRODUCTION

Extrapolations from gross brain biochemical studies to nervous system function at the cellular level have been extremely difficult because of the complex interrelationships among a variety of neuronal and glial cell types. As a result, numerous attempts have been made to separate the cell types prior to biochemical analysis. For example, Lowry (1953), Hydén (1959), and Hamberger (1963) have hand-dissected glia from neurons in order to study their metabolic relationships, and Roots and Johnston (1965) have used a "sieving-fishing" method for their studies. However, although useful cell separations can be achieved this way, the yields are necessarily low. More recently, a variety of gradient centrifugation methods producing larger quantities of cells have been developed for preparing brain fractions enriched for neurons (Bocci, 1966; Satake and Abe, 1966; Satake *et al.,* 1968; Flangas and Bowman, 1968; Sellinger *et al.,* 1971), glia (Korey *et al.,* 1958; Fewster *et al.,* 1967), or both (Rose, 1967, 1969; Rose and Sinha, 1969; Freysz *et al.,* 1968; Blomstrand and Hamberger, 1969; Norton and Poduslo, 1970). However, although these preparations have yielded valuable biochemical information, the enrichments are only partial and the cell viability is uncertain, thus precluding many important experiments.

Established clonal lines in tissue culture have several advantages over either cell separations from whole brain or primary cell cultures. Clonal lines

This work was supported by grants from the National Institutes of Health, No. NSca 10861–01, and the American Cancer Society, No. VC 124–A.

permit one to work with functionally and genetically homogeneous, viable cell populations in quantities sufficient for most biochemical studies. They have proved invaluable in stuides of a variety of organs such as the adrenal gland (Buonassisi *et al.,* 1962), pituitary gland (Tashjian *et al.,* 1968), and, more recently, the nervous system. For example, Sato and coworkers have developed clonal lines of rat astrocytes (Benda *et al.,* 1968; Lightbody *et al.,* 1970) and mouse neuroblastoma (Augusti-Tocco and Sato, 1969), and Pfeiffer and Wechsler (1972) have isolated a clonal line of rat Schwann cells (see below). These cell lines have been used to study a variety of specialized neuronal functions including neurotransmitter synthesis, electrical and chemical membrane excitability, action-potential generation, and neurite formation (Augusti-Tocco and Sato, 1969; Nelson *et al.,* 1969; Schubert *et al.,* 1969, 1971*a, b;* Seeds *et al.,* 1970; Blume *et al.,* 1970; Minna *et al.,* 1971, 1972; Rosenberg *et al.,* 1971; Kates *et al.,* 1971; Schubert and Jacob, 1970; Prasad and Hsie, 1971; Furmanski *et al.,* 1971; Gilman and Nirenberg, 1971*a;* Prasad, 1972), as well as glial functions including synthesis of S100 protein (Pfeiffer *et al.,* 1970; Herschman, 1971) and response to catecholamines (Schimmer, 1971; Gilman and Nirenberg, 1971*b;* Clark and Perkins, 1971).

In view of the success of these early studies, Dr. Wolfgang Wechsler of the Max Planck Institute of Brain Research at Cologne and I have embarked on a program to develop numerous clonal lines of cells of the nervous system, all of which will preferably be from the same species and strain. It is expected that such a family of cell lines will be valuable for the study of both the normal and diseased cell biology of the nervous system, including the cell communication occurring among the various glial and neuronal species.

II.   ISOLATION OF CLONAL LINES

A.   General Approach

Following principles set down by Sato and coworkers, the general approach we use for establishing tumor cell lines of the nervous system which retain the ability to carry out organ-specific biochemical functions in tissue culture involves five principal steps:

1. Recognition of an organ-specific biochemical function expressed at the cellular level.
2. Development of a relatively rapid and sensitive assay for this function (usually biochemical or immunological).
3. Development of tumors (preferably transplantable) of the organ under investigation which express the chosen organ-specific functions.

4. Development of cell strains in culture that retain this function.

5. Selection of clonal lines that retain this function.

Each of these steps will now be considered in more detail.

B. Specific Approach

1. Cellular Organ Specific Biochemical Function

Numerous biochemical processes unique to nervous system tissue are now recognized. However, two "marker" proteins in particular, S100 protein and 2', 3'-cyclic nucleotide-3'-phosphohydrolase, have proved to be especially useful for choosing appropriate material to introduce into tissue culture.

a. *S100 Protein.* In 1965, Moore (1965) isolated a highly acidic protein from beef brain in the course of experiments designed to identify proteins restricted to nervous tissue. This protein, which appeared to be absent in liver, he promptly named "S100" in recognition of its unusual solubility in 100% saturated ammonium sulfate at neutral pH (Moore, 1965; Moore and McGregor, 1965). Subsequently, Levine and Moore (1966) used the serological technique of microcomplement fixation (Levine, 1967a) to kindle further interest in this protein by confirming the suspicion that here was a protein unique to the nervous system.

S100 protein has since been quantitatively assayed in various anatomical sites in the central nervous system: it is present in higher concentration in cerebral white matter than in gray matter but is found in equal concentrations in the spinal white and gray (Kessler *et al.*, 1968; Moore *et al.*, 1968). In developing human and rat brain, the period of most rapid rise in S100 protein parallels morphological and electrophysiological maturation (Moore and Perez, 1968; Zuckerman *et al.*, 1970).

Although the function of S100 protein is still unknown, strict nervous system specificity, the immunological similarity among a wide variety of vertebrate species, which implies evolutionary stability (Levine, 1967b; Levine and Moore, 1966; Moore and Perez, 1968), the effects of calcium, potassium, and sodium ions on conformation changes of S100 protein (Calissano *et al.*, 1969; Kessler *et al.*, 1968), and changes brought about by S100 protein on cation diffusion across lipid membranes (Calissano and Bangham, 1971) provide intriguing material for speculation as to its biochemical role in the nervous system.

b. *2',3'-Cyclic Nucleotide-3'-Phosphohydrolase (CNPase).* Several lines of evidence have suggested that CNPase may be unique to nervous tissue, specifically myelin. For example, its specific activity is considerably greater in white matter than gray matter (Drummond *et al.*, 1962; Kurihara and

TABLE I

2′,3′-Cyclic Nucleotide-3′-Phosphohydrolase (CNPase) Activity in Tumor Cell Lines

| Cell line | | | | CNPase |
Name	Reference	Tissue of origin	Species	Specific activity[a]
C6	Benda et al. (1968)	CNS glioma	Rat	0.9
C21	Benda et al., (1968)	CNS glioma	Rat	1.4
C3	Benda et al. (1968)	CNS glioma	Rat	0.07
RN1	Pfeiffer et al. (1972)	PNS neurinoma	Rat	0.04
RN2	Pfeiffer et al. (1972)	PNS neurinoma	Rat	1.2
RN3	Pfeiffer et al. (1972)	PNS neurinoma	Rat	0.06
RN4	Pfeiffer et al. (1972)	PNS neurinoma	Rat	0.05
NB41A	Augusti-Tocco and Sato (1969)	Neuroblastoma	Mouse	0.03
I10A	Yasumura et al. (1966b)	Leydig cell tumor	Rat	0.06
AT20	Yasumura et al. (1966b)	Pituitary tumor	Mouse	0.05
Mel	Yasumura et al. (1966b)	Melanoma	Mouse	0.05
Y1	Yasumura et al. (1966a)	Adrenal tumor	Mouse	0.02

[a]Micromoles substrate converted/min/mg total protein in reaction as described by Glastris and Pfeiffer (1972).

Tsukada, 1967), it fractionates with myelin (Kurihara and Tsukada, 1967), and its first appearance and subsequent increase in specific activity occur in a time sequence similar to that for myelination (Kurihara and Tsukada, 1968). Furthermore, mutant mice with genetic defects resulting in subnormal myelination have only low levels of CNPase activity (Olafson *et al.*, 1969; Kurihara *et al.*, 1969, 1970, 1971). However, more recent investigations have identified this enzymatic activity in apparently myelin-free neuronal membrane preparations (Morgan *et al.*, 1971), astrocytoma cells in culture (Zanetta *et al.*, 1972), human erythrocyte membranes (Sudo *et al.*, 1972), and several biochemically differentiated tumor cell lines of both nervous system and non-nervous system origin (Pfeiffer and Wechsler, 1972) (Table I). However, non-neurogenic tissues have on the average only 0.04 times the activity found in normal CNS and PNS tissues and in glial cultures. Thus CNPase appears to be an excellent glial cell marker by virtue of its higher specific activity in this cell type. The observation that CNP is present in high concentrations in astrocytes as well as Schwann cells raises some interesting questions in regard to earlier work linking this activity with myelin. Possibly, astrocytes participate in myelination in a previously unsuspected fashion. Additionally, it may be useful as a more general membrane marker for many other cell types. Preliminary studies have suggested that although CNPase is restricted to membrane fractions, it is probably not localized strictly in a single membrane species. For example, although 5'-nucleotidase (an activity often used as a plasma membrane marker; Glastris and Pfeiffer, 1972) and CNPase activities increased in parallel during early stages of plasma membrane isolation from rat Schwann cells, in later stages CNPase activity remained constant or decreased somewhat while 5'-nucleotidase activity continued to increase (Table II).

2. Rapid and Sensitive Assay for Function

In other to apply a marker function to the development of clonal lines, one must have an assay for that function which is both rapid and sensitive. The requirement for reasonable rapidity stems largely from the need (1) to screen numerous tumors initially and (2) to make constant checks for retention of function during and after the clonal isolation procedures. Sensitivity is a consequence of the small amount of material available for assay, particularly during the early stages of adaptation to tissue culture.

Fortunately, immunogical and enzymatic criteria can often meet these requirements. For example, S100 protein is routinely measured by microcomplement fixation as described by Levine (1967a). S100 protein concentrations of 0.01 µg/ml can easily be measured, and greater sensitivity can be obtained. It is noteworthy that microcomplement fixation is particularly well adapted to the assay of particulate cellular antigens, since no precipitation phenomena are involved in the reaction (Pfeiffer *et al.,* 1971). Thus it should prove useful to studies of organ-specific surface functions. Similarly, 2', 3'-cyclic nucleotide-3'-phosphohydrolase can be assayed by, for example, thin layer chromatographic separation of substrate and product at sensitivities approaching 0.01 unit specific activity (Glastris and Pfeifier, 1972).

What are missing, unfortunately, in most cases are assays meeting the requirements for rapidity and sensitivity that can be applied at the single-cell level directly to a monolayer culture with retention of cell viability. Assays of this type would provide a means of picking directly from mixed cell population colonies possessing the ability to carry out the desired biochemical process.

3. Development of Differentiated Tumors

Although tumors may be induced in a variety of ways, two are of particular current interest and practical applicability because they allow a large measure of control over the organ in which tumor induction occurs.

The first of these is that developed by Dr. Jacob Furth (1968) and recently applied by Sato and coworkers to the development of hormone-dependent lines (Sato *et al.,* 1970). The tissue of interest is induced to undergo abnormal cellular proliferation, often by tampering with the animal's physiology in such a way as to upset normal growth controls. In the early stages, the cells are not malignant, insofar as complete reversion to normal proliferative controls would occur if the stimulatory agent were removed. However, sustained stimulation often results in irreversible, unrestrained neoplastic proliferation, presumably as a result of a genetic mutation. Such a mutation can be either "spontaneous" or made more probable by experimental intervention via ap-

TABLE II

Relative Specific Activities of CNPase and 5'-Nucleotidase at Five Stages of Purification of Plasma Membranes from Rat Schwann Cells[a]

Stage of purification	Relative specific activity			
	CNPase		5'-Nucleotidase	
	Expt. 1	Expt. 2	Expt. 1	Expt. 2
1[b]	1.0	1.0	1.0	1.0
2	1.3	1.0	1.2	1.1
3	2.5	1.9	3.4	1.6
4	5.7	4.2	5.5	7.0
5	5.1	4.1	11.9	8.6

[a]Enzyme activities were assayed by the methods described by Glastris and Pfeiffer (1972).
[b]Stage 1 corresponds to the crude homogenate.

plication of, for example, drugs or X-ray. One drawback to this approach is, of course, that it usually requires some rather detailed prior knowledge of the normal physiology in order to apply the experimental pressure needed to encourage hyperplasia. Although such information is available for the endocrine organs, for example, the approach to take in the case of the nervous system is less obvious.

A second general approach is to administer to experimental animals carcinogens capable of inducing neoplastic growth in specific organs. For example, the extensive work of Druckrey and coworkers (Druckrey *et al.,* 1965, 1966, 1967, 1972) and the investigations at the Max Planck Institute of Brain Research in Cologne (Wechsler *et al.,* 1969; Zülch and Mennel, 1970; Wechsler, 1972) have shown that substituted nitrosourea compounds will produce tumors in rats; the target organ is determined to a large extent by the nature of the alkyl group. The compound methylnitrosourea (MNU) or ethylnitrosourea (ENU) is administered either to young adult rats intravenously, orally, intraperitoneally, or subcutaneously or to prenatal rats transplacentally (Wechsler *et al.,* 1969; Koestner *et al.,* 1971, 1972; Swenberg *et al.,* 1971). Neurological signs and weight loss are sufficient to identify animals with tumors. As a rule of thumb, rats develop tumors 6–18 months after treatment (on a dose-dependent scale) with a high specificity for the central and peripheral nervous systems. Although the majority of these tumors have been considered to be different types of gliomas with predominant but varying patterns of astrocytomas, oligodendrogliomas, and ependymomas in the central nervous system, and malignant neurinomas in the peripheral nervous system, rare meningiomas and fibrosarcomas have been found, and the rare occurrence of neuronal tumors (neuroblastoma or gangliocytoma) has not been ruled out and has been indicated from ongoing tissue culture studies in our laboratory.

4. Cell Strains

a. Background. The loss of specific phenotypic traits from cells grown in culture long perplexed investigators and led to the idea of *in vitro* dedifferentiation. Presumably, the conditions of cell culture, while allowing for cell proliferation, were not sufficiently close to the *in vivo* environment to allow continued exhibition of the more critically balanced differentiated function. In contrast to this idea, however, was posed the alternative hypothesis of overgrowth of the cultures by fibroblasts (Sato and Yasumura, 1966). In this view, the fibroblasts would have a selective advantage in culture and quickly outpopulate the cells displaying an organ-specific function. The problem in this case would be one of dilution rather than genetics.

By studying the conditions under which cultures of biochemically differentiated, transplantable adrenal tumor cells lost the ability to synthesize ketosteriods, Sato and coworkers demonstrated (1) that fibroblastic overgrowth was indeed a major problem and (2) that when loss of phenotypic traits did occur even in clonal lines, injection of the cells back into an animal in order to form a new tumor would in some cases restore the lost trait. In addition, a general technique for initiating lines of differentiated cells was developed, the technique of alternate-animal-culture passage.

  b. Alternate-Animal-Culture Passage. Alternate-animal-culture passage (Buonassisi *et al.*, 1962) may be of value in establishing a new cell line from a tumor previously not exposed to cell culture conditions. Tumor cells displaying the differentiated function of interest are dissociated from solid tumor chunks, plated into culture, and allowed to attach and hopefully grow for a few days. Cells that survive the initial effects of *in vitro* conditions are then harvested and injected back into an animal of the same strain in order to form a new tumor (in the event that injection of the cells back into an animal of the same strain is not practical, e.g., when working with human tumors, the highly vascularized lining of the cheek pouches of cortisone-treated hamsters are sometimes used). Tumors arising from these cells are checked for retention of differentiated function and again put back into culture. The survivors from this second passage in culture are then injected back into another animal to form another tumor and so forth. In this way, at each passage cells that are better able to grow in culture are selected and saved before they too succumb to the unaccustomed rigors of *in vitro* growth. Only tumor cells are expected to benefit from this selective process, since stromal elements that survive the culture period should not participate in the process of the new tumor formation. Eventually, tumors may be obtained that can readily be plated into culture. The final step would then be to select for cells that express the function of interest.

  c. Enrichment Techniques. There are several ways in which one can enrich for a particular cell type. For example, some cell types (especially fibroblasts) attach to tissue culture dishes faster than others (and will often attach to bacteriological plates). Alternatively, some attach better to gelatin- or collagen-coated plates. Thus appropriate choices of substrate, combined with transfers of the medium and unattached cells to new culture dishes at short intervals after the initial plating, can effect crude separations of cell types.

  Other potentially useful procedures are suggested by the methods used for separating particular cell types from brain tissue (see Introduction) and the elegant unit gravity sedimentation method described by Miller and Phillips (1969) for separating various cell types involved in the immune response. Although these procedures have not been applied widely as a preliminary enrichment technique, the results obtained with normal tissue cell separations warrant their use with tumors.

5. Clonal Lines

Methods for the isolation of the descendants of a single cell, i.e., clonal populations, offer means to isolate a particular type of cell from a mixed population (Puck *et al.*, 1956). This may be isolation of a genetic variant from among generally similar cells (e.g., the establishment of a subline), isolation of the hybrid cells from parental and homotypic hybrid cells, or, in the present case, isolation of one phenotype from several (e.g., the isolation of differentiated astrocytes from fibroblasts).

Several approaches to cloning cells have been developed, including growth in soft agar (Sanders and Burford, 1964; MacPherson and Montagnier, 1964; Pluznik and Sachs, 1965), use of feeder layers of lethally irradiated cells (Puck and Marcus, 1955), plating of cells onto small pieces of coverslip (Schenck and Moskowitz, 1958; Freeman *et al.*, 1964), culture of cells in capillary tubes (Sanford *et al.*, 1948, 1961) or in single drops of medium (Lwoff *et al.*, 1955), and use of small cylinders to select monolayer colonies (Puck *et al.*, 1956). In each approach, the key technical problem is to plate cells at sufficiently low density to allow isolation of single cells (or the progeny of single cells) and yet to provide an environment in which the cells can still proliferate. The primary limitation in this endeavor is a nutritional one (Fisher *et al.*, 1958, 1959; Zaroff *et al.*, 1961). Because of inadequacies in the growth medium for many cell types, cross-feeding among cells is an important source of metabolites in culture. For example, Lockhart and Eagle (1959) demonstrated that at low densities "nonessential" amino acids were necessary for the growth of single human cells in culture. Thus cells have been grown in capillary tubes (Sanford *et al.*, 1961) in microdrops in order to reduce the volume of medium through which important diffusible cellular products would become distributed. In the feeder layer technique (Puck and Marcus, 1955; Stoker and Sussman, 1965), cells are plated on monolayers of cells that have been previously sterilized by exposure to X-irradiation. Irradiated cells remain attached to the petri dish, continue to metabolize, and often divide several times before dying off. During this period, the irradiated cells provide nutritional support for the unirradiated cells, helping them to become attached and begin proliferation.

However, regardless of the method used for separating a single cell type from a mixed population and growing it up to a genetically homogeneous population, it must be closely coupled to assays for biochemical functions unique to or at least highly characteristic of the cell type of interest.

III. CELLULAR LOCATION OF S100 PROTEIN

Several investigations have attempted to determine which cell types of the nervous system synthesize S100 protein. Perez *et al.* (1970) and Cicero *et al.*

(1970) used degeneration experiments to obtain evidence that glia made S100 protein. Although it has been suggested that nerve cells contain S100 protein (Hydén and McEwen, 1966; Perez and Moore, 1968), a mouse neuroblastoma does not synthesize this protein (Augusti-Tocco and Sato, 1969), and it is generally agreed that S100 is a glial protein (Nelson and Ruddle, 1971).

A. S100 Protein in Experimental Rat Tumors

Similar results have been obtained from studies of S100 protein in experimentally induced rat tumors (Benda, 1968a; Wechsler et al., 1973). In order to further assess the utility of S100 protein for studies of the nervous system, specifically nervous system malignancies, we assayed for the presence of this protein in 40 neurogenic and 11 nonneurogenic tumors produced in rats by injection of methyl- and ethylnitrosourea (Wechsler et al., 1973). Of 17 CNS tumors, 15 had S100 protein; of 22 PNS tumors, 19 had S100. No S100 could be detected in nine nonneurogenic neoplasms produced in the same series of experiments. We concluded from these experiments (1) that S100 protein is present in the great majority of MNU- and ENU-induced rat tumors of the central and peripheral nervous systems and (2) that the presence of S100 protein is a definitive sign for the presence of neural cells in a tumor.

B. S100 Protein in Human Tumors

The study of S100 protein in numerous human tumors of the nervous system has helped to further define the cells responsible for S100 production. In human tumors, S100 has been identified by sereological techniques in many tumors defined histologically as glioblastomas and astrocytomas and in a single oligodendroglioma, but not in those classified as meningiomas or in a medulloblastoma (Benda, 1968b; Haglid and Carlsson, 1971; Kornblith, Pfeiffer, Herschman, and Levine, work in progress).

In addition, we have studied a series of human acoustic neurinomas (Pfeiffer et al., 1972), tumors of the eighth cranial nerve whose cell of origin has long been controversial. Some investigators have held that these tumors are neural in origin, arising specifically from Schwann cells (Verocay, 1908; Masson, 1932; Murray and Stout, 1940; Stout, 1949; Zülch and Milhaud, 1960; Luse, 1960; Lumsden, 1963; Pineda, 1964; Wechsler and Hossman, 1965; Cravioto, 1969). In contrast, others have contended that since this tumor produces collagenous elements and reticulin fibers, it must be mesodermal in origin, arising specifically from fibroblasts (Penfield, 1932; Cox and Crange, 1937; Bailey and Hermann, 1938, Tarlov, 1940; Zimmerman et al., 1956; Raimondi and Beckman, 1967). Since both of these viewpoints have been derived largely from electron microscopy and tissue culture, it appeared that a new approach was needed to resolve the controversy. Thus we have assayed a series of benign human acoustic neurinomas for S100 protein. Every one of 15 such tumors examined was found to contain S100 protein, in some cases in unusually high amounts (Pfeiffer *et al.*, 1972). Thus we conclude that neural cells are at least a major component of these tumors. The cells that make the collagen which is also present in these tumors are yet to be defined, of course. However, since we have recently demonstrated the synthesis of collagen and procollagen by a clonal line of rat Schwann cells (see below), we postulate that at least a major fraction of the collagen in these tumors is made by the neural cells (Church *et al.*, 1973).

C. S100 Protein in Clonal Cell Lines

Since both spontaneous and chemically induced tumors of the nervous system tend to exhibit varying degrees of cellular heterogeneity, the presence of S100 protein in homogeneous clonal cell lines offers a potentially more definitive identification of cell types involved in its synthesis. There are at least four such cells. Two of them, named C6 and C21, were derived from MNU-induced cerebral gliomas in rats (Benda *et al.*, 1968); they are generally considered to be astrocytes. A third, named CHB, was originally thought to have been derived from a grade II–III cerebral astrocytoma (Lightbody *et al.*, 1970). However, Stuhlmüller *et al.* (personal cummunication) later discovered that the karyotype was similar to that of a rat. This discrepancy is probably not a simple case of the contamination of the original line with rat glial cells, since line CHB differs significantly from the only other glial lines capable of synthesizing S100 protein (C6 and C21) which have been cultured in the same laboratories. These differences include their morphological appearance in monolayer culture, growth control parameters, control and extent of S100 protein synthesis, lack of cortisol induction of glycerol phosphate dehydrogenase, surface antigens (Lightbody *et al.*, 1970), and the extent to which 3', 5'-cyclic AMP levels can be stimulated by norepinephrine (Gilman and Nirenberg, 1971*b*). A fourth line that synthesizes S100 protein was derived from a rat peripheral neurinoma (RN2) and is described in more detail below (Pfeiffer and Wechsler, 1972).

IV. STUDIES OF MYELINATION IN VITRO

A. Demyelinating Disease

1. Experimental Allergic Encephalomyelitis

Experimental allergic encephalomyelitis (EAE) is an experimentally induced inflammatory and demyelinating disease of the central nervous system

(Patterson, 1966; Adams and Leibowitz, 1969) that occurs when an animal is injected with central nervous system tissue or a basic protein from central nervous system myelin (Einstein *et al.,* 1962; Kies, 1965; Eylar *et al.,* 1969). This condition appears to be mediated primarily by cell-bound antibodies, although circulating antibodies appear also in later stages of the disease (Adams and Leibowitz, 1969). EAE has been studied for many years as an animal model for autoimmune disease in man (Kabat *et al.,* 1947; Carnegie *et al.,* 1967); it is similar both clinically and histologically to certain human demyelinating diseases such as multiple sclerosis (Patterson, 1969).

The chemical identity of the encephalitogenic agent was discovered by the demonstration that it (1) was a myelin component (Laatsch *et al.,* 1962), (2) was a basic protein constituting 30% of the total myelin protein (Alvord, 1968; Kies, 1965), and (3) was localized in relatively small peptides obtained by both peptic and tryptic (Hashim and Eylar, 1969; Carnegie and Lumsden, 1967) digests of this basic protein. These peptides were then shown to include the same unique region surrounding the single tryptophan residue (Hashim and Eylar, 1969; Eylar *et al.,* 1970) Phe-Ser-*Trp*-Gly-Ala-Glu-Gly-*Gln-Lys,* in which Trp . . . Gln, Lys are required for encephalitogenic activity. Although the basic protein of bovine central nervous system is similar in size and shape to histones (molecular weight 18,400; Eylar, 1970), it differs from histones in its higher content of histidine and proline (Carnegie *et al.,* 1967).

In spite of the above information, however, the pathogenetic mechanisms involved in EAE are not completely understood. Nor is the role of myelin basic protein in human multiple sclerosis firmly established, although several laboratories have found degradation of the basic protein in the plaques and purified myelin of multiple sclerosis patients (Hallpike and Adams, 1969; Riekkinen *et al.,* 1971). The unraveling of initial lesion from secondary response remains to be accomplished, with the hypothesis of virally induced multiple sclerosis held tenable.

2. *Experimental Allergic Neuritis*

Idiopathic polyneuritis (IP) (or Landry-Guillain-Barré-Strohl syndrome) is a demyelinating disease of the peripheral nervous system which is distinguished by perivenous inflammation in nerves and spinal roots with release of protein and destruction of adjacent medulated fibers (Arnason, 1969). Like its CNS counterpart multiple sclerosis, the etiology (particularly the initial event) of IP is unknown. Nevertheless, autoimmune disease is strongly implicated here, too, largely through the study of an immunologically induced neuritis in animals called "experimental allergic neuritis" (EAN) (Waksman and Adams, 1956), an inflammatory, demyelinating disease of the peripheral nervous tissue (Arnason, 1969). At least two basic proteins can be isolated from the peripheral myelin of several species (Eng *et al.,* 1968; Mihl and Wolfgram, 1969; Brostoff *et al., 1972*). Recently, Eylar and coworkers have succeeded in producing both EAE and EAN in guinea pigs by injecting either of two basic proteins that they have purified from rabbit sciatic nerves and named P_1 and P_2 (Brostoff *et al., 1972*; Brostoff, 1972). P_1 is similar in both size and charge to the basic protein from bovine brain. In contrast, the P_2 protein is smaller (molecular weight 11,000–12,000) and more basic, due largely to the greater number of amidated acidic amino acids.

B. Primary Tissue Culture Systems

Availability of primary tissue culture systems has already provided the basis for important advances in numerous areas of medicine. P. Y. Patterson (1966) has summarized the impact of *in vitro* systems for experimental autoimmune disease:

> A major advance in the experimental autoimmune disease field has been the development of *in vitro* systems in which serum or cells from sensitized animals can be observed to interact directly with "tissue targets." The targets have consisted of cell suspensions or living cultures of tissue corresponding to that to which the animal has been sensitized. The assay systems are sensitive and have led to the recognition of circulating antibodies or the presence of immune activity associated with sensitized cells not previously detected with standard *in vitro* serological techniques.

Several of these systems are described here.

Among the most successful of the tissue culture systems to which Patterson (1966) refers is that of Bornstein and coworkers (Bornstein and Murray, 1958, and below). Neonatal or embryonic rat or mouse central nervous system tissue can be maintained in tissue culture with myelination occurring within 2–3 weeks. Treatment of these myelinated cultures with sera from animals with latent or acute EAE causes reversible demyelination with no apparent damage to axons (Bornstein and Appel, 1961), while premyelination treatment of the primary cultures prevents myelination from occurring at all (Bornstein and Raine, 1970); 7S γ-globulin and complement seem to be the necessary causative agents (Appel and Bornstein, 1964). Upon removal of the disease sera, remyelination often occurs, an observation pertinent to the remitting course seen often in multiple sclerosis and occasionally in EAE. It has been shown that sera from patients with active demyelinating neurological diseases such as multiple sclerosis also exert toxic effects on the myelin and glia in these cultures which are indistinguishable from those obtained with EAE sera (Bornstein, 1963). This last finding has provided some of the best evidence that EAE and human demyelinating diseases may share common immunological mechanisms. Recently, Fry *et al.* (1971) have found a correspondence between myelination and the synthesis of sulfatides in these cultures.

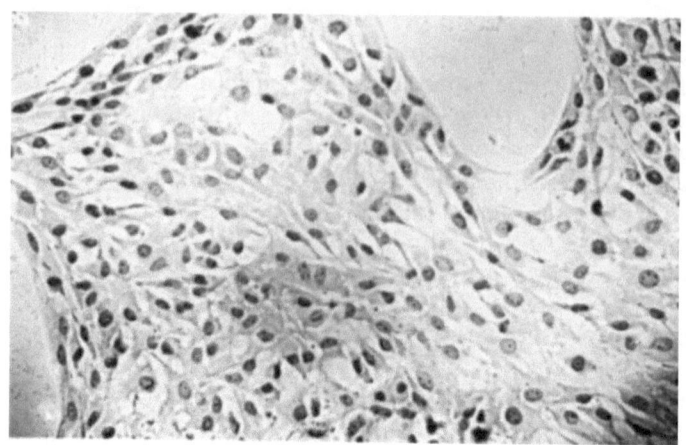

Fig. 1.   Photomicrograph of RN2 cells stained with toluidine blue. × 300.

Koprowski and Fernandes (1962) obtained lymph node cells from rats immunized with guinea pig spinal cord. These cells, when added to tissue culture monolayers of puppy brain, became aggregated around the glia, causing their destruction. Lymph node cells from normal rats did not have this effect unless they were first incubated in serum from a sensitized animal. However, the serum from a sensitized animal by itself had no such effect. Although the relationship to myelin breakdown was not as clear as in the work of Bornstein and coworkers, the indication of a role for both serum and lymphocytes is important.

Berg and Kallen (1962) used cultures of neonatal rat brain in plasma clots to demonstrate rapid toxic effects on glia by sera from guinea pigs and rabbits with EAE.

Winkler (1965) observed a similar phenomenon for the peripheral nervous system. Lymph node cells from rats with experimental allergic neuritis caused demyelination of cultures of fetal rat trigeminal ganglion within 2–3 days. Demyelination also occurred when serum from rats with manifest, but not latent, EAN was used. In both cases, axons were apparently unaffected.

Bunge and coworkers (Bunge, 1971) have studied a variety of experimentally induced myelin degenerations of rat dorsal ganglion cells in long-term tissue culture. Different patterns are observed among Wallerian degeneration, cyanide treatment, glycerol exposure, trypsin treatment, and diphtheria toxin. For example, diphtherial toxin induces a segmental demyelination in which only some segments are destroyed; the Schwann cell itself is uninjured when its myelin is destroyed. In fact, the Schwann cells appear to clean up the myelin debris in about a week, after which remyelination may occur. Trypsin treatment causes the myelin to pull away from the nodes and undergo a considerable distortion in 3 hr, while the axons remain unaffected. The myelin is not broken down but rather pulls back from the node, allowing a new Schwann cell to move into the area to invest the bare axon.

C. Clonal Line of Rat Peripheral Neurinoma Cells

1. Isolation of Clone RN2

The possibility of using S100 protein as a marker for Schwann cells has recently been put to use in the development of a clonal line of rat peripheral neurinoma cells (Pfeiffer and Wechsler, 1972). This line was derived from an ethylnitrosourea-induced, transplantable cervical root neurinoma (Wechsler and Ramadan, 1971). Several criteria including the *in vivo* location of the primary tumor, its histological classification as a malignant neurinoma, and the presence of S100 protein had suggested that this tumor might be of Schwann cell origin. The tumor was introduced into tissue culture by methods described above, and four morphologically distinct clonal lines were isolated and named RN1, RN2, RN3, and RN4. Since only RN2 synthesizes S100 protein, our subsequent studies with Dr. Wechsler have concentrated on this line in view of our prejudice for the need for biochemical criteria to correlate cell cultures with a specific cell type.

2. General Characteristics of Line RN2

RN2 is generally grown in monolayer culture (Fig. 1); it has a doubling time of about 20 hr and a low-density plating efficiency of about 50%. The cell

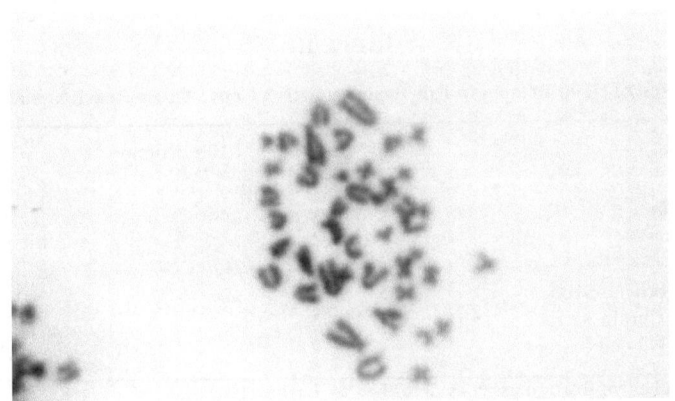

Fig. 2. Chromosome spread from line RN2.

population is quite homogeneous, with bipolar or stellate cells with long un-branched processes.

The mean chromosome number is 43, one extra relative to the number in the normal rat. The extra chromosome is probably a small teleocentric. Otherwise, the chromosome morphologies are normal for rat (Fig. 2).

3. S100 Protein

RN2 cultures have been assayed repeatedly for S100 protein. They have contained amounts of S100 ranging from 0.01 to 0.2% of the soluble protein, depending on the age of the culture (it appears that stationary-phase con-ditions are required for S100 accumulation by the cells). Serological studies (microcomplement fixation) have indicated that the S100 protein from RN2 cells is closely related serologically to S100 protein from rat brain (Table III); a comparison of the maximum percent complement fixation attained at a fixed antibody concentration by a group of antigens is a measure of the degree of serological similarity (cross-reaction) of these antigens (Levine, 1967a). The maxima displayed by S100 protein in crude homogenates of rat brain and RN2 cells are nearly equal when assayed with antiserum prepared against purified beef-brain S100 protein (kindly provided by Dr. L. Levine, Brandeis University).

4. 2′,3′-Cyclic Nucleotide-3′-Phosphohydrolase

Cell line RN2 also has 2′,3′-cyclic nucleotide-3′-phosphohydrolase activity at levels characteristic of glia (Table I) (Pfeiffer and Wechsler, 1972).

TABLE III

Comparison of S100 Protein in Rat Brain and RN2 Cells: Cross-Reaction and Amount

Material	S100 protein[a]	
	Cross-reaction: maximum complement fixation, %[b]	Amount: % total soluble protein[c]
Purified bovine S100	95	100
Crude rat brain extract	74	0.4
Crude RN2 cell extract	77	0.1

[a]Microcomplement fixation assay as described by Levine (1967a).
[b]At a constant antibody titer of 1/1200.
[c]Supernatant after Dounce homogenization and centrifugation at 35,000 × g for 20 min.

5. Myelin Encephalitogenic Proteins

The presence of S100 protein and the high levels of CNPase indicate that line RN2 is of neural origin (see above). In view of its derivation from a peripheral neurinoma, RN2 cultures are currently being analyzed for biochemical functions that would be indicative of Schwann cells. Since a major role of Schwann cells is to form the myelin sheath around peripheral axons from an extension of their plasma cell membranes (Geren, 1954; Robertson, 1955), biochemical properties unique to myelin should provide excellent markers for Schwann cells. It must be recognized, however, that plasma membranes from cells that are not actively myelinating an axon (i.e., forming a multilayered myelin sheath) may be more closely related to the "immature" myelin from young rats described by Cuzner and Davison (1968) than to adult myelin. "Immature" myelin is characterized by a lower content of cerebrosides, basic protein, and cholesterol but elevated amounts of gangliosides (Cuzner and Davison, 1968; Agrawal *et al.,* 1970; Davison, 1971).

The specificity of the encephalitogenic (basic) proteins of myelin makes them excellent biochemical indicators of myelin synthesis. Recently, we have purified a basic protein from RN2 cells that appears to be closely related to the central nervous system encephalitogenic protein from bovine and rat brain, and to one of the peripheral myelin proteins, by virtue of its molecular weight (estimated by acrylamide gel electrophoresis in sodium dodecylsulfate) and amino acid composition (Pfeiffer and Wechsler, 1972). In addition, immunological studies were carried out using antiserum prepared against either bovine myelin basic protein (kindly provided by Dr. Helene Rausch, Stanford University) or guinea pig myelin basic protein (kindly provided by Dr. Marion Kies, National Institutes of Health). Positive reactions were obtained by both passive cutaneous anaphylaxis and a microprecipitin reaction (Sundar Raj, work in progress). Experiments are in progress to further characterize the cross-reacting basic protein and to study its synthesis and fate in the cell cultures.

6. Procollagen and Collagen Synthesis by RN2 Cells

The presence of collagen fibers in tissues composed predominantly of neuroectoderm has suggested that neuroectodermal cells may themselves synthesize collagen. In particular, many discussions have centered around the collagen fibrils observed in human peripheral neurinomas (see Section IIIB). For those who accept the morphological (Murray and Stout, 1940, Pineda, 1965; Cravioto and Lockwood, 1968) and biochemical (Pfeiffer *et al.,* 1972) evidence for the neural origin of these tumors, these collagen fibers have provided the basis for concluding that cells of neural origin can synthesize collagen. In contrast, others have taken the opposite view, namely, that the very presence of these collagen fibers indicates that these tumors must be fibroblastic in origin rather than neural. Thus it is of interest that we have recently been able to demonstrate collagen synthesis in the peripheral neurinoma clonal line RN2 (Church *et al.*, 1973). The evidence for this is twofold.

a. Proline Hydroxylation. First, experiments were carried out to determine if RN2 cells were capable of hydroxylating proline to hydroxyproline, a modification thought to occur only in collagen molecules (Green and Goldberg, 1965). Stationary-phase cultures of RN2 were grown in medium lacking serum in the presence of proline-H^3 for 2–3 days, after which the ratio of hydroxyproline-H^3 to proline-H^3 was determined both for the proteins excreted into the medium and for the cell-layer proteins. On the average, 14.1 % of the total tritium-labeled proline (proline plus hydroxyproline) in medium proteins was hydroxylated, and 1.3 % in cell-layer proteins. By comparison, similar experiments with 3T6 fibroblasts have yielded analogous values of 20 % and 12 %, respectively. In contrast, only very low values of proline hydroxylation (less than 1 %) were reported for several nonfibroblastic lines studied by Green and Goldberg (1965).

b. Collagenase Sensitivity. Second, samples of the proteins excreted by RN2 cells into the medium were electrophoresed on SDS–acrylamide gels with and without prior treatment with protease-free collagenase. One of the protein bands present in the "untreated" gel was absent in the "collagenase-treated" gel. Its molecular weight of approximately 155,000 (in contrast to collagen α_1 or α_2 molecules of molecular weight around 95,000) suggests its role as a precursor of tropocollagen. Studies are underway to ascertain its functional role (Church *et al.*, ongoing research).

These data show that cells of neural origin can in fact synthesize collagen and suggest further that Schwann cells themselves may be responsible for a large part of the collagen seen in peripheral neurinomas.

7. Current Work

Current work with clone RN2 is centered around experiments designed to assess the ability of these cells to produce myelin-like membranes. These experiments include assays for galactosylceramides (Mokrasch *et al.*, 1971), further studies of myelin basic protein synthesis, studies of a methylase which specifically methylates arginine 107 in the bovine encephalitogenic protein (Carnegie and Baldwin, 1971; Paik *et al.*, 1972; Sundar Raj and Pfeiffer, 1973), and attempts to demonstrate the presence of myelin proteolipid protein in these cells (Tenenbaum and Folch-Pi, 1966; Wolfgram and Kotori, 1968; Mokrasch, 1972). Of particular interest, of course, will be attempts to induce the RN2 cells to actually myelinate primary cultures of peripheral nerve root ganglia axons.

This work is also being extended to a study of myelinating cells of the central nervous system. Methyl- and ethylnitrosourea induced brain tumors have been introduced into tissue culture and cloned and are being analyzed in a fashion similar to that used for line RN2. In addition to several glial cell types, evidence is accumulating for the presence of possible neuronal cell types.

V. PROSPECTUS

The neuroglia, i.e., the oligodendroglia and astrocytes of the CNS and the Schwann cells of the PNS, are now recognized to be more than structural elements in the nervous system. Numerous studies have suggested that they facilitate neuronal function in a variety of ways. For example, they concentrate (and possibly inactivate via nonspecific esterases) transmitter substances (Koelle, 1955; Henn and Hamberger, 1971) and control the ionic environment surrounding neurons (Kuffler and Nicholls, 1966). Amino acid uptake studies have led to the hypothesis that glia form metabolic substrates for neurons (Henn and Hamberger, 1971).

Of particular interest to our present discussion is the role of certain glial species in myelin formation (Mokrasch et al., 1971). CNS myelin is formed by an extension of the external plasma membrane of the oligodendroglia wrapping around the axon (e.g., Peters, 1960; Maturana, 1960), while PNS myelin is formed by a similar extension of the Schwann cell membrane (Geren, 1954; Robertson, 1955). Thus demyelination is a disorder of oligodendroglia or Schwann cells. The primary lesion resulting in demyelination could be either to the glial cell body, causing a breakdown of membrane maintenance, or to the elaborate plasma membrane directly.

The development and study of clonal lines of Schwann and oligodendroglial cells are expected to provide useful model *in vitro* systems for the study of both normal myelination and demyelinating diseases such as multiple sclerosis and idiopathic neuritis in humans and experimental allergic encephalomyelitis and neuritis in animals. From an experimental point of view, they would have several important advantages: (1) single cell type in fairly large quantities circumventing cell purification techniques; (2) established, continuously growing lines, avoiding frequent initiation of primary cultures and permitting exchange and standardization of cellular material among laboratories; and (3) open, *in vitro* systems in which experimental tools such as radioisotope-labeled metabolic precursors, drugs, and immune sera could be readily introduced and removed. Synthesis and turnover of myelin components, the course of demyelination and remyelination, and the action of cell-mediated and circulating antibodies are examples of areas of inquiry that could be readily studied in these systems. They would provide pure sources of oligodendroglia or Schwann cells for studies of the antigens involved in demyelinating disease. Finally, these cell lines might be valuable as diagnostic tools for detecting autoimmune antibodies or lymphocytes before clinical symptoms appear and conceivably as agents of treatement by remyelinating diseased nervous tissue.

VI. REFERENCES

Adams, C. W. M., and Leibowitz, S. 1969. The general pathology of demyelinating disease, pp. 309–382. *In* G. Bourne (ed.). The Structure and Function of the Nervous System, Vol. 3 Academic Press, New York.

Agrawal, H. C., Banik, N. L., Bone, A. H., Davison, A. N., Mitchell, R. F., and Spohn, M. 1970. The identity of a myelin-like fraction isolated from developing brain. *Biochem. J.* **120**:635–642.

Alvord, E. C., Jr. 1968. The etiology and pathogenesis of experimental allergic encephalomyelitis, pp. 52–70. *In* O. T. Bailey and D. E. Smith (eds.). The Central Nervous System. Williams & Wilkins, Baltimore.

Appel, S. H., and Bornstein, M. B. 1964. The application of tissue culture to the study of experimental allergic encephalomyelitis, II. *J. Exptl. Med.* **119**:303–312.

Arnason, B. G. W. 1969. Idiopathic polyneuritis and experimental allergic encephalomyelitis. A comparison, pp. 156–177. *In* L. P. Rowland (ed.). Immunologic Disorders of the Nervous System. Williams & Wilkins, Baltimore.

Augusti-Tocco, G., and Sato, G. 1969. Establishment of functional clonal lines of neurons from mouse neuroblastoma. *Proc. Natl. Acad. Sci.* **64**:311–315.

Bailey, P., and Herrmann, J. D. 1938. Role of cells of Schwann in formation of tumors of peripheral nerves. *Am. J. Pathol.* **14**:1–38.

Benda, P. 1968*a*. Protéine S100 et cellules gliales du rat. *Rev. Neurol.* **118**:364–367.

Benda, P. 1968*b*. Protéine S100 et tumers cérébrales humaines. *Rev. Neurol.* **118**:368–372.

Benda, P., Lightbody, J., Sato, G., Levine, L., and Sweet, W. 1968. Differentiated rat glial cell strain in tissue culture. *Science* **161**:370–371.

Berg, O., and Källen, B. 1962. An *in vitro* gliotoxic effect of serum from animals with experimental allergic encephalomyelitis. *Acta Pathol. Microbiol. Scand.* **54**:425–433.

Blomstrand, C., and Hamberger, A. 1969. Protein turnover in cell-enriched fractions from rabbit brain. *J. Neurochem.* **16**:1401–1407.

Blume, A., Gilbert, F., Wilson, S., Farber, J., Rosenberg, R. N., and Nirenberg, M. 1970. Regulation of acetylcholinesterase in neuroblastoma cells. *Proc. Natl. Acad. Sci.* **67**:786–792.

Bocci, V. 1966. Enzyme and metabolic properties of isolated neurones. *Nature* **212**:826–827.

Bornstein, M. B. 1963. A tissue culture approach to demyelinative disorders. *Natl. Cancer Inst. Monogr.*, No. 11, pp. 197–211.

Bornstein, M. B., and Appel, S. H. 1961. The application of tissue culture to the study of experimental "allergic" encephalomyelitis. I. Patterns of demyelination. *J. Neuropathol. Exptl. Neurol.* **20**:141–147.

Bornstein, M. B., and Murray, M. R. 1958. Serial observations on patterns of growth, myelin formation, maintenance and degeneration in cultures of new-born rat and kitten cerebellum. *J. Biophys. Biochem. Cytol.* **4**:499–504.

Bornstein, M. B., and Raine, C. S. 1970. Experimental allergic encephalomyelitis. Antiserum inhibition of myelination *in vitro*. *Lab. Invest.* **23**:536–542.

Brostoff, S. 1972. Winter Conference on Brain Research. BIS Conference Report No. 20, p. 43.

Brostoff, S., Burnett, P., Lampert, P., and Eylar, E. H. 1972. Isolation and characterization of a protein from sciatic nerve myelin responsible for experimental allergic neuritis. *Nature New Biol.* **235**:210–212.

Bunge, R. P. 1971. Myelin degeneration in tissue culture. *Neurosci. Res. Progr. Bull.* **9**: 496–498.

Buonassisi, V., Sato, G., and Cohen, A. J. 1962. Hormone producing cultures of adrenal and pituitary tumor origin. *Proc. Natl. Acad. Sci.* **48**:1184–1190.

Calissano, P., and Bangham, A. D. 1971. Effect of two brain specific proteins (S100 and 14.3.2) on cation diffusion across artificial lipid membranes. *Biochem. Biophys. Res. Commun.* **43**:504–509.

Calissano, P., Moore, B. W., and Friesen, A. 1969. Effect of calcium on S100, a protein of the nervous system. *Biochemistry* **8**:4318–4326.

Carnegie, P. R., and Baldwin, G. S. 1971. Specific enzymic methylation of an arginine in the experimental allergic encephalomyelitis protein from human myelin. *Science* **171**: 579–581.

Carnegie, P. R., and Lumsden, C. E. 1967. Fractionation of encephalitogenic polypeptides from bovine spinal cord by gel filtration in phenol–acetic acid–water. *Immunology* **12**: 133–145.

Carnegie, P. R., Bencina, B., and Lamoureau, G. 1967. Experimental allergic encephalomyelitis. *Biochem. J.* **105**:559–568.

Church, R. L., Tanzer, M. L., and Pfeiffer, S. E. 1973. Procollagen and collagen synthesis by a clonal line of rat Schwann cells. *Proc. Natl. Acad. Sci.* **70**:1943–1946.

Cicero, T. J., Cowan, W. M., Moore, B. W., and Suntzeff, V. 1970. The cellular localization of the two brain specific proteins, S100 and 14-3-2. *Brain Res.* **18**:25–34.

Clark, R. B., and Perkins, J. P. 1971. Regulation of adenosine 3′,5′-cyclic monophosphate concentration in cultured human astrocytoma cells by catecholamines and histamine. *Proc. Natl. Acad. Sci.* **68**:2757–2760.

Cox, L. B., and Cranage, M. L. 1937. Studies on the tissue culture of intracranial tumors. *J. Pathol. Bacteriol.* **45**:477–499.

Cravioto, H. 1969. The ultrastructure of acoustic nerve tumors. *Acta Neuropathol.* **12**: 116–140.

Cravioto, H., and Lockwood, R. 1969. The behavior of acoustic neuroma in tissue culture. *Acta neuropathol. (Berl.)* **12**:141–157.

Cuzner, M. L., and Davison, A. N. 1968. The lipid composition of rat brain myelin and subcellular fractions during development. *Biochem. J.* **106**:29–34.

Davison, A. N. 1971. Myelinogenesis. Chemical aspects. *Neurosci. Res. Progr. Bull.* **9**: 465–470.

Druckrey, H., Ivankovic, S., and Preussman, R. 1965. Selektive Erzeugung maligner Tumoren im Gehirn and Rükenmark von Ratten durch N-Methyl-N-nitroscharnstoff. *Z. Krebsforsch.* **66**:389–408.

Druckrey, H., Ivankovic, S., and Preussman, R. 1966. Teratogenic and carcinogenic effects in the offspring after single injection of ethylnitrosourea to pregnant rats. *Nature* **210**:1378–1379.

Druckrey, H., Preussman, R., Ivankovic, S., and Schmähl, D. 1967. Organotrope carcinogene Wirkungen bei 65 verschiedenen *N*-Nitroso-Verbindungen an BD-Ratten. *Z. Krebsforsch.* **69**:103–201.

Druckrey, H., Ivankovic, S., Preussman, R., Zülch, K. J., and Mennel, H. D. 1972. Selective induction of malignant tumors of the nervous system by resorptive carcinogens, pp. 85–147. *In* The Experimental Biology of Brain Tumors, Thomas, Springfield, Ill.

Drummond, G. I., Iyer, N. T., and Keith, J. 1962. Hydrolysis of ribonucleoside 2′, 3′-cyclic phosphates by a diesterase from brain. *J. Biol. Chem.* **237**:3535–3539.

Einstein, E. R., Robertson, D. M., Di Caprio, J., and Moore, W. 1962. The isolation from bovine spinal cord of a homogeneous protein with encephalitogenic activity. *J. Neurochem.* **9**:353–361.

Eng, L., Chao, F., Gerstl, B., Pratt, D., and Tavaststjerna, M. 1968. The maturation of human white matter myelin. Fractionation of the myelin membrane proteins. *Biochemistry* **7**:4455–4465.

Eylar, E. H. 1970. Amino acid sequence of the basic protein of the myelin membrane. *Proc. Natl. Acad. Sci.* **67**:1425–1431.

Eylar, E. H., Salk, J., Beveridge, G., and Brown, L. 1969. Experimental allergic encephalomyelitis. *Arch. Biochem. Biophys.* **132**:34–48.

Eylar, E. H., Caccam, J., Jackson, J. J., Westall, F., and Robinson, A. B. 1970. Experimental allergic encephalomyelitis: Synthesis of disease-inducing site of basic protein. *Science* **168**:1220–1223.

Fewster, M. E., Scheibel, A. B., and Mead, J. F. 1967. The preparation of glial cells from rat and bovine white matter. *Brain Res.* **6**:401–408.

Fisher, H. W., Puck, T. T., and Sato, G. 1958. Molecular growth requirements of single mammalian cells. The action of fetuin in promoting cell attachment to glass. *Proc. Natl. Acad. Sci.* **44**:4–10.

Fisher, H. W., Puck, T. T., and Sato, G. 1959. Molecular growth requirements of single mammalian cells, III. *J. Exptl. Med.* **109**:649–659.

Flangas, A. L., and Bowman, R. E. 1968. Neuronal perikarya of rat brain isolated by zonal centrifugation. *Science* **161**:1025–1027.

Freeman, A. A., Ward, T. G., and Wolford, R. G. 1964. A simplified method for the cloning of heteroploid and diploid mammalian cells. *Proc. Soc. Exptl. Biol.* **116**:339–343.

Freysz, L., Bieth, R., Judes, C., Sensenbrenner, M., Jacog, M., and Mandel, P. 1968. Distribution quanitative des divers phospholipides dans les neurons et les cellules gliales isoles du cortex cerebral de rat adulte. *J. Neurochem.* **15**:307–313.

Fry, J. M., Lehrer, G. M., and Bornstein, M. B. 1971. Abst. Papers 11th Ann. Meet. Am. Soc. Cell. Biol., New Orleans, Nov. 17–20, 1971. Abst. No. 183, p. 96.

Furmanski, P., Silverman, D. J., and Lubin, M. 1971. Expression of differentiated functions in mouse neuroblastoma mediated by dibutyryl-cyclic adenosine monophosphate. *Nature* **233**:413–415.

Furth, J. 1968. Hormones and neoplasia, pp. 131–151. *In* A. Engel, and T. Larsson, (eds.). Thule International Symposium on Cancer and Aging. Nordiska Bokhandelus Förlieg, Stockholm.

Geren, B. B. 1954. The formation from the Schwann cell surface of myelin in the peripheral nerves of chick embryos. *Exptl. Cell Res.* **7**:558–562.

Gilman, A. G., and Nirenberg, M. 1971a. Regulation of adenosine 3′,5′-cyclic monophosphate metabolism in cultured neuroblastoma cells. *Nature* **234**:356–357.

Gilman, A. G., and Nirenberg, M. 1971b. Effect of catecholamines on the adenosine 3′,5′-cyclic monophosphate concentrations of clonal satellite cells of neurons. *Proc. Natl. Acad. Sci.* **68**:2165–2168.

Glastris, B., and Pfeiffer, S. E. 1973. Mammalian membrane marker enzymes: Sensitive assay for 5′-nucleotidase and assay for mammalian 2′,3′-cyclic-nucleotide-3′-phosphohydrolase. *In* S. Fleischer, L. Packer, and R. W. Estabrook (eds.). Methods in Enzymology—Biomembranes, Chap. VII. 15, Academic Press, New York (in press).

Green, H., and Goldberg, B. 1965. Synthesis of collagen by mammalian cell lines of fibroblastic and nonfibroblastic origin. *Proc. Natl. Acad. Sci.* **53**:1360–1365.

Haglid, K. G., and Carlsson, C. A. 1971. An immunological study of some human brain tumors concerning the brain specific protein S100. *Neurochirurgia* **14**:24–27.

Hallpike, J. F., and Adams, C. W. M. 1969. Proteolysis and myelin breakdown: A review of recent histochemical and biochemical studies. *Histochem. J.* **1**:559–578.

Hamberger, A. 1963. Difference between isolated neuronal and vascular glia with respect to respiratory activity. *Acta Physiol. Scand.* **58**:1–58 (Suppl. 203).

Hashim, G. A., and Eylar, E. H. 1969. Allergic encephalomyelitis: Isolation and characterization of encelphalitogenic peptides from the basic protein of bovine spinal cord. *Arch. Biochem. Biophys.* **129**:645–654.

Henn, F. A., and Hamberger, A. 1971. Glial cell function: Uptake of transmitter substances. *Proc. Natl. Acad. Sci.* **68**:2686–2690.

Herschman, H. R. 1971. Synthesis and degradation of a brain specific protein (S100 protein) by cloned cultured human glial cells. *J. Biol. Chem.* **246**:7569–7571.

Hydén, H. 1959. Quantitative assay of compounds in isolated, fresh nerve cells and glial cells from control and stimulated animals. *Nature* **184**:433–435.

Hydén, H., and McEwen, B. S. 1966. A glial protein specific for the nervous system. *Proc. Natl. Acad. Sci.* **55**:354–358.

Kabat, E. A., Wolf, A., and Bezer, A. 1947. The rapid production of acute disseminated encephalomyelitis in rhesus monkeys by injection of heterologous and homologous brain tissue with adjuvants. *J. Exptl. Med.* **85**:117–129.

Kates, J. R., Winterton, R., and Schlessinger, K. 1971. Induction of acetylcholinesterase activity in mouse neuroblastoma tissue culture cells. *Nature* **229**:345–347.

Kessler, D., Levine, L., and Fasman, G. D. 1968. Some conformational and immunological properties of a bovine brain acidic protein. *Biochemistry* **7**:758–764.

Kies, M. W. 1965. Chemical studies on an encephalitogenic protein from guinea pig brain. *Ann. N.Y. Acad. Sci.* **122**:161–170.

Koelle, G. B. 1955. The histochemical identification of acetylcholinesterase in cholinergic, adrenergic and sensory neurons. *J. Pharmacol. Exptl. Therap.* **114**:167–184.

Koestner, A., Swenberg, J. A., and Wechsler, W. 1971. Transplacental production with ethylnitrosourea of neoplasms of the nervous system in Sprague-Dawley rats. *Am. J. Pathol.* **63**:37–50.

Koestner, A., Swenbert, J. A., and Wechsler, W. 1972. Experimental tumors of the nervous system induced by resorptive *N*-nitroso-urea compounds, pp. 9–30. *In* W. G. Bingham (ed.). Progress in Experimental Tumor Research, Vol. 17. Karger, Basel.

Kaprowski, H., and Fernandez, M. V. 1962. Autosensitization reaction *in vitro. J. Exptl. Med.* **116**:467–476.

Korey, S. R., Orchen, M., and Brotz, M. 1958. Study of white matter, I. *J. Neuropathol. Exptl. Neurol.* **17**:430–438.

Kuffler, S. W., and Nicholls, J. G. 1966. The physiology of neuroglial cells. *Ergeb. Physiol. Biol. Chem. Exptl.* **57**:1–90.

Kurihara, T., and Tsukada, Y. 1967. The regional and subcellular distribution of 2′, 3′-cyclic nucleotide 3′-phosphohydrolase in the central nervous system. *J. Neurochem.* **14**:1167–1174.

Kurihara, T., and Tsukada, Y. 1968. 2′, 3′-Cyclic nucleotide 3′-phosphohydrolase in the developing chick brain and spinal cord. *J. Neurochem.* **15**:827–832.

Kurihara, T., Nussbaum, L., and Mandel, P. 1969. 2′3′-Cyclic nucleotide 3′-phosphohydrolase in the brain of the "Jimpy" mouse, a mutant with deficient myelination. *Brain Res.* **13**:401–403.

Kurihara, T., Nussbaum, L., and Mandel, P. 1970. 2′-3′-Cyclic nucleotide 3′-phosphohydrolase in brains of mutant mice with deficient myelination. *J. Neurochem.* **17**:993–997.

Kurihara, T., Nussbaum, J. L., and Mandel, P. 1971. 2′-3′-Cyclic nucleotide 3′-phosphohydrolase in purified myelin from brain of "Jimpy" and normal young mice. *Life Sci.* **10**:421–429 (Part II).

Laatsch, R. H., Kies, M. W., Gordon, S., and Alvord, E. C., Jr. 1962. The encephalitogenic activity of myelin isolated by ultracentrifugation. *J. Exptl. Med.* **115**:777–788.

Levine, L. 1967a. Microcomplement fixation, pp. 709–719. *In* D. M. Weir (ed.). Handbook of Experimental Immunochemistry. Blackwell Scientific Publications, Oxford.

Levine, 1967b. Immunochemical approaches to the study of the nervous system, pp. 220–230. *In* G. C. Quarton, T. Melnechuk, and F. O. Schmitt (eds.). The Neurosciences. Rockefeller University Press, New York.

Levine, L., and Moore, B. W. 1966. Structural relatedness of a vertebrate brain acidic protein as measured immunologically, pp. 454–458. *In* F. O. Schmitt and T. Melnechuk (eds.). Neurosciences Research Symposium Summaries, Vol. 1. Press, Cambridge, Mass.

Lightbody, L., Pfeiffer, S. E., Kornblith, P. L., and Herschman, H. R. 1970. Biochemically differentiated clonal glial cells in tissue culture. *J. Neurobiol.* **1**:411–417.

Lockhart, R. Z., Jr., and Eagle, H. 1959. Requirements for growth of single cells. *Science* **129**:252–254.

Lowry, O. H. 1953. The quantitative histochemistry of the brain. *J. Histochem. Cytochem.* **1**:420–428.

Lumsden, C. E. 1963. Tissue culture in relation to tumors of the nervous system, pp. 317–322. *In* D. S. Russell and L. J. Rubenstein (eds.). Pathology of Tumors of the Nervous System. Williams & Wilkins, Baltimore.

Luse, S. A. 1960. Electron microscopic studies of brain tumors. *Neurology* **10**:881–905.

Lwoff, A., Dulbecco, R., Vogt, M., and Lwoff, M. 1955. Kinetics of release of poliomyelitis virus from single cells. *Virology* **1**:128–139.

MacPherson, I., and Montagnier, L. 1964. Agar suspension cultures for the selective assay of cells transformed by polyoma virus. *Virology* **23**:291–294.

Masson, P. 1932. Experimental and spontaneous schwannomas (peripheral gliomas). *Am. J. Pathol.* **8**:367–415.

Maturana, H. R. 1960. The fine anatomy of the optic nerve of anurans—An electron microscope study. *J. Biophys. Biochem. Cytol.* **7**:107–119.

Mihl, E., and Wolfgram, F. 1969. Myelin types with different protein components in the same species. *J. Neurochem.* **16**:1091–1097.

Miller, R. G., and Phillips, R. A. 1969. Separations of cells by velocity sedimentation. *J. Cell. Physiol.* **73**:191–202.

Minna, J., Nelson, P., Peacock, J., Glazer, D., and Nirenberg, M. 1971. Genes for neuronal properties expressed in neuroblastoma × L cell hybrids. *Proc. Natl. Acad. Sci.* **68**: 234–239.

Minna, J., Glazer, D., and Nirenberg, M. 1972. Genetic dissection of neural properties using somatic cell hybrids. *Nature New Biol.* **235**:225–231.

Mokrasch, L. C. 1972. Preparation and properties of animal proteins in organic solvents. *Prep. Biochem.* **2**:1–19.

Mokrasch, L. C., Bear, R. S., and Schmitt, F. O. 1971. Myelin. *Neurosci. Res. Progr. Bull.* **9**:440–598.

Moore, B. W. 1965. A soluble protein characteristic of the nervous system. *Biochem. Biophys. Res. Commun.* **19**:739–744.

Moore, B. W., and McGregor, D. 1965. Chromatographic and electrophoretic fractionation of soluble proteins of brain and liver. *J. Biol. Chem.* **240**:1647–1653.

Moore, B. W., and Perez, V. S. 1968. Specific acidic proteins of the nervous system, pp. 343–359. *In* F. D. Carlson (ed.). Physiological and Biochemical Aspects of Nervous Integration. Prentice-Hall, Englewood Cliffs, N. J.

Moore, B. W., Perez, V. J., and Gehring, M. 1968. Assay and regional distribution of a soluble protein characteristic of the nervous system. *J. Neurochem.* **15**:265–272.

Morgan, I. G., Wolfe, L. S., Mandel, P., and Gombos, G. 1971. Isolation of plasma membranes from rat brain. *Biochem. Biophys. Acta* **241**:737–751.

Murray, M. R., and Stout, A. P. 1940. Schwann cell versus fibroblast as the origin of the specific nerve sheath tumor. *Am. J. Pathol.* **16**:41–60.

Nelson, P. G., and Ruddle, F. H. 1971. Contributions of clonal systems to neurobiology. *Neurosci. Res. Progr. Bull.* (In preparation from notes at a meeting of NRP work session, Brookline, Mass.)

Nelson, P., Ruffner, W., and Nirenberg, M. 1969. Neuronal tumor cells with excitable membranes grown *in vitro. Proc. Natl. Acad. Sci.* **64**:1004–1010.

Norton, W. T., and Poduslo, S. E. 1970. Neuronal soma and whole neuroglia of rat brain: A new isolation technique. *Science* **167**:1144–1146.

Olafson, R. W., Drummond, G. I., and Lee, J. F. 1969. Studies on 2′, 3′-cyclic nucleotide-3′-phosphohydrolase from brain. *Can. J. Biochem.* **47**:961–966.

Paik, W. K., Kim, S., and Lee, H. W. 1972. Protein methylation during the development of the brain. *Biochem. Biophys. Res. Commun.* **46**:933–941.

Patterson, R. Y. 1966. Experimental allergic encephalomyelitis and autoimmune disease. *Advan. Immunol.* **5**:131–208.

Patterson, R. Y. 1969. Immune processes and infectious factors in central nervous system disease. *Ann. Rev. Med.* **20**:75–100.

Penfield, W. 1932. Tumors of the sheaths of the nervous system, pp. 955–990. *In* W. Penfield (ed.). Cytology and Cellular Pathology of the Nervous System. Hoeber, New York.

Perez, V. J., and Moore, B. W. 1968. Wallerian degeneration in rabbit tibial nerve: Changes in amounts of the S100 protein. *J. Neurochem.* **15**:971–977.

Perez, V. J., Olney, J. W., Cicero, T. J., Moore, B. W., and Bahu, B. A. 1970. Wallerian degeneration in rabbit optic nerve: Cellular localization in the central nervous system of the S100 and 14-3-2 protein. *J. Neurochem.* **17**:511–519.

Peters, A. 1960. The formation and structure of myelin sheaths in the central nervous system. *J. Biophys. Biochem. Cytol.* **8**:431–446.

Pfeiffer, S. E., and Wechsler, W. 1972. A biochemically differentiated line of Schwann cells. *Proc. Natl. Acad. Sci.* **69**:2885–2889.

Pfeiffer, S. E., Herschman, H. R., Lightbody, J. E., Sato, G., and Levine, L. 1971. Modification of cell surface antigenicity as a function of culture conditions. *J. Cell. Physiol.* **78**:145–151.

Pfeiffer, S. E., Herschman, H. R., Lightbody, J., and Sato, G. 1970. Synthesis by a clonal line of rat glial cells of the protein unique to the nervous system. *J. Cell. Physiol.* **75**: 329–340.

Pfeiffer, S. E., Kornblith, P. L., Levine, L., Cares, H. L., and Seals, J. 1972. S100 protein in human acoustic neurinomas. *Brain Res.* **41**:187–193.

Pineda, A. 1964. Submicroscopic structure of acoustic tumors. *Neurology* **14**:171–184.

Pluznik, D. H., and Sachs, L. 1965. The cloning of normal mast cells in tissue culture. *J. Cell. Comp. Physiol.* **66**:319–324.

Prasad, K. N. 1972. Morphological differentiation induced by prostaglandin in mouse neuroblastomas cells in culture. *Nature New Biol.* **326**:49–52.

Prasad, K. N., and Hsie, A. W. 1971. Morphologic differentiation of mouse neuroblastoma cells induced *in vitro* by dibutyryl adenosine 3',5'-cyclic monophosphate. *Nature New Biol.* **233**:141–142.

Puck, T. T., and Marcus, P. I. 1955. A rapid method for viable cell titration and clone production with HeLa cells in tissue culture. *Proc. Natl. Acad. Sci.* **41**:432–437.

Puck, T. T., Marcus, P. I., and Cieciura, S. J. 1956. Clonal growth of mammalian cells *in vitro*. *J. Exptl. Med.* **103**:273–283.

Raimondi, A. J., and Beckman, F. 1967. Perineural fibroblastomas: Their fine structure and biology. *Acta Neuropathol.* **8**:1–23.

Riekkinen, P. J., Palo, J., and Arstila, A. U. 1971. Protein composition of multiple sclerosis myelin. *Arch. Neurol.* **24**:545–549.

Robertson, J. D. 1955. The ultrastructure of adult vertebrate peripheral myelinated nerve fibers in relation to myelinogenesis. *J. Biophys. Biochem. Cytol.* **1**:271–278.

Roots, B. I., and Johnston. P. V. 1965. Lipids of isolated neurons. *Biochem. J.* **94**:61–63.

Rose, S. P. R. 1967. Preparations of enriched fractions from cerebral cortex containing isolated, metabolically active neuronal and glial cells. *Biochem. J.* **102**:33–43.

Rose, S. P. R. 1969. Neurons and glia: Separation techniques and biochemical interrelationships, pp. 183–239. *In* A. Lajtha (ed.). Handbook of Neurochemistry, Vol. 2. Plenum Press, New York.

Rose, S. P. R., and Sinha, A. K. 1969. Some properties of isolated neuronal cell fractions. *J. Neurochem.* **16**:1319–1328.

Rosenberg, R. M., Vandeventer, L., DeFrancesco, L., and Friedkin, M. E. 1971. Regulation of the synthesis of choline-*O*-acetyltransferase and thymidylate synthetase in mouse neuroblastoma in cell culture. *Proc. Natl. Acad. Sci.* **68**:1436–1440.

Sanders, F. K., and Burford, B. O. 1964. Ascites tumors from BHK. 21 cells transformed *in vitro* by polyoma virus. *Nature* **201**:786–789.

Sanford, K. K., Earle, W. R., and Likely, D. G. 1948. The growth *in vitro* of single isolated tissue cells. *J. Natl. Cancer Inst.* **9**:229–246.

Sanford, K. K., Covalesky, A. B., Dupress, L. T., and Earle, W. R. 1961. Cloning of mammalian cells by a simplified capillary technique. *Exptl. Cell Res.* **23**:361–372.

Satake, M., and Abe, S. 1966. Preparation and characterization of nerve cell perikaryon from rat cerebral cortex. *J. Biochem.* **59**:72–75.

Satake, M., Hasegawa, S., Abe, S., and Tanaka, R. 1968. Preparation and characterization of nerve cell perikaryon from pig brain stem. *Brain Res.* **11**:246–250.

Sato, G. H., and Yasumura, Y. 1966. Retention of differentiated function in dispersed cell cultures. *Trans. N.Y. Acad. Sci. II.* **28**:1063–1079.

Sato, G., Augusti-Tocco, G., Posner, M., and Kelly, P. 1970. Hormone-secreting and hormone-responsive cell cultures, pp. 539–546. *In* E. B. Astwood (ed.). Recent Progress in Hormone Research, Vol. 26. Academic Press, New York.

Schenck, D. M., and Moskowitz, M. 1958. Method for isolating single cells and preparation of clones from human bone marrow cultures. *Proc. Soc. Exptl. Biol. Med.* **99**: 30–33.

Schimmer, B. P. 1971. Effects of catecholamines and monovalent cations on adenylate cyclase activity in cultured glial tumor cells. *Biochem. Biophys. Acta* **252**:567–573.

Schubert, D., and Jacob, F. 1970. 5-Bromodeoxyuridine-induced differentiation of a neuroblastoma. *Proc. Natl. Acad. Sci.* **67**:247–254.

Schubert, D., Humphreys, S., Baroni, C., and Cohn, M. 1969. *In vitro* differentiation of a mouse neuroblastoma. *Proc. Natl. Acad. Sci.* **64**:316–323.

Schubert, D., Tarikas, H., Harris, A. J., and Heinemann, S. 1971a. Induction of acetylcholinesterase activity in a mouse neuroblastoma. *Nature New Biol.* **233**:78–80.

Shubert, D., Humphreys, S., de Vitry, F., and Jacob, F. 1971b. Induced differentiation of a neuroblastoma. *Develop. Biol.* **25**:514–546.

Seeds, N. W., Gilman, A. G., Amano, T., and Nirenberg, M. 1970. Regulation of axon formation by clonal lines of a neural tumor. *Proc. Natl. Acad. Sci.* **66**:160–167.

Sellinger, O. Z., Azcurra, J. M., Johnson, D. E., Ohlsson, W. G., and Locin, Z. 1971. Independence of protein synthesis and drug uptake in nerve cell bodies and glial cells isolated by a new technique. *Nature New Biol.* **230**:253–256.

Stoker, M., and Sussman, M. 1965. Studies on the action of feeder layers in cell culture. *Exptl. Cell Res.* **38**:645–653.

Stout, A. P. 1949. Atlas of Tumor Pathology, Sect. II, Fasc. 6, pp. 15–30. American Registry of Pathology, A.F.I.P., Washington, D.C.

Sudo, T., Kikuno, M., and Kurihara, T. 1972. 2′,3′-Cyclic nucleotide 3′-phosphohydrolase in human erythrocyte membranes. *Biochem. Biophys. Acta* **255**:640–646.

Sundar Raj, N., and Pfeiffer, S. E. 1973. Myelin basic protein arginine methyltransferase: Wide distribution among both neurogenic and non-neurogenic tissues. *Biochem. Biophys. Res. Comm.* **52**:1039–1045.

Swenberg, J. A., Koestner, A., and Wechsler, W. 1971. Induction of tumors of the nervous system in adult rats with intravenous methylnitrosourea. *J. Neuropathol. Exptl. Neurol.* **30**:122.

Tashjian, A., Yasumura, Y., Levine, L., Sato, G., and Parker, M. 1968. Establishment of clonal strains of rat pituitary tumor cells that secrete growth hormone. *Endocrinology* **82**:342–352.

Tarlov, I. M. 1940. Origin of the perineural fibroblastoma. *Am. J. Pathol.* **16**:33–40.

Tenenbaum, D., and Folch-Pi, J. 1966. The preparation and characterization of water soluble proteolipid protein from bovine brain white matter. *Biochem. Biophys. Acta* **115**:141–147.

Verocay, J. 1908. Multiple Geschwulste als Systemerkrankung am nervosen Apparate, pp. 378–415. *In* Festschrift Hans Chiari aus Anlasz seines 25 Jahringer Professoren—Jubilaums gewidmet, W. Braumuller, Vienna and Leipzig.

Waksman, B. H., and Adams, R. D. 1956. A comparative study of experimental allergic neuritis in the rabbit, guinea pig, and mouse. *J. Neuropathol. Exptl. Neurol.* **15**:293–314.

Wechsler, W. 1972. Old and new concepts of oncogenesis in the nervous system of man and animals, pp. 219–278. *In* W. G. Bingham (ed.). Progress in Experimental Tumor Research, Vol. 17. Karger, Basel.

Wechsler, W., and Hossman, K. A. 1965. Zur Feinstruktur menschlicher Acusticusneuri-
nome. *Beitr. Pathol. Anat.* **132**:319–343.

Wechsler, W., and Ramadan, M. A. 1971. Ethyl-nitrosourea-induced transplantable
tumors of the peripheral nervous system in inbred rats. *Naturwissenschaften* **58**:577–
578.

Wechsler, W., Kleihues, P., Matsumoto, S., Zülch, K. J., Ivankovic, S., Preussman, R.,
and Druckrey, H. 1969. Pathology of experimental neurogenic tumors chemically-
induced during prenatal and postnatal life. *Ann. N.Y. Acad. Sci.* **159**:360–408.

Wechsler, W., Pfeiffer, S. E., Swenberg, J. A., and Koestner, A. 1972. S100 protein in
experimental rat tumors of the central and peripheral nervous system. *Naturwissenschaften* **59**:370–371.

Wechsler, W., Pfeiffer, S. E., Swenberg, J. A., and Koestner, A. 1973. S100 protein in
methyl- and ethylnitrosourea induced tumors of the rat nervous system. *Acta Neuropathol. (Berl.)* **24**:287–303

Winkler, G. F. 1965. *In vitro* demyelination of peripheral nerve induced with sensitized
cells. *Ann. N.Y. Acad. Sci.* **122**:287–296.

Wolfgram, F., and Kotori, K. 1968. The composition of the myelin proteins of the central
nervous system. *J. Neurochem.* **15**:1281–1290.

Yasumura, Y., Buonassasi, V., and Sato, G. H. 1966a. Clonal analysis of differentiated
function in animal cell cultures. *Cancer Res.* **26**:529–535.

Yasumura, Y., Tashjian, A. H., and Sato, G. H. 1966b. Establishment of four functional,
clonal strains of animal cells in culture. *Science* **154**:1186–1189.

Zanetta, J. P., Benda, P., Gombos, G., and Morgan, I. G. 1972. The presence 2′,3′-cyclic
AMP 3′-phosphohydrolase in glial cells in tissue culture. *J. Neurochem.* **19**:881–883.

Zaroff, L., Sato, G., and Mills, S. E. 1961. Single cell platings from freshly isolated mammalian tissue. *Exptl. Cell Res.* **23**:565–575.

Zimmerman, H. M., Netsky, M. G., and Davidoff, L. M. 1956. Atlas of Tumors of the
Nervous System, Lea and Febiger, Philadelphia.

Zückerman, J. E., Herschman, H. R., and Levine, L. 1970. Appearance of a brain specific
antigen (the S100 protein) during human foetal development. *J. Neurochem.* **17**:247–
251.

Zulch, K. J., and Milhaud, M. 1960. Etude de la fibre du neurimone. Son origine Schwan-
nienne et sa nature neuroectodermique. *Rev. Neurol.* **103**:541–555.

Zülch, K. J., and Mennel, H. D. 1970. Recent results on chemically induced tumors of the
nervous system, pp. 60–83. In Sixth International Congress of Neuropathology.
Masson, Paris.

Chapter 10

Induction of Enzymes by Glucocorticoids and Catecholamines in a Rat Glial Cell Line

Jean de Vellis

Laboratory of Nuclear Medicine and Radiation Biology
and Department of Anatomy
University of California, Los Angeles, California

and

Gary Brooker

Department of Pharmacology
School of Medicine
University of Virginia, Charlottesville, Virginia

I. INTRODUCTION

The rat brain glial tumor cell line RGC6 was originally selected for its high content of S100, a nervous tissue–specific protein (Benda *et al.*, 1968). Subsequently, this cell line was shown to have retained other characteristic properties of brain tissue, such as the glycerol phosphate dehydrogenase induction by cortisol (de Vellis and Inglish, 1969). Although not all tissues have been tested, this induction appears to be brain specific (de Vellis and Inglish, 1968). In addition, de Vellis and Inglish found that catecholamines induced lactic dehydrogenase in RGC6 cells but not in several other cell lines (de Vellis and Inglish, 1969; de Vellis *et al.*, 1971*b*). Catecholamines, as we shall see later, also cause a large increase in the intracellular concentration of cyclic AMP. The magnitude of the response appears to be unique to

This work was supported by USPHS Grants HD–05615, HD–04612, HE–1330, USAEC and American Heart Assoc.

nervous tissue, which has the highest level of adenylcyclase and phosphodiesterase (for review, see Robison *et al.*, 1971). The function of cyclic AMP in the nervous system remains largely speculative. More generally, the role of hormones in the acquisition and maintenance of differention and functions of nervous tissue is still far from being understood (de Vellis and Clemente, 1970). In this chapter, we will discuss RGC6 cells as target cells for glucocorticoids and catecholamines, a rather unique opportunity to contrast the mechanisms of action of these two hormones in the same cell line. Furthermore, studies of these hormonal factors and, of course, S100 protein may provide insights into the functions of glial cells, which are essentially unknown except for the role of oligodendrocytes and Schwann cells in myelination of axons.

II. MATERIALS AND METHODS

RGC6 cells, originally given by Dr. Gordon Sato, are grown as monolayers in T-30 or T-250 Falcon plastic flasks. The culture medium is 3 ml for T-30 flasks and 10 ml for T-250 flasks of Ham's F10 (Gibco) containing 10% virus-screened fetal calf serum (Reheis) without antibiotics. Penicillin and streptomycin may stop bacterial contamination but cannot prevent mycoplasma infection, which often occurs simultaneously with the introduction of bacteria. It is thus better to occasionally lose flasks contaminated with bacteria. Since mycoplasma infection will often occur and go unnoticed until tested for, RGC6 cells and their subclones are cured of mycoplasma by heating cultures at 45°C for 30 min. All clones obtained are still diploid, and their karyotypes are undistinguishable from those of normal rat cells. Virus C particles have not been seen in electron micrographs (de Vellis *et al.*, 1971a). Clones are kept at a low passage number by freezing the stock of cells at liquid nitrogen temperature. Then continuing stocks are passed every 6–8 months. All cultures are kept at 37°C in incubators gassed with an air–CO_2 mixture.

III. INDUCTION OF GLYCEROL PHOSPHATE DEHYDROGENASE BY CORTISOL

Glycerol phosphate dehydrogenase (GPDH) (E.C. 1.1.1.8) is a soluble cytoplasmic enzyme which is NAD^+ dependent. GPDH catalyzes the conversion of dihydroxyacetone phosphate to glycerol phosphate. The reaction is reversible, but its equilibrium favors glycerol phosphate. Mitochondrial glycerol phosphate dehydrogenase, a very different protein, is a flavoprotein which converts glycerol phosphate to dihydroxyacetone phosphate. This reaction is irreversible and uses oxygen. These two enzymes can work together to form the glycerol phosphate cycle, net result of which is generation of NAD^+ from NADH. NAD^+ is required for glycolysis. Another function of cytoplasmic GPDH is to provide precursors for phospholipids, since glycerol phosphate can be converted to phosphatidic acid. It should be mentioned that the brain has no glycerokinase. Mitochondrial glycerol phosphate dehydrogenase is not under hormonal control in the brain (de Vellis and Inglish, 1968), and in the ensuing discussion GPDH refers only to the cytoplasmic enzyme. GPDH has been purified from rat brain, characterized, and injected into rabbits to obtain GPDH antisera. A given amount of GPDH antibody inactivates GPDH equally from control and induced animals or cultures, indicating that GPDH is identical in all four preparations. Therefore, enzyme activity represents enzyme concentration (McGinnis and de Vellis, 1973).

The concentration of glycerol phosphate dehydrogenase in the rat brain is controlled by glucocorticoids. de Vellis and Inglish (1968) observed that following hypophysectomy or adrenalectomy of adult rats GPDH activity decreased to about 35% of control after 3 weeks. Hypophysectomy of 20-day-old rats stopped the developmental increase of GPDH. In both instances, several other enzymes and brain protein content remained unchanged, indicating that cortisol regulates specifically GPDH. Injection of cortisol to adrenalectomized rats and ACTH (or cortisol) to hypophysectomized rats restored GPDH level to normal. As it can be expected from the above results, thyroidectomy and gonadectomy of adult rats had no effect on GPDH concentration. The hormonal specificity was confirmed in studies with RGC6 cells. Thyroid hormones, insulin, growth hormone, estradiol, testosterone, progesterone, and catecholamines cannot induce GPDH. Furthermore, cortisol can even induce in cells maintained in serum-free medium (de Vellis et al., 1971b). Therefore, in vivo as in vitro, the presence of a glucocorticoid appears to be the only hormonal requirement for GPDH induction.

TABLE I

Basal Level and Induction of GPDH in Various Subclones of RGC6 Cells[a]

Clone	Control (units/mg protein)	Cortisol (% control)
C6	50.8 ± 7.1 (15)	171.0 ± 9.8 (15)
G10	9.50 ± 0.21 (3)	170.1 ± 8.6 (3)
9F	17.2 ± 1.2 (4)	152.3 ± 11.5 (4)
11D	52.0 ± 2.9 (3)	268.1 ± 35.5 (3)
9E	65.4 ± 11.9 (4)	188.9 ± 5.8 (4)
2B	51.0 ± 4.1 (6)	300.5 ± 15.4 (6)

[a]Cortisol succinate was added at a final concentration of 2.76×10^{-6} M to the culture medium. Enzyme activity was measured 24 hr later. Cultures were 11 days old and in stationary phase for the last 4 days. Number of cultures is given in parentheses. Data are expressed ± SD.

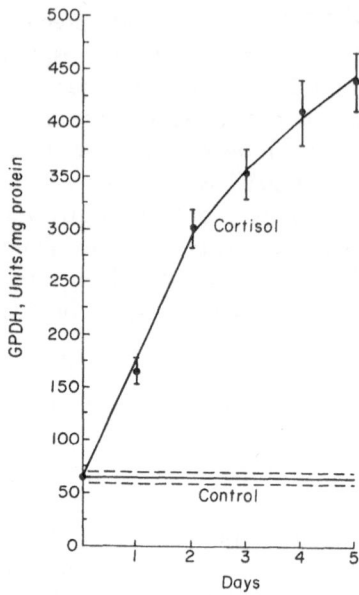

Fig. 1.   Time course of GPDH induction by cortisol in RGC6 cells. Cortisol was added at a final concentration of 5×10^{-7} M. The culture medium was changed every 24 hr. GPDH was assayed as previously indicated (de Vellis and Inglish, 1968).

TABLE II

Effect of Norepinephrine(NE), Cortisol, and Dibutyryl Cyclic AMP (DBcAMP) on GPDH and LDH Inductions in RGC6 Cells[a]

Treatments	GPDH (units/mg protein, % control)	LDH (units/mg protein, % control)
Control	100 ± 4.1	100.0 ± 5.0
DBcAMP, 10^{-4} M	90.1 ± 1.9	98.1 ± 5.8
DBcAMP, 5×10^{-4} M	100.1 ± 6.0	160.0 ± 3.8
DBcAMP, 10^{-3} M	103.4 ± 9.1	207.1 ± 13.5
NE, 10^{-6} M	100.1 ± 5.1	208.2 ± 10.6
Cortisol, 1.38×10^{-6} M	350.0 ± 30.1	108.1 ± 4.6
NE $\times$ cortisol	345.1 ± 20.1	205.6 ± 8.1

[a]Compounds were added to the culture medium at the indicated final concentrations. GPDH and LDH were assayed at 24 hr. Specific activity is expressed as percent control $\pm$ SD.

The basal activity of GPDH in some subclones of RGC6 cells is shown in Table I. The inducibility of GPDH at 24 hr does not correlate with basal activity, indicating that basal and induced activities are under separate control. A time course of the induction is shown in Fig. 1. A new steady state usually 10–18 times higher than the basal level is reached 5 days after addition of cortisol. The effect of cortisol concentration on GPDH induction is shown in Fig. 2. Saturation is reached at 10^{-7} M. Dexamethasone induces and saturates at lower concentrations. The corticosterone dose–response curve is similar to that of cortisol. Studies with these three hormones labeled with H^3 showed that there was an immediate nuclear uptake and retention of the hormone added to the culture medium (McEwen and de Vellis, unpublished data). In a variety of experimental conditions, GPDH induction correlated with nuclear binding of the hormone, suggesting an action of glucocorticoids at the nuclear, hence transcriptional, level. This conclusion is in agreement with the inhibitory effect of actinomycin D. Inhibitors of protein synthesis, such as puromycin, acetoxycycloheximide, and cycloheximide, inhibit GPDH induction, indicating that de novo protein synthesis is required (de Vellis et al., 1971b). A further discussion of nuclear events will be presented in Section V.

Unlike LDH, GPDH is not inducible by dibutyryl cyclic AMP (Table II). This is in agreement with the fact that cortisol does not cause a rise in cyclic AMP in RGC6 cells (Table III). The addition of both norepinephrine and cortisol gives a GPDH induction identical to that obtained with cortisol alone, suggesting that cyclic AMP does not even have a secondary effect on GPDH induction. S100 protein accumulation in RGC6 cells starts only after cultures have reached confluency (Benda et al., 1968; Pfeiffer et al., 1970). Unlike S100 protein, GPDH induction was observed in cultures during logarithmic growth as well as in stationary phase. In the original C6 clone, little variation in inducibility of GPDH was observed with age of the culture (de Vellis and Inglish, 1969; de Vellis et al., 1971a). However, clones 11D and 2B, which display high inducibility (Table I), induce maximally 8–10 days after passage (Fig. 3). On each side of this point, there is a marked drop in inducibility. These results confirm the observation of Davidson and Benda (1970), who used a subclone of RGC6 cells. The rise and fall of inducibility of GPDH with age correlate with hormonal receptor activity (de Vellis and Inglish, 1973).

Glucocorticoids have other effects on RGC6 cells. The transport of amino acids and glucose is reduced. This effect is time dependent, following a time course which is a mirror image of GPDH induction (Shinwari and de Vellis, 1972). The dose–response curves for cortisol effects on transport are similar to that for GPDH induction, showing a saturation at approximately 10^{-7} M (Fig. 2). Another effect of cortisol is to modify the appearance of dense bodies (de Vellis et al., 1971a) which we now have identified as lysosomes since

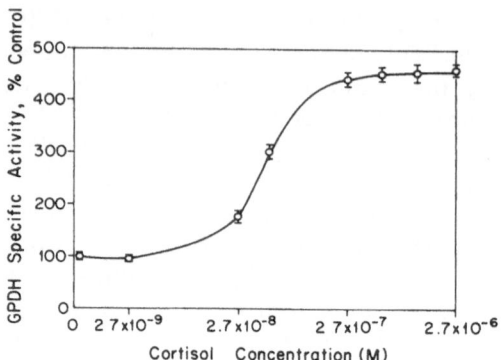

Fig. 2. Effect of cortisol concentration on GPDH induction. Cortisol was dissolved in ethanol and added in 10 μl. Cultures (2B clone) were assayed 24 hr later.

they contain acid phosphatase. The decrease in electron density of lysosomes is not seen in several other cell lines and may, therefore, be a property of cells responsive to cortisol (de Vellis et al., 1971b). HeLa cells, which are target cells for cortisol, show a response similar to that of RGC6 cells.

IV. EFFECT OF CATECHOLAMINES ON CYCLIC AMP AND LACTIC DEHYDROGENASE

Lactic dehydrogenase (LDH) (E.C. 1.1.1.27) is inducible by catecholamines but not by cortisol and several other hormones in RGC6 cells (de Vellis and Inglish, 1969; de Vellis et al., 1971b). The question arose as to

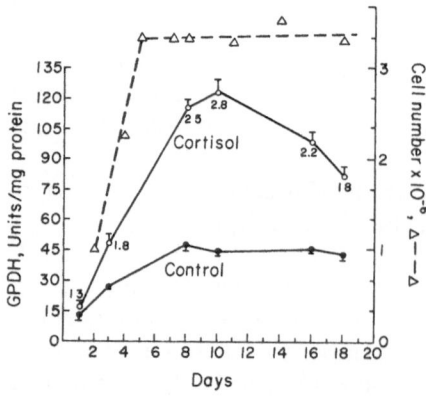

Fig. 3. Inducibility of GPDH in RGC6 cell cultures at various ages. Filled circles represent the basal level of GPDH in the 11D subclone. Open circles represent the level of GPDH after a 24-hr induction by cortisol, and the number near each symbol represents the increase over basal level. The average cell numbers in each flask are given by triangles. Each point represents the average of four cultures ± SD.

whether cyclic AMP would induce LDH, since many effects of catecholamines are known to be mediated by cyclic AMP. When dibutyryl cyclic AMP was used at concentrations up to 10^{-4} M, it had no effect on LDH. This result was rather surprising, since dibutyryl cyclic AMP is thought to penetrate cells fairly well. Actually, RGC6 cells and many other cells are not very permeable to this compound, although more than to cyclic AMP. Higher concentrations (millimolar) induced LDH maximally (de Vellis, 1971) (Table II). de Vellis and Brooker (1972) showed that cyclic AMP mediates the action of catecholamines on LDH.

The time course of LDH induction is shown in Fig. 4. After a lag of approximately 4 hr, there is a rapid rise in LDH activity which reaches a plateau after 20 hr. Preceding the rise in LDH is a large transient rise in the intracellular level of cyclic AMP. The correlation between cyclic AMP levels in cells and LDH induction can be seen in Fig. 5, which shows dose–response curves obtained with epinephrine and isoproterenol. At 3×10^{-9} M, isoproterenol causes a threefold increase in cyclic AMP and induces LDH half maximally. At 3×10^{-8} M, isoproterenol causes a thirtyfold increase in cyclic AMP and a full induction of LDH. Epinephrine is less potent than isoproterenol and requires concentrations 10 times higher to show the same effects. These results agree with well-known physiological effects of these compounds in other tissues. Several compounds which may increase cyclic AMP levels in brain tissues (for review, see Robison *et al.*, 1971) were tested (Table III). Tyramine, dopamine, histamine, and adenosine have no effect on cyclic AMP level and LDH activity. Epinine, octopamine and phenylephrine, which approximately triple cyclic AMP concentration, induce LDH half maximally. These results are in agreement with those of Gilman and Nirenberg (1971), who observed that dopamine, histamine, and adenosine had no effect on cyclic AMP level of RGC6 cells. However, a human astrocytoma cell line, 1181N1, was found to be responsive to histamine and adenosine (Clark and Perkins, 1971, 1972). Finally, propranolol, a β-blocker, inhibits the rise in cyclic AMP and LDH induction, whereas dibenzyline, an α-blocker, affects neither cyclic AMP nor LDH (Table IV), indicating that the effect of catecholamines is mediated by a β-receptor. The evidence for cyclic AMP as mediator of the catecholamine induction of LDH may be summarized in the following manner: (1) only the compounds which cause a rise in intracellular concentration of cyclic AMP induce LDH, (2) the rise in cyclic AMP precedes LDH induction, (3) cyclic AMP and dibutyryl cyclic AMP mimic the action of the active hormones, and (4) compounds which block the rise in cyclic AMP inhibit the induction.

LDH induction appears to require *de novo* protein and RNA synthesis, since addition of actinomycin D, acetoxycycloheximide, or puromycin at the same time as the hormone results in complete inhibition of the induction

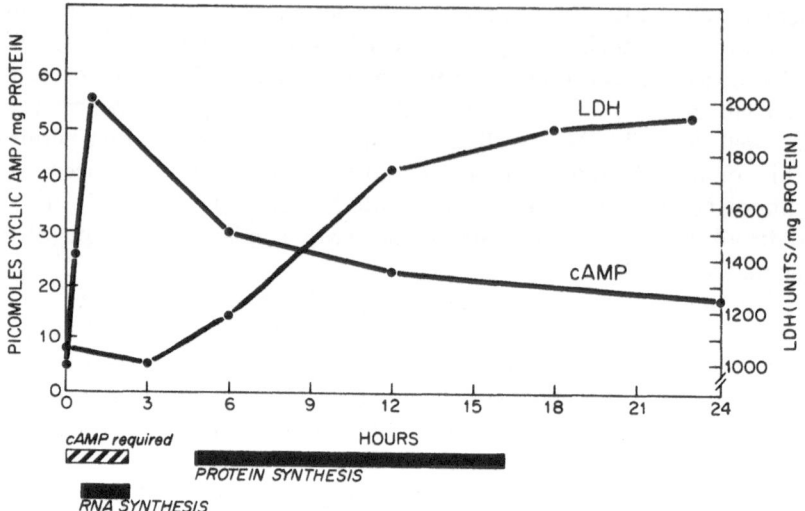

Fig. 4. Time course of cyclic AMP level and LDH induction in RGC6 cells following the addition of norepinephrine to the culture medium. Norepinephrine was added at a final concentration of 3×10^{-5} M. Cyclic AMP was measured using high-pressure anion exchange liquid chromatography (Brooker, 1970). LDH was assayed as previously indicated (de Vellis and Inglish, 1968). For other details, see text.

TABLE III

Effect of Catecholamines and Other Compounds on Cyclic AMP Level and LDH Activity in RGC6 Cells[a]

Treatment	Cyclic AMP (pmoles/mg protein, % control)	LDH (units/mg protein, % control)
Control	100	100
Tyramine, 3×10^{-5} M	90 ± 5	96 ± 3
Dopamine, 3×10^{-5} M	90 ± 6	98 ± 7
Histamine, 10^{-4} M	100 ± 8	101 ± 4
Adenosine, 1.25×10^{-4} M	100 ± 7	99 ± 3
Epinine, 3×10^{-5} M	400 ± 100	148 ± 11
Octopamine, 3×10^{-5} M	300 ± 80	141 ± 5
Phenylephrine, 3×10^{-5} M	320 ± 30	146 ± 5
Norepinephrine, 3×10^{-5} M	3500 ± 180	185 ± 9
Cortisol, 2.7×10^{-6} M	108 ± 10	110 ± 6

[a] All compounds were added to the culture medium at the indicated final concentrations. Cyclic AMP was measured 45 min later. LDH activity was determined at 24 hr in another set of cultures. For other details, see Fig. 4.

TABLE IV

Effect of α- and β-Blockers on the Action of Norepinephrine on RGC6 Cells

Treatments[a]	Cyclic AMP (pmoles/mg protein)	LDH (units/mg protein, % control)
Control	7 ± 3	100
NE	337 ± 32	213 ± 8
NE + propranolol	7 ± 2	117 ± 12
NE + dibenzyline	327 ± 95	225 ± 15

[a]All compounds were added to the culture medium at a final concentration of 3×10^{-5} M. Cyclic AMP was measured 45 min later. LDH activity was determined at 24 hr in another set of cultures. For other details, see Fig. 4. The effects of epinine, octopamine, and phenylephrine on cyclic AMP and LDH were similarly blocked by propranolol but not by dibenzyline.

(de Vellis *et al.*, 1971*b*). The periods during which RNA synthesis and protein synthesis are required are shown at the bottom of Fig. 4. Time zero represents the time of addition of norepinephrine. Actinomycin D was added at several points between 0 and 6 hr. Up to 30 min, blockage of LDH induction (measured at 24 hr) was total. At later times the inhibition decreased, and it disappeared at 2.5 hr. However, addition of acetoxycycloheximide, an inhibitor of protein synthesis, inhibited totally the induction when added at 5 hr. The requirement for protein synthesis parallels the rise in LDH activity. To find out the period during which cyclic AMP is required (Fig. 4), the following experiment was performed: The medium containing norepinephrine was removed at various times and replaced by fresh medium containing propranolol. This procedure was found to decrease the intracellular concentration of cyclic AMP to basal level in a few minutes. LDH was assayed at 24 hr. When the propranolol washout procedure was done after 2.5 hr, LDH induction was maximal, but at earlier times there was inhibition of the induction, suggesting that an elevated level of cyclic AMP is necessary only during the first 2.5 hr., i.e., during the *de novo* RNA synthesis period and not during the period of protein synthesis. Therefore, it appears that the magnitude of the LDH induction depends not only on the magnitude of the rise in cyclic AMP but also on its duration. In other words, a transient rise in cyclic AMP of very short duration would not result in LDH induction.

The isoenzymes of LDH present in RGC6 cells are V (MMMM), IV, and III. The induction by catecholamines shifts this pattern further toward V so that the increase in activity is the result of accumulation of more M than H subunits (Yu and de Vellis, 1973).

Catecholamines have other metabolic effects on RGC6 cells. The uptake of amino acid analogues, such as aminoisobutyric acid, is increased. The effect appears to be mediated by cyclic AMP (Shinwari and de Vellis, 1972). Another metabolic effect was reported by Opler and Makman (1972): norepinephrine increases glycogenolysis in RGC6 cells. Histamine has a similar effect, but its action, unlike that of norepinephrine, is not blocked by propranolol. These results are rather interesting, since Gilman and Nirenberg (1971) and de Vellis and Brooker (1972) did not find an effect of histamine on cyclic AMP level.

V. DIFFERENTIAL SENSITIVITY OF GPDH AND LDH INDUCTIONS TO INHIBITORS OF RNA SYNTHESIS

Roeder and Rutter (1969, 1970) showed that three types of RNA polymerases may be separated from rat liver and sea urchin embryo nuclei on the basis of chromatographic properties and sensitivity to ions. RNA polymerase I is localized in the nucleolus and is responsible for the synthesis of ribosomal RNA. RNA polymerases II and III are situated in the nucleoplasm and synthesize giant nuclear heterogeneous RNA (Zylber and Penman, 1971). In

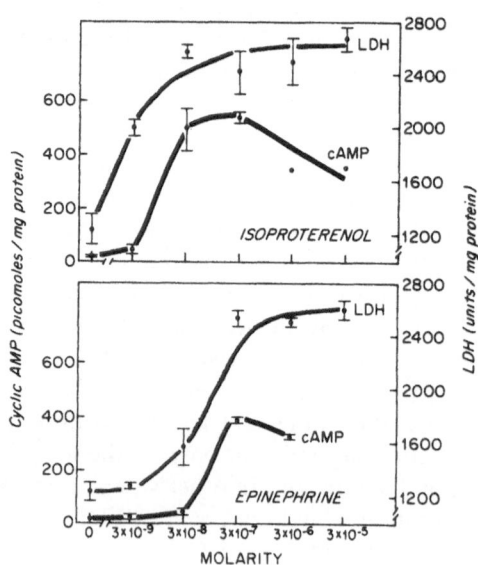

Fig. 5.   Effect of isoproterenol and epinephrine concentration on cyclic AMP and LDH levels of RGC6 cells. Cyclic AMP was measured 45 min after addition to the culture medium of the indicated concentrations of epinephrine and isoproterenol. LDH activity was measured at 24 hr on another set of cultures.

isolated nuclei of RGC6 cells, we showed the presence of three RNA polymerases (de Vellis and Inglish, 1972) using the method of Zylber and Penman
(1971). The existence of specific inhibitors of the RNA polymerases made it
possible to ask which polymerase(s) synthesizes the RNA required for GPDH
and LDH inductions. RNA polymerase II is specifically inhibited by
α-amanitin, while the other two enzymes are not affected even at very high
concentrations (Lindell et al., 1970). A low level of actinomycin D(AMD), 0.04
μg/ml, inhibits ribosomal RNA synthesis but not giant nuclear heterogeneous
RNA (Penman et al., 1968).

GPDH induction is inhibited by α-amanitin, whereas LDH induction is
totally insensitive (Table V). Inhibition of ribosomal RNA synthesis reduces
GPDH induction but not LDH. This leaves RNA polymerase III to synthesize
RNA necessary for LDH induction. That RNA is required for LDH induction
is indicated not only by the inhibitory effect of actinomycin D added at 1
μg/ml but also by that of cordycepin, an inhibitor of mRNA synthesis
(Penman et al., 1970). Ethidium bromide, an inhibitor of mitochondrial
RNA synthesis (Zylber et al., 1969), has no effect on GPDH or LDH induction. The sensitivity of GPDH induction of low levels of actinomycin D
suggests that either GPDH induction requires de novo rRNA synthesis in
addition to mRNA synthesis or that the genes coding for GPDH have a high
affinity for actinomycin D, like rRNA genes.

The interpretation of results obtained with inhibitors of RNA and
protein synthesis depends on their presumed specificity of action. Therefore,
several important parameters of the two inductions were studied. Inhibitors
had no effect on the nuclear uptake and retention of cortisol-H^3, a prerequisite

TABLE V

Effect of Inhibitors of RNA Synthesis on LDH and GPDH Induction in RGC6 Cells[a]

Treatments	GPDH (units/mg protein, % control)	LDH (units/mg protein, % control)
Control	100	100
Induced (NE + cortisol)	350 ± 30	205 ± 20
α-Amanitin (10^{-5} M)	145 ± 11	210 ± 25
AMD (0.05 μg/ml)	165 ± 5	207 ± 12
AMD (1 μg/ml)	101 ± 6	98 ± 7
Cordycepin (2 × 10^{-4} M)	180 ± 8	145 ± 12
Ethidium bromide (1 μg/ml)	360 ± 1	213 ± 8

[a]Compounds were added to the culture medium at the indicated final concentrations. NE and cortisol were added as in Table II. GPDH and LDH were assayed at 24 hr. AMD = actinomycin D.

for the induction of GPDH. Inhibitors did not prevent the rise in cyclic AMP caused by addition of catecholamines. The effect of inhibitors on incorporation of leucine-1-C^{14} and uridine-C^{14} correlated with their presumed action. In conclusion, our results suggest that *de novo* RNA synthesis for GPDH is transcribed by RNA polymerase II and that for LDH by RNA polymerase III (de Vellis and Inglish, 1972). The RNAs may be transcribed from the structural or the regulatory genes of these two enzymes. At the present time, it is not possible to distinguish between these two alternatives.

VI. CONCLUSIONS

The RGC6 cell line may be put to further use to compare and contrast the mechanisms of action of glucocorticoids and catecholamines, which represent two classes of hormones since the latter but not the former acts via cyclic AMP. It is not known where glucocorticoids bind in cell nuclei and what is the sequence of events which finally results in enzyme induction. The model of Jacob and Monod for enzyme induction in bacteria has not been proven for hormones in mammalian cells. Because of this, Tomkins *et al.* (1969) proposed a model which is based on a modification of mRNA turnover. By some unknown mechanism, the inducer would increase the stability of mRNA. Direct evidence for this scheme is still lacking. As for catecholamines, it would be important to determine if LDH (or other enzymes) induction is the result of activation of protein kinase(s) by cyclic AMP (or of some unknown effect of cyclic AMP). If the cyclic AMP effect is mediated by a protein kinase, how is specificity achieved? Is it by phosphorylation of a histone or an acidic protein? The diversity of acidic proteins could provide specificity in activation of genes.

It has not been established yet that the effects of catecholamines on human and rat glial tumor cell lines represent functions of normal glial cells *in vivo*. However, it is tempting to speculate that these functions, like S100 protein and GPDH induction, represent specialized properties of nervous tissue which have been retained by cultured tumor cells. A glial adenylcyclase sensitive to one and perhaps several compounds known to be present in neurons would provide a mechanism to coordinate glial metabolism with that of neurons.

The loss of inducibility of GPDH in somatic cell hybrids (RGC6–3T3 cells) (Davidson and Benda, 1970) and when cells are grown in medium containing bromodeoxyuridine (Lyons and de Vellis, unpublished data) shows that GPDH induction shares many of the general characteristics of differentiated functions.

GPDH induction is probably a function of glial cells, for the following reasons: First, the induction occurs in all brain regions, a property more consistent with the fact that glial cells appear to be the same everywhere in the brain while neurons vary greatly morphologically and functionally. Second, cortisol-H³ binding has been seen by autoradiography in only a few types of neurons (McEwen *et al.*, 1970; Gerlach and McEwen, 1972). Neurons in all brain regions should have shown uptake of cortisol if GPDH induction were to be neuronal. Glial cell nuclei show concentration of cortisol-H³ in autoradiograms (Gasser, personal communication). Third, GPDH induction occurs in RGC6 cells, which have no property of neurons but contain S100 protein, a putative glial marker. Finally, GPDH development occurs late following glial proliferation. Its developmental pattern (de Vellis *et al.*, 1967) resembles that of S100 protein (Herschman *et al.*, 1971) and carbonic anhydrase (Millichop, 1957). Carbonic anhydrase is also considered a glial marker (Giacobini, 1964). However, RGC6 cells do not appear to have this enzyme.

VII. REFERENCES

Benda, P., Lightbody, L., Sato, G., Levine, L., and Sweet, W. 1968. Differentiated rat glial cell strain in tissue culture. *Science* **161**:370.

Brooker, G. 1970. Determination of picomole amounts of enzymatically formed adenosine 3',5'-cyclic monophosphate by high pressure anion exchange chromatography. *Anal. Chem.* **42**:1108–1110.

Clark, R. B., and Perkins, J. P. 1971. Regulation of adenosine 3', 5'-cyclic monophosphate concentration in cultured human astrocytoma cells by catecholamines and histamine. *Proc. Natl. Acad. Sci.* **68**:2757–2760.

Clark, R. B., and Perkins, J. P. 1972. The effect of adenosine on the formation of cyclic AMP in cultured human astrocytoma cells. *Fed. Proc.* **31**:513 (abst.).

Davidson, R. L., and Benda, P. 1970. Regulation of specific functions of glial cells in somatic hybrids, II. Control of inducibility of glycerol-3-phosphate dehydrogenase. *Proc. Natl. Acad. Sci.* **67**:1870–1877.

de Vellis, J. 1971. *In* Contributions of Clonal Systems to Neurobiology. Neuroscience Research Program, March 1971 (in press).

de Vellis, J., and Brooker, G. 1972. Effect of catecholamines on cultured glial cells: Correlation between cyclic AMP levels and lactic dehydrogenase induction. *Fed. Prod.* **31**:513.

de Vellis, J., and Clemente, C. D. 1970. Neural cell differentiation, pp. 529–574. *In* O. A. Schjeide and J. de Vellis (eds.). Cell Differentiation. Van Nostrand Reinhold, New York.

de Vellis, J., and Inglish, D. 1968. Hormonal control of glycerolphosphate dehydrogenase in the rat brain. *J. Neurochem.* **15**:1061–1070.

de Vellis, J., and Inglish, D. 1969. Glycerolphosphate dehydrogenase induction in a cloned glial cell culture by glucocorticoids, pp. 151–152. Second Internat. Meet. Soc. Neurochem., Milan, Italy.

de Vellis, J., and Inglish, D. 1972. Hormonal induction of enzymes in cultured glial cells: Differential inhibition by α-amanitin, cordycepin, and actinomycin D. *In Vitro* **7**:247.

de Vellis, J., and Inglish, D. 1973. Age-dependent changes in the regulation of glycerolphosphate dehydrogenase in the rat brain and in a glial cell line. *Progr. Brain Res.* **40**.

de Vellis, J., Schjeide, O. A., and Clemente, C. D. 1967. Protein synthesis and enzymic patterns in the developing brain following head X-irradiation of newborn rats. *J. Neurochem.* **14**:499–511.

de Vellis, J., Inglish, D., and Galey, F. 1971a. Effects of cortisol and epinephrine on glial cells in culture, pp. 23–32. *In* D. Pease (ed.). Cellular Aspects of Growth and Differentiation in Nervous Tissue. ULCA Forum in Medical Sciences, No. 14, University of California Press, Berkeley.

de Vellis, J., Inglish, D., Cole, R., and Molson, J. 1971b. Effects of hormones on the differentiation of cloned lines of neurons and glial cells, pp. 25–39. *In* D. Ford (ed.). Influence of Hormones on the Nervous System. Karger, Basel.

Gerlach, J. L., and McEwen, B. S. 1972. Rat brain binds adrenal steroid hormone: Radioautography of hippocampus with corticosterone. *Science* **175**:1133–1136

Giacobini, E. 1964. Metabolic relations between glia and neurons studied in single cells, pp. 15–38. *In* M. M. Cohen and R. S. Snider (eds.). Morphological and Biochemical Correlates of Neural Activity. Harper & Row, New York.

Gilman, A. G., and Nirenberg, M. 1971. Effect of catecholamines on the adenosine 3', 5' cyclic AMP concentrations of clonal satellite cells of neurons. *Proc. Natl. Acad. Sci.* **68**:2165–2168.

Herschman, H. R., Levine, L., and de Vellis, J. 1971. Appearance of a brain-specific antigen (S-100 protein) in the developing rat brain. *J. Neurochem.* **18**:629–633.

Lindell, T. J., Weinberg, F., Morris, P. W., Roeder, R. G., and Rutter, W. J. 1970. Specific inhibition of nuclear RNA polymerase II by α-amanitin. *Science* **170**:447–449.

McEwen, B. S., Weiss, J. M., and Schwartz, L. S. 1970. Retention of corticosterone by cell nuclei from brain regions of adrenalectomized rats. *Brain Res.* **17**:471–482.

McGinnis, J. F. and de Vellis, J. 1973. Purification and hormonal regulation of brain glycerolphosphate dehydrogenase *in vivo* and in a rat glial cell line. Fed. Proc. **32**(3): 604.

Millichop, J. G. 1957. Development of seizure patterns in newborn animals. Significance of brain carbonic anhydrase. *Prod. Soc. Exptl. Biol. Med.* **96**:125–129.

Opler, L. A., and Makman, M. H. 1972. Mediation by cyclic AMP of hormone-stimulated glycogenolysis in cultured rat astrocytoma cells. *Biochem. Biophys. Res. Commun.* **46**: 1140–1145.

Penman, S., Vesco, C., and Penman, M. 1968. Localization and kinetics of formation of nuclear heterodisperse RNA, cytoplasmic heterodisperse RNA and polyribosome-associated messenger RNA in HeLa cells. *J. Molec. Biol.* **34**:49–69.

Penman, S., Rosbach, M., and Penman, M. 1970. Messenger and heterogenous nuclear RNA in HeLa cells: Differential inhibition by cordycepin. *Proc. Natl. Acad. Sci.* **67**: 1878–1885.

Pfeiffer, S. E., Herschman, H. R., Lightbody, J., and Sato, G. 1970. Synthesis by a clonal line of rat glial cells of a protein unique to the nervous system. *J. Cell. Physiol.* **75**: 329–340.

Robison, G. A., Butcher, R. W., and Sutherland, E. W. 1971. Cyclic AMP. Academic Press, New York.

Roeder, R. G., and Rutter, W. J. 1969. Multiple forms of DNA-dependent RNA polymerase in eukaryotic organisms. *Nature* **224**:234–237.

Roeder, R. G., and Rutter, W. J. 1970. Specific nucleolar and nucleoplasmic RNA polymerases. *Proc. Natl. Acad. Sci.* **65**:675–682.

Shinwari, M. A., and de Vellis, J. 1972. Effects of cortisol and norepinephrine on the uptake of analogs of amino acids and glucose into cultured glial cells, p. 121, Third Meet. Am. Soc. Neurochem., Seattle.

Tomkins, G. M., Gelehrter, T. D., Granner, D., Martin, D., Samuels, H. H., and Thompson, E. B. 1969. Control of specific gene expression in higher organisms. *Science* **166**:1474–1480.

Yu, G. and de Vellis, J. 1973. The effect of norepinephrine and dibutyryl cyclic AMP on lactate dehydrogenase isozymes in a rat glial cell line. *Trans. 3rd Meeting Amer. Soc. Neurochem.* P. 145, Columbus, Ohio.

Zylber, E. A., and Penman, S. 1971. Products of RNA polymerases in HeLa cell nuclei. *Proc. Natl. Acad. Sci.* **68**:2861–2865.

Zylber, E., Vesco, C., and Penman, S. 1969. Selective inhibition of the synthesis of mitochondria-associated RNA by ethidium bromide. *J. Molec. Biol.* **44**:195–204.

Chapter 11

The Metabolism of Glycosphingolipids and Glycosaminoglycans

Allen C. Stoolmiller, Glyn Dawson, and Albert Dorfman

Departments of Pediatrics and Biochemistry, LaRabida–
University of Chicago Institute
and
Joseph P Kennedy, Jr. Mental Retardation Research Center
Pritzker School of Medicine
University of Chicago, Chicago, Illinois

I. INTRODUCTION

The role of complex carbohydrate-containing substances in cell physiology has attracted increased attention as a result of the appreciation of their importance in cell-surface phenomena and the existence of a large number of heritable diseases characterized by defects in degradation of these substances. In general, the hexosamine-containing macromolecules of eukaryotic cells may be classified as glycosphingolipids, glycoproteins, and glycosaminoglycans. Since there is no available information concerning the synthesis of glycoproteins by clonal lines derived from the nervous system in tissue culture, the metabolism of this class of substances will not be considered in this chapter.

The extensive literature regarding the glycosphingolipids of the central nervous system has been reviewed many times (Svennerholm, 1964; O'Brien and Sampson, 1965; Ledeen, 1966; Sweeley and Dawson, 1969; Stoffel, 1971). Despite the numerous investigations of glycosphingolipid composition, struc-

Original investigations referred to in this chapter were supported by grants from the following sources: USPHS No. AM-05996, USPHS No. HD-04583, USPHS No. HD-06426, State of Illinois, Department of Mental Health No. 116–13-RD, and USPHS Training Grant 5-TO5-GM-01939. G. D. is a Joseph P. Kennedy, Jr. Scholar.

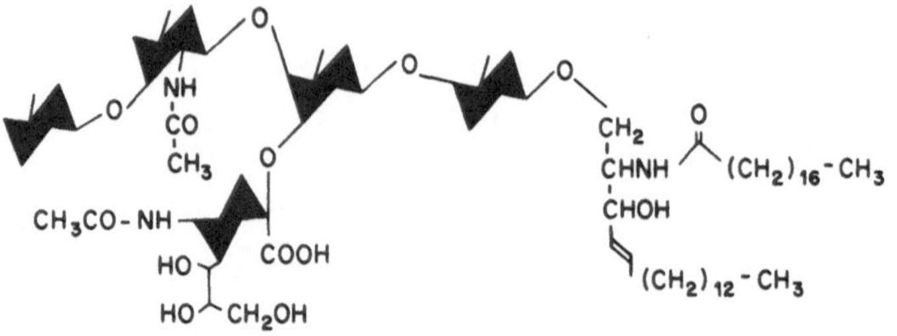

Gal β (1→3) GalNAc β (1→4) Gal β (1→4) Glc - Ceramide (G_{M1})

$$\alpha \begin{pmatrix} 3 \\ \uparrow \\ 2 \end{pmatrix}$$

neuNAc

Fig. 1. Structure of the major brain monosialoganglioside, G_{M1}.

ture, and biosynthesis in neural tissues, there is as yet little specific information regarding localization (with the exception of cerebrosides in myelin), cells of origin, and physiological functions of this group of compounds. In the case of the glycosaminoglycans, only recently have satisfactory data been accumulated with respect to the nature and concentration of glycosaminoglycans in the nervous system. The availability of clonal cell strains makes possible the study of the cell of origin, the intracellular localization, and possibly the functions of the both glycosaminoglycans and glycosphingolipids. Studies reported in this chapter have been carried out with cell strains derived from tumors and are therefore subject to the same limitations that have been extensively discussed elsewhere in this volume. In general, such studies on tumors reveal the potentiality of cells to carry out synthetic reactions, but negative results must be interpreted with caution both because the cells are derived from tumors and because studies are performed under conditions which may not permit expression of all of the biochemical potential of the cells in question.

II. GLYCOSPHINGOLIPIDS

A. Glycosphingolipids of the Nervous System

Of the two major types of glycosphingolipids associated with the central nervous system, cerebroside (galactosylceramide) and its sulfate ester, sulfatide, are characteristic of white matter, and gangliosides of gray matter. Both of these types of glycosphingolipids are virtually absent from extraneural tissues and therefore have potential value as markers for cells of neural origin in tissue culture.

Galactosylceramide has the structure galactosyl-β-(1→1)-N-acylsphingosine (Shapiro and Flowers, 1961) and together with sulfatide is a major component of the myelin sheath. However, apart from its strong haptenic properties (Rapport and Graf, 1969), little is known of its biological role. In common with most brain lipids, it is rapidly metabolized during myelination. An inherited deficiency of galactosylceramide-β-D-galactosidase (globoid cell leukodystrophy) leads to rapid neurological degeneration and demyelination (Suzuki and Suzuki, 1970). This condition is simulated experimentally by the intracerebral injection of galactosylceramide to produce the so-called globoid-cell response (Austin and Lehfeldt, 1965). Studies on whole brain and purified myelin suggest that galactosylceramide and sulfatide are important metabolic products of glial cells and, more specifically, oligodendroglial cells (Poduslo and Norton, 1972; O'Brien and Sampson, 1965).

Gangliosides share a common lipid moiety (ceramide) with galactosylceramide, but the more complex oligosaccharide chain is linked through glucose instead of galactose and contains N-acetylneuraminic acid (sialic acid) and N-acetylgalactosamine. Gangliosides were first isolated by Klenk (see Svennerholm, 1964; Ledeen, 1966). The structures of at least eight different gangliosides, whose basic structure is that of monosialoganglioside, G_{M1}[1] (Fig. 1), have now been established in a number of laboratories (Ledeen, 1966; Wiegandt, 1970). The presence of from one to three sialic acid residues confers hydrophilic properties on gangliosides. They are assumed to be bound to the plasma membrane, but there is recent evidence that they are rapidly transported along axons in goldfish (Forman and Ledeen, 1972). A role in neuronal function has been suggested by their relatively high concentration in gray matter (tenfold that in white matter), their enrichment in synaptosomal membrane fractions, and the intraneuronal accumulation of G_{M1} and G_{M2} in certain inherited storage diseases. In contrast to this association of gangliosides with neuronal perikarya and dendrites, myelin has a very low ganglioside content, probably restricted to G_{M1} ganglioside (Suzuki et al., 1968). Further, glial cells in diseases such as Tay-Sachs disease do not appear to store appreciable levels of gangliosides until late in the disease process.

[1]Abbreviations used are Cer, ceramide; Gal, galactose; GalNAc, N-acetylgalactosamine; Glc, glucose; GlcNAc, N-acetylglucosamine; GlcUA, glucuronic acid; IdUA, iduronic acid; neuNAc, N-acetylneuraminic acid (sialic acid); PAPS, phosphoadenylylsulfate; Xyl, xylose; G_{M3}, neuNAc-(2 → 3)-Gal-(1→4)-Glc-Cer; G_{M2}, neuNAc-(2→3)-[GalNAc-(1→4)-] Gal-(1→4)-Glc-Cer; G_{M1}, neuNAc-(2→3)-[Gal-(1→3)-GalNAc-(1→4)-] Gal-(1→4)-Glc-Cer; G_{D1a}, neuNAc-2(→3)-[neuNAc-(2→3)-Gal-(1→3)-GalNAc-(1→4)-]Gal-(1→4)-Glc-Cer; G_{D2}, neuNAc-(2→8)-neuNAc-(2→3)-[GalNAc-(1→4)-] Gal-(1→4)-Glc-Cer; G_{D3}, neuNAc-(2→8)-neuNAc-(2→3)-Gal-(1→4)-Glc-Cer.

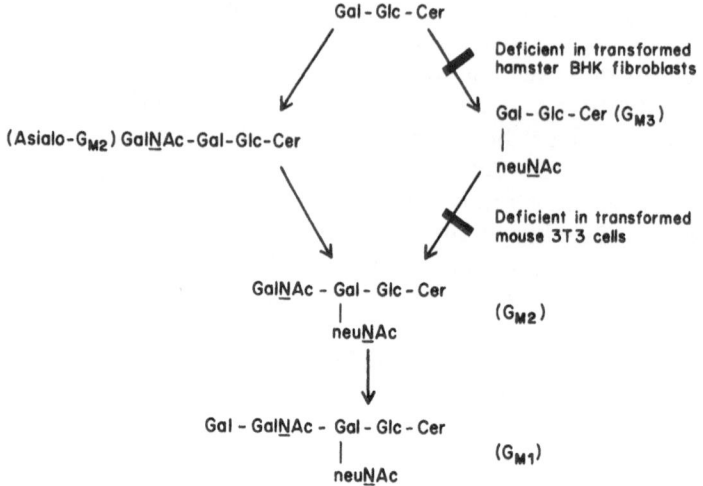

Fig. 2. Metabolic scheme for pathways of ganglioside biosynthesis.

B.   Biosynthesis of Glycosphingolipids

Considerable progress has been made in delineating the mechanism of biosynthesis of glycosphingolipids. Figure 2 shows the presently accepted pathways, largely derived from *in vitro* studies on chick, rat, and frog brain (Kaufman *et al.*, 1967; Maccioni *et al.*, 1972; DiCesare and Dain, 1972). It is generally accepted that multienzyme complexes are involved in their synthesis, and although there is evidence for the existence of specific transferases, studies of this kind actually involve the transfer of monosaccharide to purified glycolipid acceptor by crude particulate enzyme fractions in the presence of detergent.

Two alternative pathways theoretically exist for the synthesis of G_{M2} ganglioside from lactosylceramide, and both the intermediates, G_{M3} and asialo-G_{M2} are found in NB41A and NB2a neuroblastoma cell strains. *In vitro* studies on whole brain indicate that G_{M3} is the most likely intermediate even though chemically it is virtualy undetectable in normal gray or white matter. In contrast, G_{M3} is often the major glycosphingolipid in extraneural tissue. For this reason, we have defined a "ganglioside" as a glycolipid containing both hexosamine and sialic acid in order to specifically exclude G_{M3} from this classification. However, in many previous reports, the term "ganglioside" is used ambiguously and often refers to the sialic acid extractable by lipid solvents and may even contain glycoprotein. One possible distinction between tissue of neural origin and that of visceral origin may therefore reside in the presence or absence of gangliosides. However, this apparent distinction is complicated by the report that mouse 3T3 cells contain significant levels of G_{M2} G_{M1}, and G_{D1a} gangliosides. Following transformation by oncogenic viruses, these cells become deficient in G_{M3}: N-acetylgalactosaminyltransferase (Fig. 2) (Mora *et al.*, 1969; Fishman *et al.*, 1972) and the ganglioside level is greatly reduced (Yogeeswaran *et al.*, 1972). The cell type from which mouse 3T3 cells were derived is unknown and could conceivably be of neurological origin. In contrast, a similar viral transformation of baby hamster (BHK) fibroblasts resulted in a deficiency of the lactosylceramide: sialotransferase (Den *et al.*, 1971) as shown in Fig. 2; BHK fibroblasts do not contain gangliosides (Dawson *et al.*, 1972a).

Galactosylceramide biosynthesis reaches a maximum at the time of myelination, and the glycolipid is probably all derived from the transfer of galactose from UDP-galactose to ceramide (Radin, 1970). The alternative pathway involving initial galactosylation of sphingosine to form psychosine followed by condensation with acyl CoA is possible (Radin, 1970), but this reaction has not been convincingly demonstrated.

C.   Catabolism of Glycosphingolipids

Catabolism occurs by means of a pathway which is essentially the reverse of the biosynthetic pathway (Fig. 3), but the enzymes involved are, for the most part, soluble lysosomal hydrolases with an acid pH optimum of 4.0–5.0.

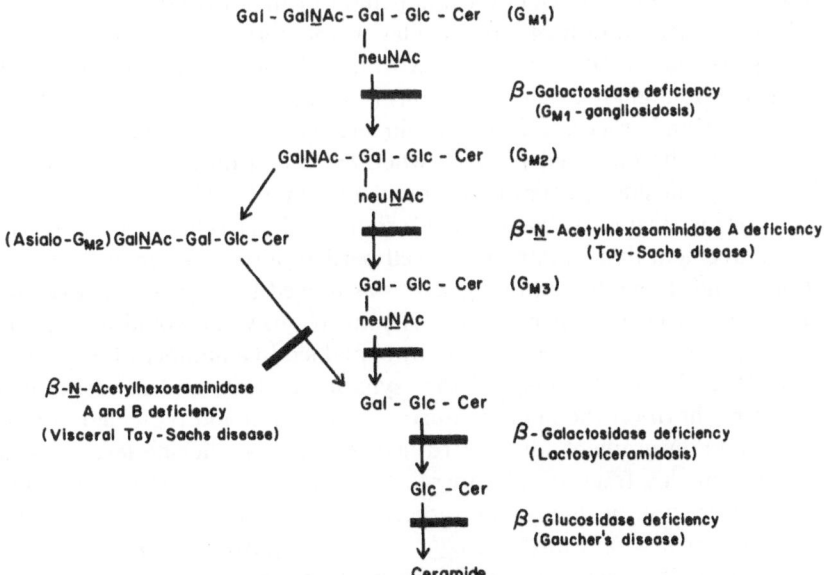

Fig. 3.   Scheme for the catabolism of gangliosides showing sites of metabolic blocks in certain inherited storage diseases.

There is considerable interest in the degradation of gangliosides because inherited defects (structural gene mutations) result in the virtual absence of activity of one of the hydrolases (Brady *et al.*, 1971), causing severe mental retardation and early death. Five of these are shown in Fig. 3, namely, G_{M1}-gangliosidosis, the two variants of Tay-Sachs disease, lactosylceramidosis, in which the neurons are grossly ballooned with storage material, and Gaucher's disease. There are two major white matter diseases involving glycolipids in which the myelin is destroyed, galactosylceramide-β-D-galactosidase deficiency (globoid cell leukodystrophy) and arylsulfatase A deficiency (metachromatic leukodystrophy).

D. Metabolism of Glycosphingolipids in Normal Nerve Cells

Because of the heterogeneity of the brain, it is essential to obtain preparations of pure cell types in order to study sites of synthesis and degradation and the biological role of brain-specific glycosphingolipids.

In recent years, improved techniques have permitted the bulk isolation of neuronal- and glial-rich fractions from normal whole brain. Derry and Wolfe (1967) isolated neurons and glia from Deiters' vestibular nucleus of the ox brain stem by the procedure of Hydén and Pigon (1960) and reported that the ganglioside concentration was highest in the neuropil and the membranes of the axon terminals and endings. This was confirmed by Wiegandt (1967), Lapetina *et al.* (1967) and Dekiremenjian and Burnngraber (1969), who found the highest concentration of gangliosides in the nerve endings, especially in the synaptosomal membranes and microsomes. However more recent studies on neuronal- and glial-enriched fractions (Norton and Poduslo, 1971; Tamai *et al.*, 1970; Hamberger and Svennerholm, 1971) did not show enrichment of ganglioside in the neuronal fraction when expressed on the basis of micromoles of "ganglioside" per gram of protein, percent of sialic acid per total lipid content, or picograms of "ganglioside" sialic acid per cell, respectively. The general agreement that isolated nerve cell perikarya (referred to as "neuronal fractions" and shown to be homogeneous as judged by microscopic examination) are not enriched in gangliosides is contrary to what would be expected from analyses of gray matter but may be explained in a number of ways. Norton and Poduslo (1971) observed that synaptic endings and dendrite membranes were shorn off the neurons during purification and remained in a discrete layer upon gradient ultracentrifugation; the ganglioside level was not determined in this fraction. Hamberger and Svennerholm (1971) also considered the possibility that ganglioside-rich membranes or free gangliosides were lost either mechanically or enzymically during isolation. However, they did not detect either gangliosides in the medium or evidence of catabolism.

Because of the use of trypsin in the isolation procedure and the absence of any physiological or biochemical evidence that these neuronal fractions contain viable neurons (electrical activity, biogenic amine synthesis, etc.), the reports of low ganglioside levels in neurons and relatively high levels in glial cells are not definitive. Further, attempts to culture these neuronal-rich fractions have been unsuccessful.

Fractionation techniques have been used by Norton and Poduslo (1971) and Hamberger and Svennerholm (1971) to isolate astroglia from rat brain. Both groups reported a very low "galactolipid" content for these cell preparations and a ganglioside content which was greater than that of neuronal perikarya. They ascribed this latter finding to the high ratio of surface membrane to mass in the astrocytes and concluded that gangliosides are normal glial cell constituents. In contrast, oligodendroglia preparations from bovine brain (Poduslo and Norton, 1972) had a high "galactolipid" content (10.9% of total lipids) but contained low levels of ganglioside. This is in keeping with the low level of gangliosides in white matter. However, the finding of gangliosides in astrocytes raises important questions about the concept of their localization in neurons which many not be explainable on the basis of contamination by axons and neuronal membranes. In all these studies, G_{M3}, which we exclude from our definition of a ganglioside, was included in the ganglioside fraction. As will be seen later, these results are also at variance with studies on normal and malignant astrocytes in tissue culture.

Many laboratories have been successful in culturing nervous tissue for short periods of time, but few studies of lipid metabolism in such cultures have been reported. Sourander et al. (1966) cultured retina cells and cerebellum from 2- to 14-day-old rats and observed a basal monolayer growth of large, thin mesenchymal cells, on the surface of which could be seen various neuroectodermal cells (neurons, astrocyte glial cells, rods, etc.). After 2 weeks, the retinal cultures were characterized by rapid and extensive outgrowth and flattening; cultures always showed the same type of stratification and cellular pattern. After 12 days, cells were exposed to emulsions or suspensions of various glycosphingolipids. Addition of glucosylceramide or galactosylceramide resulted in the appearance within 24 hr of mono- and multinucleated cells with an irregularly shaped, granulated cytoplasm. After 2–3 days, the cytoplasm became distended by an increasing number of granules, and the cells detached from the glass surface, became spherical, and often floated free in the nutrient medium. The accumulation of glycosphingolipid (demonstrated by PAS staining) was confined to the mesenchymal cell layer presumably derived mainly from the walls of the blood vessels, no PAS-positive cytoplasmic granules being observed in neurons, neuroglial cells, or rods.

The addition of emulsions of sulfatide to such cultures also resulted in an extensive PAS-positive reaction in the mesenchymal cell monolayer. These mesenchymal cells tended to float freely and then clump together; metachromatic granules were still seen in these cells up to 3 weeks after the addition of sulfatide. Although some astroglial cells occasionally showed metachromasia, such granules were seldom seen within the cytoplasm of neurons.

These experiments support the concept that in white matter diseases such as globoid cell leukodystrophy and metachromatic leukodystrophy the galactosylceramide and sulfatide, respectively, are stored in phagocytizing cells of mesenchymal origin (microglial cells and histiocytes). The inability of neurons to phagocytize these glycolipids is in agreement with histological studies on pathological tissue derived from patients with globoid cell leukodystrophy and metachromatic leukodystrophy. This series of experiments illustrates the usefulness of cultured nervous tissue in the study of certain aspects of glycosphingolipid metabolism. Provided that one can use specific histological stains, or the material is found in great excess, the problem of heterogeneity can be overcome by microscopic examination. However, the paucity of viable material is severely limiting for any kind of biochemical study of lipid metabolism, as evidenced by a recent report by Andrews et al. (1971) which illustrated the difficulties of attempting labeling studies with isotopic precursors.

The most successful approach for culturing "normal" cells of neurological origin has been that of Shein et al. (1970), who developed techniques for producing subcutaneous "normal" astroglial cell nodules in newborn hamsters and for preparing pure cultures of normal untransformed immature astrocytes in gram quantities. Identification was based on morphological and staining characteristics. When compared with the average cell of rat white matter, the average astroglial cell of the nodule contained 1/40 as much water-insoluble glycolipid (lipid hexose) and 1/19 as much ganglioside (measured only as lipid sialic acid). Similar comparison of astroglial cells with rat gray matter gave values of 1/16 for glycolipid and 1/44 for ganglioside. From these studies, it was concluded that oligodendrocytes (and therefore myelin) are the only type of neural elements which contain appreciable amounts of galactosylceramide and sulfatide and that neurons and their processes are the principal loci of gangliosides. This conclusion is at variance with the analyses of astroglial- and oligoderdroglial-rich fractions from rat brain but in agreement with our studies on tumor cell lines in culture.

Since tumors presumably arise from a single cell or "clone" of cells, analysis of glial tumors may reflect the composition of a normal glial cell. On the basis of thin layer chromatographic analysis, Christensen-Lou et al. (1965) reported that galactosylceramide was present in all samples of normal brain and in most glioblastomas but was absent from one of two astrocytomas and from all meningiomas, neurilemmomas, and metastatic tumors of the breast and cervix (Gopal et al., 1964). Studies by Slagel et al. (1967) revealed variable levels of galactosylceramide in a number of glioblastomas but showed for the first time that gangliosides (assayed by determination of hexosamine and sialic acid content) were constituents of both an astrocytoma and a glioblastoma. The ganglioside content was either equal to or less than the level in the surrounding tissue (no ganglioside enrichment). These studies were extended to include oligodendrogliomas by Christensen-Lou and Clausen (1968). When expressed as percent of the total polar lipids, the ceramide "monohexoside" (presumably galactosylceramide) content of four oligodendrogliomas was 23.5%, that of ten astrocytomas 12.6%, and that of ten glioblastomas 8.6%, whereas in white matter the content was 38.6%. Although no enrichment of galactosylceramide was found, these results tend to corroborate the involvement of oligodendroglia in myelin formation, but it is difficult to assess the significance of the lower levels in astrocytes. This report indicated that gangliosides and inositides were minor (3–5%) components of the polar lipid fraction.

In contrast to the considerable number of studies carried out on gliomas, little information is available on the glycolipid composition of neuroblastomas. We have recently examined a liver biopsy specimen containing neuroblastoma metastases. No attempt was made to excise the numerous tumor nodules from the surrounding hepatic tissue, but comparison with normal liver (Table I) revealed a significantly higher ganglioside content in the pathological liver, a finding consistent with the specific association of gangliosides with neurons.

E. Glycosphingolipid Metabolism in Cultured Cell Strains of Nervous System Origin

Difficulties in developing cell culture lines of neural origin have hampered study of the metabolism of specific cell types of the nervous system. The establishment of a cell strain from a chemically induced rat astrocytoma (Benda et al., 1968) and of a neuroblastoma cell line from a spontaneously occurring mouse neuroblastoma (Augusti-Tocco and Sato, 1969), described extensively in other portions of this volume, have facilitated the study of glycosphingolipid metabolism. More recently, a chemically induced schwannoma (Pfeiffer and Wechsler, 1972), described in Chapter 9, has also become available.

A study of the glycosphingolipid composition of the rat astrocytoma (RGC6) was conducted to determine the glycosphingolipid composition. Rat astrocytoma cells, grown in monolayer culture using modified Eagle's medium supplemented with fetal calf serum (10%), contained hematoside (G_{M3}) as the major glycosphingolipid and only small amounts of glycosylceramide, lactosylceramide, and disialohematoside (G_{D3}) (Dawson et al., 1971). The amount of G_{M3} per gram dry weight of cells was twofold greater at low cell density (2–3×10^6 per plate) than at high cell density (15×10^6 per plate), as shown

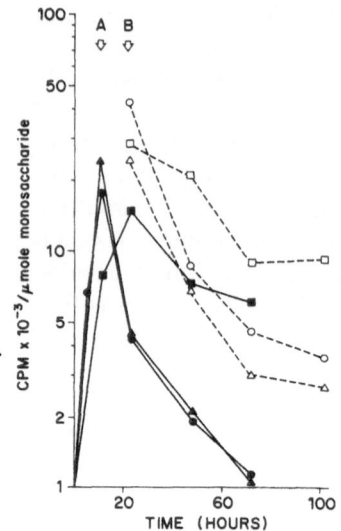

Fig. 4. Semilogarithmic plot showing incorporation of glucose-U-C^{14} into glucosylceramide (GL-1a, circles), lactosylceramide (GL-2a, triangles), and hematoside (G$_{M3}$, squares) of RGC6 astrocytoma cells grown in monolayer culture (modified Eagle's medium plus 10% fetal calf serum). In experiment A (open symbols), the labeled medium was replaced by normal medium after 12 hr. In experiment B (filled symbols), the labeled medium was replaced by fresh labeled medium after 12 hr and by normal medium after 24 hr.

in Table II. Biosynthetic studies (Fig. 4) have established the *de novo* synthesis of all three glycosphingolipids from glucose-C^{14}, thus eliminating the possibility that the glycosphingolipids found in these cells could be absorbed from the fetal calf serum. Subsequent studies (Embree *et al.*, 1972; Synder *et al.*, 1970) on rat "astrocytoma" cells and normal immature hamster brain astroglia cultured *in vitro* confirmed that G$_{M3}$ was the major glycosphingolipid in cultured astrocytes and that gangliosides, as we define them, were absent. Further, these authors concluded that if normal astrocytes *in vivo* are similar to the tumor astrocytes, they must contain about twice as much phospholipid as cholesterol (on a molar basis) and be low but not totally lacking in gangliosides and water-insoluble glycolipids such as galactosylceramide. This is in essential agreement with our studies on RGC6 and CHB4 (Stoolmiller *et al.*, 1972) astrocytoma cell strains.

The results seem to indicate that glial cells resemble fibroblasts in composition, as evidenced by the presence of relatively large amounts of G$_{M3}$ (hematoside) but little of the hexosamine-containing higher gangliosides. Interpretation of results with tumor-derived glial cells must again be tempered by considering the finding of Mora *et al.* (1969) and Yogeeswaran *et al.* (1972) that mouse 3T3 fibroblasts contain G$_{M2}$, G$_{M1}$, and G$_{D1a}$ but that after transformation with oncogenic virus the level of G$_{M3}$: hexosaminyltransferase activity is reduced and G$_{M3}$ becomes the major glycosphingolipid, as we find in RGC6.

In contrast to these results with RGC6, analyses of two cloned cell lines from a C1300 mouse neuroblastoma, NB41A and NB2a, showed the major glycosphingolipids to be the gangliosides G_{M2}, G_{M1}, and G_{D1a}. Previous studies on chick brain, rat brain, and mouse 3T3 fibroblasts (Kaufman *et al.*, 1967; Mora *et al.*, 1969; Maccioni *et al.*, 1971; Roseman, 1970) showed that G_{M3} is the intermediate in the biosynthesis of gangliosides from lactosylceramide. Initially, enzymic studies with NB41A particulate fractions were consistent with the existence of both pathways (Dawson *et al.*, 1972a), and evidence from chemical analysis supported this (Table III). However, the specific activities of these two enzymes altered with increasing passage number (up to 20) of the cells, the activity of the lactosylceramide-sialotransferase increasing (Stoolmiller and Bittner, 1972) and that of the lactosylceramide-hexosaminyl transferase declining. This could be attributed to differences in culture conditions (serum, etc.) and was confirmed by analysis of the glycosphingolipid con-

TABLE I

Glycosphingolipids in Liver Metastasized with Neuroblastoma

Glycolipid	Control[a]	NB liver[a]
Glucosylceramide	5	7
Galactosylceramide	<0.5	0.5
Lactosylceramide	6	8
Trihexosylceramide	3	2
Globoside	2	1
G_{M3}	15	14
G_{M2}	0	3
G_{M1}	0	3
G_{D3}	2	3
G_{D2}	0	6
G_{D1a}	0	12

[a]Expressed as μmoles/100g fresh weight.

TABLE II

Effect of Cell Density on the Glycosphingolipid Content[a] of
RGC6 Astrocytoma Cells in Culture

Glycolipid	Days in subculture[b]		
	4	7	10
Glucosylceramide	0.82	0.56	0.53
Lactosylceramide	0.63	0.35	0.25
G_{M3}	4.70	2.05	1.80

[a]In μmoles/g dry weight.
[b]Cell densities were approximately 2×10^6, 10×10^6, and 15×10^6 cells/100-mm Falcon dish. Approximately the same weight of cells was used for each determination.

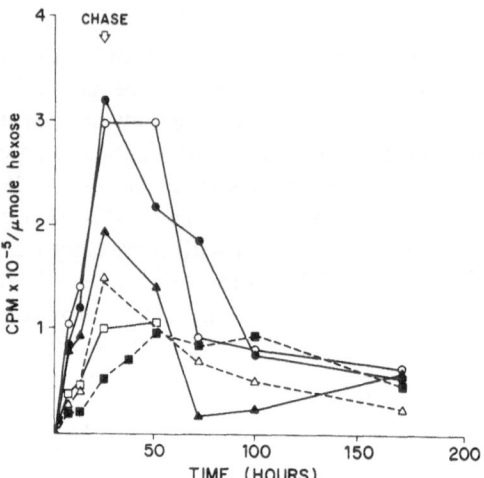

Fig. 5.　Incorporation of glucose-U-C[14] into glucosylceramide (GL-1a) and lactosylcer-amide (GL-2a) (open squares), asialo-G_{M2} (filled squares), G_{M3} (open triangles), G_{M2} (filled triangles), G_{M1} (open circles), and G_{D1a} (filled circles) of C1300 mouse NB41A cells grown in monolayer culture (modified Eangle's medium plus 10% fetal calf serum). The C[14] label was removed after 24 hr.

TABLE III

Effect of High Passage Number on the Glycosphingolipid Content[a] of NB41A
Neuroblastoma Cells and Its Partial Reversal by Cyclic AMP
and Serum-Free Medium

Glycolipid	NB41A (low passage)	NB41A (high passage)	NB41A (high passage + cyclic AMP)	NB41A (high passage in serum-free medium)
Glucosylceramide	0.25	0.13	0.27	0.41
Lactosylceramide	0.14	0.12	0.23	0.18
Asial-G_{M2}	0.35	0.06	0.32	0.20
Tetrahexosylceramide	0.49	0.08	0.17	0.13
G_{M3}	0.05	0.27	0.18	0.30
G_{M2}	0.43	0.33	0.68	0.82
G_{M1}	0.06	0.09	0.19	0.19
G_{D1a}	0.29	0.21	0.38	0.40
G_{D2}	0.06	0.03	0.06	0.06

[a]In μmoles/g dry weight.

tent of the cells (Table III). The phenomenon was partly reversed (Table III) by culture in serum-free modified Eagle's medium or in normal medium containing dibutyryl cyclic AMP (5×10^{-5} M), both of which have been observed to increase neurite formation. This increased degree of neurite formation appeared to be accompanied by an increased ganglioside concentration, which can be explained by the increased ratio of surface area to cell volume. Such observations emphasize the care required in carrying out metabolic studies with cell strains in continuous culture.

In vivo labeling studies using glucose-C^{14} as precursor have failed to resolve the question of the alternative pathways for ganglioside synthesis, since the specific activity of both G_{M3} and asialo-G_{M2} failed to equal that of the more complex gangliosides (G_{M2}, G_{M1}, or G_{D1a}), as shown in Fig. 5. This apparent inability to detect precursor–product relationships can be explained if one assumes that the pool size of an intermediate in a multienzyme reaction complex is small and that a separate multienzyme complex exists for the synthesis of each ganglioside. Such an explanation has been proposed by Maccioni *et al.* (1971) on the basis of biosynthetic studies using rat brain preparations. The advantage of using neuroblastoma lines for these studies appears to lie in the presence in the cells of likely precursors (glucosylceramide, lactosylceramide, G_{M3}, and asialo-G_{M2}), whereas in mammalian brain G_{M1} is often the simplest ganglioside present in significant amounts and G_{M2} is often less than 2% of the total ganglioside.

The studies carried out on RGC6 and NB41A cell strains have indicated that glycosphingolipids containing both sialic acid and *N*-acetylgalactosamine (gangliosides) are typical of neurons and do not occur to any significant extent in astrocytes. Recent preliminary studies on a rat schwannoma cell line, RN2 (Pfeiffer and Wechsler, 1972), have indicated a lack of gangliosides and the presence of G_{M3}, as found in RGC6. In addition, large amounts of the myelin-specific glycolipid galactosylceramide (together with smaller amounts of sulfatide) were found (Pfeiffer and Dawson, 1972), which is in keeping with the schwannoma cell origin of peripheral myelin. These observations have been complemented by a recent study on ganglioside biosynthesis in neuronal-enriched and glial-enriched fractions of rat brain (Jones *et al.*, 1972). It was found that *N*-acetyl neuraminic acid-4-C^{14} was incorporated into gangliosides to a far greater extent in neuronal-enriched fractions. In contrast, sterol synthesis was almost negligible in neuronal-rich fractions compared to glial-rich fractions.

Such studies point out the usefulness of tissue culture of individual nerve cell types in the study of glycosphingolipid metabolism in the brain. The major task to be overcome is the resolution of discrepanicies in glycosphingolipid analysis of neuronal- glial-, and oligodendroglial-rich fractions *vs.* cloned cell strains in tissue culture.

TABLE IV

Composition of Glycosaminoglycans

Name	Sugar constituents	O-Sulfate	N-Sulfate	Linkage Uronidic	Linkage Hexosaminidic	Glycosidic linkage to protein
Hyaluronic acid	D-Glucuronic acid N-Acetyl-D-glucosamine	−	−	β 1→3	β 1→4	
Chondroitin-4-sulfate	D-Glucuronic acid N-Acetyl-D-galactosamine	+	−	β 1→3	β 1→4	Xyl-Ser
Chondroitin-6-sulfate	D-Glucuronic and L-iduronic acids N-Acetyl-D-galactosamine	+	−	β 1→3	β 1→4	Xyl-Ser
Deramtan sulfate	D-Glucuronic and L-iduronic acids N-Acetyl-D-galactosamine	+		α 1→3	β 1→4	Xyl-Ser
Heparan sulfates and heparin	D-Glucuronic and L-iduronic acids N-Acetyl-D-glucosamine	+	Few	β 1→4 α 1→4	α 1→4	Xyl-Ser
Keratan sulfate I[a]	D-Galactose N-Acetyl-D-glucosamine	Few	+	β 1→4	β 1→4	GlcNAc-AspNH₂
Keratan sulfate II[a]	D-Galactose N-Acetyl-D-glucosamine N-Acetyl-D-galactosamine	+	−	β 1→4	β 1→4	GalNAc-Thr GalNAc-Ser

[a] In addition to the principal monosaccharides, mannose, fucose, and sialic acid also occur.

III. GLYCOSAMINOGLYCANS

A. Chemistry of Glycosaminoglycans

Glycosaminoglycans occur singly or in mixtures together with other macromolecules of the matrix of connective tissues. The long-standing uncertainty regarding the extracellular compartment of the central nervous system has beclouded the interpretation of studies of the glycosaminoglycan composition. However, recent studies leave little doubt as to the presence of specific types of glycosaminoglycans in the brain.

The substances in animal tissues most often classified as glycosaminoglycans include the following: hyaluronic acid, chondroitin-4- and -6-sulfates, dermatan sulfate, keratan sulfates I and II, heparan sulfates, and heparin. The monosaccharide constituents of the glycosaminoglycans and their known linkages are given in Table IV. Hyaluronic acid is a polymer composed of alternating units of D-glucuronic acid and N-acetylglucosamine. The repeating disaccharides of the chondroitin-4- and -6-sulfates are comprised of D-glucuronic acid and N-acetyl-D-galactosamine and differ from each other only with respect to the positions of the ester-sulfate on the hexosamine moeity. Dermatan sulfate is unlike the chondroitin sulfates in that its predominant uronosyl moieties are L-iduronic acid, although D-glucuronic acid is present in variable amounts (Fransson and Rodén, 1967a, b). The keratan sulfates, which contain no uronic acid, are composed principally of repeating disaccharide units of N-acetylglucosamine and galactose. At least two types of keratan sulfate have been distinguished, type I in cornea and type II in skeletal tissues. In addition to the principal monosaccharides, mannose, fucose, sialic acid, and N-acetylgalactosamine have been found in keratan sulfates, although the last sugar has been found only in keratan sulfate II. Sulfate is present in variable amounts in ester linkage on C-6 of both galactose and the hexosamine. A good deal is known about the physical properties of glycosaminoglycans and their structural heterogeneity (Mathews, 1967). Some heterogeneity is due to variation in length of polysaccharide chains, extent of sulfation, position of sulfate esters, relative proportion of the two uronic acids in dermatan sulfate, heparin, and heparan sulfates, and linkage to protein in keratan sulfates. Additional details concerning the occurrence, structure, and chemistry of these glycosaminoglycans may be found elsewhere (Rodén, 1970; Dorfman and Matalon, 1972; Rodén et al., 1972).

There is a growing realization that heparan sulfate may play an important biological role. Accordingly, it seems worthwhile to review current knowledge of the structure of heparan sulfates and of heparin. D-Glucosamine and D-glucuronic acid are constituents of heparan sulfates and heparin, but both polysaccharides contain L-iduronic acid as well (Cifonelli and Dorfman, 1962).

Heparan sulfate and heparin differ from other sulfated glycosaminoglycans in that the uronosyl linkage is 1→4 rather than the 1→3 linkage characteristic of the other glycosaminoglycans.[2] The configuration of glycosidic bonds in heparan sulfate and heparin had been thought to be exclusively α, in contrast to the other glycosaminoglycans which contain only β-linkages or stereochemically equivalent bonds as in the case of α-L-iduronosyl moieties in dermatan sulfate (Pigman, 1957). Recently, Helting and Lindahl (1971) have shown that most or perhaps all of the glucuronidic linkages are actually of β-configuration. Heparin may more accurately be depicted with alternating α- and β-glycosidic linkages (noting that the glycosidic linkages of β-D-glucuronic acid and α-L-iduronic acid are stereochemically identical), thereby providing an explanation for the fact that the optical rotation of heparin is lower than theoretically expected for a polymer composed exclusively of a-linkages (Brimacombe and Webber, 1964).

The chondroitin sulfates and dermatan sulfate bear ester sulfate groups on the C-4 and C-6 positions of hexosamines and on iduronosyl residues. Heparan sulfates and heparin contain sulfamide linkages, not encountered in other glycosaminoglycans. The N-sulfated disaccharides in heparan sulfate are interspersed between regions of more numerous N-acetylated residues (Cifonelli, 1968) but are not present in the vicinity of the protein–polysaccharide linkage region (see below) (Knecht et al., 1967; Cifonelli, 1968). The structural heterogeneity of the heparan sulfates has made it difficult to establish the detailed structure for these compounds. Heparin contains approximately 2.5 sulfate groups per disaccharide unit. The amino groups of almost all hexosamine residues except those proximal to the linkage region are bound in sulfamide linkage (Lindahl, 1966; Cifonelli, 1968). Additionally, ester sulfate is present at C-6 of glucosamine and at C-2 of iduronic acid residues (Lindahl, 1970; Lindahl and Axelsson, 1971).

Both heparan sulfates and heparin can be degraded with nitrous acid, which reacts with the N-sulfated hexosamine groups to form 2,5-anhydromannose and concomitantly cleaves adjacent hexosaminidic linkages (Cifonelli, 1968). Since only some hexosamine groups are N-sulfated in heparan sulfates, oligosaccharide fragments of varying size are produced upon nitrous acid degradation. The principal products obtained by degradation of fully sulfated heparin are disaccharides and oligosaccharide fragments with anhydromannose at their reducing ends and inorganic sulfate (Cifonelli, 1968). This technique has proven extremely useful in the detection and characterization of small quantities of heparan sulfates in a variety of cells[3] and tissues (Dorfman

[2]Keratan sulfate also has 1→4 glycosidic linkages at an analogous position within its repeating disaccharide; however, this disaccharide lacks uronic acid and is composed principally of N-acetylglucosamine and galactose.

[3]Small amounts of heparan sulfates have been found in normal, Hurler's, and Sanfilippo's fibroblasts (Matalon and Dorfman, unpublished results).

and Ho, 1970; Kraemer, 1971b). In culture, a variety of cells synthesize heparan sulfates (Kraemer, 1971b), and a substantial portion seems to be either located intracellularly or associated with cell-surface materials (Kraemer, 1971a; Kraemer and Tobey, 1972). These findings suggest that heparan sulfates may have a ubiquitous distribution and play some role other than that of the extracellular glycosaminoglycans.

Heparin and heparan sulfates were formerly thought to be metabolically distinct. The former compound, which possesses anticoagulant and lipo-proteinlipase activating activity, is present in blood vessel wall, largely as an intracellular constituent of mast cells (Schiller and Dorfman, 1959). Heparan sulfates were believed to be primarily an extracellular component, since large quantities were isolated from aorta and amyloid (Linker et al., 1958). Because of the structural similarities between heparan sulfates and heparins, it seems likely that these glycosaminoglycans comprise a family of related compounds. Studies on the biosynthesis have begun to furnish a picture of the processes by which heparin may be formed from heparan sulfate proteoglycan (Lindahl, 1970). The modifications necessary for this transition include the substitution of N-sulfate groups for N-acetyl groups (Balasubramanian and Bachhawat, 1964; Eisenman et al., 1967; Silbert, 1967), epimerization of β-D-glu-curonosyl moieties to α-L-iduronosyl moieties (Lindahl and Backstrom, 1972), and scission of protein-linked polysaccharide to yield heparin chains ranging in molecular weight from 9000 to 30,000 (Lindahl, 1970). Limited degradation of a proteoglycan may be catalyzed by an endoglycosidase and account for the finding that many heparin chains do not contain xylose and presumably are not covalently bound to protein (Lindahl, 1970). Horner (1971) views rat-skin heparin as a branched-chain carbohydrate complex with a molecular weight of over 10^6 in which heparin chains (molecular weight 36,000), each terminating in a linkage-to-protein region, are attached to a central heparan sulfate chain. Enzymic depolymerization of "macromolecu-lar heparin" may be of physiological importance in the regulation of lipo-protein lipase activity (Horner, 1972).

Most of the sulfated mucopolysaccharides are covalently linked to protein through the neutral trisaccharide, galactosylgalactosylxylose, which is glycosidically linked to the hydroxyl groups of serine residues (Rodén, 1968). The linkage structure is illustrated in Fig. 6 and has been identified in the chondroitin-4- and -6-sulfates, dermatan sulfate, heparan sulfates, and heparin. Keratan sulfate II appears to be linked to protein by an O-glycosidic linkage between N-acetyl-D-galactosamine and the hydroxy amino acids serine and threonine (Bhavanandan and Meyer, 1968), while a N-glycosidic linkage between N-acetylglucosamine and asparagine is found in corneal keratan sulfate (Baker et al., 1969). The latter linkage occurs frequently in glycoproteins (Marshall, 1972). Whether hyaluronic acid is linked to protein in mammalian tissues is not certain. Hamerman et al. (1966) suggested that

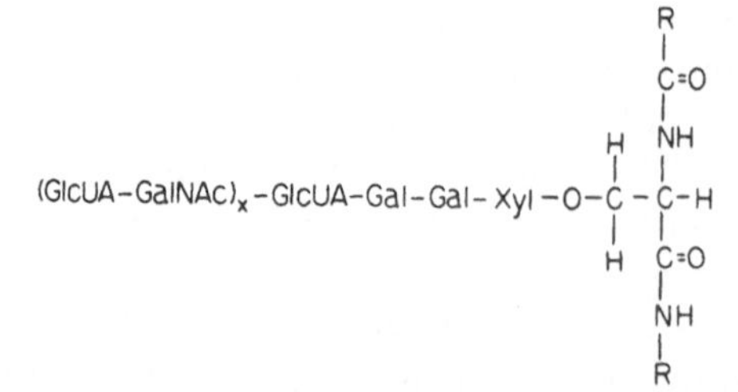

$$\text{(GlcUA-GalNAc)}_x\text{-GlcUA-Gal-Gal-Xyl} -O-\underset{\underset{\text{H}}{|}}{\overset{\overset{\text{H}}{|}}{C}} -\underset{\underset{\underset{\underset{R}{|}}{NH}}{\overset{|}{\overset{C=O}{|}}}}{\overset{\overset{\overset{\overset{R}{|}}{C=O}}{\overset{|}{NH}}}{\overset{|}{C}}}-\text{H}$$

Fig. 6. Structure of the neutral sugar linkage region in several glycosamino-glycan–protein complexes including chondroitin (illustrated), chondroitin sulfates, dermatan sulfate, heparan sulfates, and heparin.

this mucopolysaccharide is linked to protein through a glycopeptide containing glucose and galactose. Wardi *et al.* (1969) claimed that arabinose is involved in a linkage of hyaluronate with protein, but a study by Katzman (1971) indicated that the probability that arabinose is involved in a covalent linkage is extremely low. The possibility that hyaluronic acid is covalently linked to protein is an attractive hypothesis and is supported by some experimental evidence (Hamerman, 1970; Scher and Hamerman, 1972), but a linkage fragment has not been isolated.

B. Biosynthesis of Glycosaminoglycans

The glycosaminoglycans are synthesized by mechanisms involving metabolic pathways of widespread occurrence. Monosaccharide units are derived from D-glucose by a series of reactions which alter steric configuration, state of oxidation, length of carbon skeletons, and transfer of amino groups. Amino sugar formation occurs at the level of hexose-6-phosphate, but the other monosaccharide transformations involve uridine nucleotide sugars, compounds from which glycosyl residues are subsequently transferred to acceptors. The pathways of formation of uridine nucleotide sugars required for the synthesis of glycosaminoglycans are illustrated in Fig. 7. With the exception of iduronic acid, the transfer of sugars from their uridine nucleotides to intermediates of glycosaminoglycans has been demonstrated. The epimerization of UDP-glucuronic acid to UDP-iduronic acid was discovered by Jacobson and Davidson (1962) and has been confirmed in a more recent study (Fransson, 1970). It had been assumed that UDP-iduronic acid is an intermediate in the synthesis of dermatan sulfate, heparan sulfates, and heparin, but the discovery that iduronosyl residues originate at the polymer level by epimerization of glucuronosyl residues (Lindahl and Backstrom, 1972) necessitates reevaluation of the original premise. UDP-*N*-acetylglucosamine (Kornfeld *et al.,* 1964) and UDP-xylose (Neufeld and Hall, 1965) each inhibit reactions involved in their own synthesis. The notion that nucleotide sugars regulate their own synthesis by feedback inhibition has

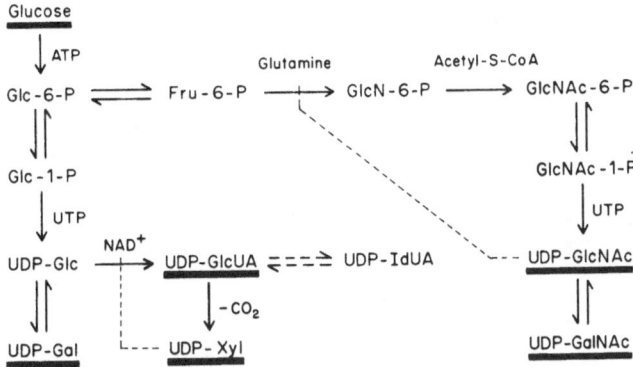

Fig. 7. The pathways of formation of uridine nucleotide sugars. Glucose and the immediate precursors involved in glycosaminoglycan formation are underlined. Two reactions subject to feedback inhibition by nucleotide sugars are indicated (these are discussed in Section IIIB).

been widely accepted, but the likelihood that UDP-N-acetylglucosamine functions in this manner under physiological conditions has been disputed by Winterburn and Phelps (1970).

Unlike protein and nucleic acid synthesis, the ordering of sugars in glycosaminoglycans is not specified by a template but rather by the specificity of glycosyltransferases with respect to both donor and acceptor groups. Carbohydrate chains grow by the sequential transfer of monosaccharide units from nucleotide sugars to the nonreducing ends of uncompleted chains. Multiglycosyltransferase systems which catalyze glycosaminoglycan formation appear to be membrane bound, although the affinity of individual enzymes may vary greatly.

The biosynthesis of the chondroitin sulfates is the most thoroughly understood example of glycosaminoglycan synthesis. The pathway of formation of chondromucoprotein is illustrated in Fig. 8. The assembly of carbohydrate chains requires six glycosyltransferases and sulfotransferase. Chondroitin sulfate chains are initiated (enzyme 1) by the transfer of xylose from UDP-xylose to appropriate serine residues of the core protein or incomplete growing core-peptides. Completion of the linkage region occurs by the transfer of two galactosyl moieties (enzymes 2 and 3) and a glucuronosyl unit (enzyme 4). Enzymes 5 and 6 act in concert, alternately transferring N-acetylgalactosamine and glucuronic acid residues until the chain is completed. The polysaccharide chain is further modified by introduction of ester sulfate by the transfer of sulfate from phosphoadenylylsulfate (D'Abramo and Lipmann, 1957). The available evidence indicates that sulfation occurs

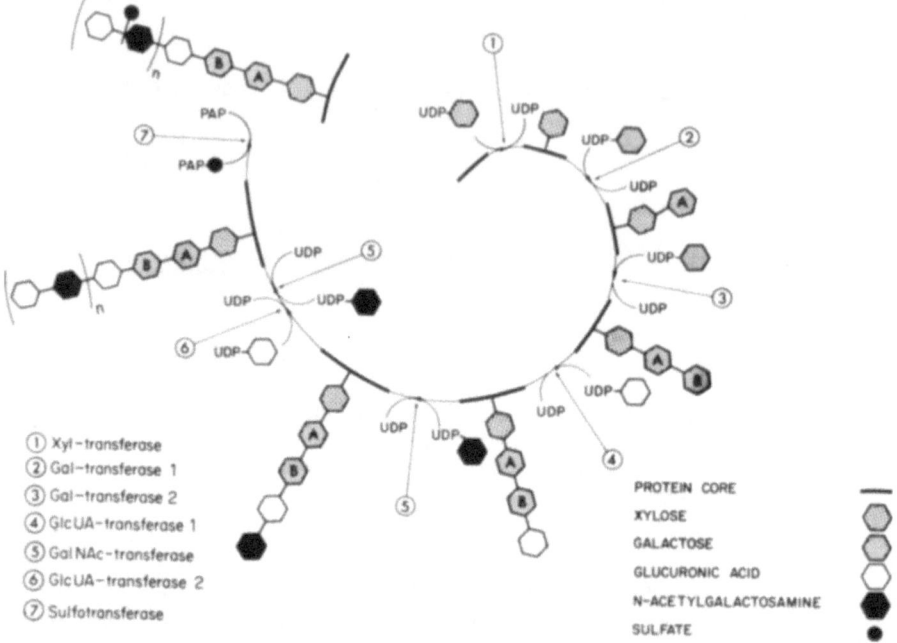

① Xyl–transferase
② Gal–transferase 1
③ Gal–transferase 2
④ GlcUA–transferase 1
⑤ GalNAc–transferase
⑥ GlcUA–transferase 2
⑦ Sulfotransferase

PROTEIN CORE

XYLOSE

GALACTOSE

GLUCURONIC ACID

N–ACETYLGALACTOSAMINE

SULFATE

Fig. 8.   The pathway of biosynthesis of chondroitin-4-sulfate.

at the macromolecular level, but the extent of sulfation during polysaccharide chain growth is not clear (Silbert and DeLuca, 1969).

A more comprehensive understanding of the mechanism of formation of glycosaminoglycans requires information concerning the individual biosynthetic reactions and a recognition of the relationship of this process to cellular structure and function. Cells engaged in chondromucoprotein synthesis contain an extensive rough endoplasmic reticulum (Godman and Porter, 1960) which appears to play a major role in the formation of glycosaminoglycans (Horwitz and Dorfman, 1968). The specific activities of the glycosyltransferases and sulfotransferase shown in Fig. 8 have been determined *in vitro* by measuring the transfer of sugars from uridine nucleotide-C^{14} sugars or sulfate from phosphoadenylyl sulfate-S^{35} to appropriate exogenous acceptors. Xylosyltransferase is assayed utilizing a protein preparation obtained by Smith degradation of bovine proteoglycan as acceptor (Baker *et al.*, 1972). The discovery of a variety of low molecular weight acceptors has enormously facilitated the assay of other glycosyltransferases involved in linkage region synthesis and polysaccharide chain elongation (Telser *et al.*,

1966; Helting and Rodén, 1968, 1969). Details concerning the activity of sulfotransferase toward different acceptors have been reviewed by Stoolmiller and Dorfman (1969) and Rodén (1970).

A study by Horwitz and Dorfman (1968) of the intracellular distribution of enzymes involved in chondromucoprotein synthesis in embryonic chick chondroblasts may be interpreted as follows: Initiation of glycosaminoglycan synthesis occurs by xylosylation of the core protein, but whether xylose addition occurs during protein synthesis while the protein core is bound to ribosomes or only after the core is completed is uncertain. The linkage region is formed primarily at the rough endoplasmic reticulum, and polysaccharide chain elongation continues and is completed as the proteoglycan proceeds through the smooth endoplasmic reticulum and the Golgi apparatus. Finally, the product is released by secretion vacuoles to the exterior. A great many factors affect glycosaminoglycan metabolism, including macromolecular materials in the extracellular milieu (Nevo and Dorfman, 1972). Elucidation of regulatory mechanisms is an area of continuing investigation.

There is presently no evidence implicating lipid-linked oligosaccharide intermediates in the synthesis of glycosaminoglycans. However, the importance of polyisoprenol-bound sugars in the formation of other heteropolysaccharides indicates that their possible involvement should not be overlooked. Biosynthetic systems known to involve lipid intermediates have been cited in numerous reports (Nikaido and Hassid, 1971; Parodi et al., 1972).

C. Glycosaminoglycans in Nervous Tissue

Because of the long-standing uncertainties concerning the nature and function of the ground substance in brain, it has been of interest to determine whether cells of the nervous system synthesize glycosaminoglycans. Prior to the availability of cultured cell strains, investigations on glycosaminoglycan synthesis in brain were conducted primarily with histochemical and biochemical techniques. Although these techniques provided convincing evidence of the existence of glycosaminoglycans, neither defined the role of particular cell types in glycosaminoglycan metabolism.

The histochemical studies of Hess (1953) led to the first suggestion that glycosaminoglycans occur in brain. This claim gained added credence from the finding that hyaluronidase promoted the diffusion of trypan blue through nervous tissue (Arteta, 1956). Abood and Abul-Haj (1956) were the first to isolate glycosaminoglycans from nervous tissue, a finding soon corroborated by Brante (1957) and Meyer et al. (1958).

The present knowledge about the glycosaminoglycan composition of brain has resulted from analytical investigations in several laboratories

(Margolis, 1969; Bachhawat et al., 1972). Hyaluronic acid, chondroitin sulfate, and heparan sulfates comprise the bulk of the glycosaminoglycans in brain of a number of animals including man, monkey, ox, sheep, rabbit, rat, and chicken (Singh et al., 1969; Margolis, 1967). The amounts range from 0.01 % in the rabbit to 0.08 % in the rat based on fresh weight. Hyaluronic acid accounts for 35–45% of the total glycosaminoglycan in all species (Szabo and Roboz-Einstein, 1962; Clausen and Hansen, 1963; Onodera et al., 1966; Margolis, 1967), and chondroitin-4- and -6-sulfates constitute from 30 to 52% in mammals but only 22% in chicken brain (Singh et al., 1969). The occurrence of heparan sulfates has been confirmed by several laboratories (Cunningham and Goldberg, 1968; Singh and Bachhawat, 1969; Singh et al., 1969; Elam et al., 1970; Margolis and Atherton, 1972). Small amounts of dermatan sulfate occur in animal brain (Cunningham and Goldberg, 1968), peripheral nerve, and probably spinal cord (Chandrasekaran and Bachhawat, 1969), but dermatan sulfate is virtually absent from the central nervous tissue of man. Heparin and the keratan sulfates do not occur in measurable quantities.

It may seem tempting to speculate on the significance of differences in the compositions of brain glycosaminoglycans in different species, but whether these variations are important is not known. Furthermore the glycosaminoglycan composition changes markedly during development and aging (Singh and Bachhawat, 1965, 1969; Mathews, 1967; Young and Custod, 1972), so data obtained from different species must be compared with caution unless it is certain that the samples are comparable.

Few studies have been conducted on the distribution of glycosaminoglycans within the nervous system, but Stary et al., (1964) and Margolis (1967) found that human and bovine gray matter contains 1.2–1.8 times more glycosaminoglycans than white matter. A similar study with sheep brain revealed no differences (Singh and Bachhawat, 1965). Spinal cord and peripheral nerve contain relatively more hyaluronic acid than brain does (Chandrasekaran and Bachhawat, 1969); however, it is likely that these neural tissues were contaminated with connective tissue to a greater degree than brain samples.

The biosynthesis of glycosaminoglycans in brain has been monitored in several mammals by the incorporation of sulfate-S^{35} (Bostrom and Odelblad, 1953; Ringertz, 1956, Guha et al., 1960; Robinson and Green, 1962; Goldberg and Cunningham, 1970). Radioactivity is incorporated more rapidly into gray matter than into white matter, in agreement with chemical studies described earlier. Balasubramanian and Bachhawat (1964) were the first to carry out in vitro studies with phosphoadenylyl sulfate-S^{35} in which the acceptor activities of different glycosaminoglycans were determined. Heparan sulfate was a good acceptor, and it has been utilized to examine the variation in extent of N- and O-sulfation during development in rat and man (George et al., 1970). No radioactive products corresponding to heparin or keratan sulfate were found (Goldberg and Cunningham, 1970). Previous to recent work to be described, the only report of glycosaminoglycan synthesis by brain tissue in culture was that of Grossfeld (1957).

D. Production of Glycosaminoglycans in Cultured Cell Strains of Nervous System Origin

The production of glycosaminoglycans was studied with three cell strains of nervous system origin: RGC6 rat astrocytoma cells (Benda et al., 1968). NB41A mouse neuroblastoma cells (Augusti-Tocco and Sato, 1969), and RN2 rat schwannoma cells (Pfeiffer and Wechsler, 1972).

1. Glia

Rat astrocytoma cells were grown under the conditions described by Dorfman and Ho (1970). The glycosaminoglycans formed during the last 24 hr of incubation were labeled by adding sulfate-S^{35} and sodium acetate-H^3 to the growth medium. The culture media from 91 plates were pooled, and the cells were removed with a rubber policeman after several rinses with isotonic salt solution. Crude glycosaminoglycans were precipitated by addition of cetylpyridinium chloride to the growth medium after dialysis and fivefold concentration. The precipitated glycosaminoglycans were dissolved in 2 M NaCl and reprecipitated with ethanol. The precipitated materials were digested with papain and the individual glycosaminoglycans isolated. The cell mass was digested with papain, and the methods outlined above were utilized to isolate the liberated glycosaminoglycans.

From 2.5 liters of media accumulated after 10 days of culture, 25 mg of glycosaminoglycans was isolated. The composition of the glycosaminoglycan mixture was determined by a differential salt solubility (Schiller et al., 1961), and the results are shown in Table V. Seventy-five percent of the uronic acid was soluble in 0.4 M NaCl, a fraction which is suspected to contain hyaluronic

TABLE V

Fractionation of Glycosaminoglycans from the Medium of RGC6 Glial Cell Cultures

Fraction	Uronic acid		Sulfate-S^{35}		Acetate-C^{14}	
	mg	%	cpm	%	cpm	%
Original	10.0	100	430,000	100	340,000	100
0.40 M	7.6	75	20,000	5	270,000	77
1.24 M	2.3	22	320,000	75	30,000	10

acid and/or chondroitin. The remainder of the uronic acid–containing material was extracted with 1.24 M NaCl. No significant amount of uronic acid was found in the 2.1-M fraction, which normally contains heparin. The 0.4-M fraction contained most of the labeled acetate, but little radioactive sulfate. In contrast, the 1.24-M fraction contained 75 % of the sulfate-S^{35} and only 10 % of the acetate-H^3.

Quantitative analyses and enzymic digestion with streptococcal hyaluronidase showed that the 0.4-M fraction consisted almost exclusively of hyaluronic acid (98 %). The 1.24-M fraction contained materials with electrophoretic mobilities corresponding to those of authentic samples of chondroitin-4-sulfate and heparan sulfates. Treatment of the 1.24-M fraction with testicular hyaluronidase and identification of the reaction products by paper chromatography confirmed the presence of chondroitin-4-sulfate. The second compound, which was hyaluronidase resistant, represented 38 % of the 1.24-M fraction and showed a uronic acid to hexosamine ratio of 1.2 and an $[\alpha]^{25}_D$ of $+ 55°$. The amino sugar was found to be solely glucosamine, 31 % of which was N-sulfated. Clearly, this compound was heparan sulfate.

From 9 ml of packed cells (3.3×10^9), approximately 15 mg of glycosaminoglycans was obtained. On salt fractionation, 63 % was recovered in the 0.4-M fraction and 37 % in the 1.24-M fraction. Electrophoresis showed the pattern of cellular glycosaminoglycans to be the same as that in the medium.

Dorfman and Ho (1970) also measured the levels of acid mucopolysaccharides in fetal calf serum and concluded that approximately 25 % of the acid mucopolysaccharides isolated from growth medium were of serum origin. On fractionation, this material was found to consist of hyaluronic acid and chondroitin-4-sulfate in a ratio of 2:1. Since these mucopolysaccharides are completely digested by testicular hyaluronidase, the heparan sulfate recovered from the growth medium was derived entirely from the glial cells.

2. Neuroblastoma

Mouse neuroblastoma cells (NB41A) were cultured under conditions similar to those employed for glial cells (Stoolmiller, 1972). The growth medium was pooled, and the cells were harvested with a rubber policeman after three rinses with isotonic saline. Glycosaminoglycans were isolated separately from the growth medium and the cells by the methods described above.

From 5.1 liters of growth medium accumulated after 9 days of culture, 12 mg of glycosaminoglycans was isolated, an amount equal to that known to be present in fetal calf serum, which was used to supplement the culture medium (Dorfman and Ho, 1970). The crude mixture was fractionated by the method of Schiller et al. (1961) and the distribution of uronic acid in the 0.4-M and

1.24-M fractions was 2:1. Both fractions were digested by testicular hyaluronidase, but they were not characterized further.

The digested neuroblastoma cell mass (12 ml) yielded only 0.3 mg of uronic acid, corresponding to approximately 0.6 mg of glycosaminoglycans. Fractionation of this mixture indicated that the sulfated glycosaminoglycans were in twofold excess over the nonsulfated ones.

In view of the low yield of glycosaminoglycans from NB41A cells, the synthesis of acid mucopolysaccharides was monitored by the incorporation of radioactivity from sulfate-S^{35} or acetate-C^{14}, and the radioactive products were isolated and characterized after addition of authentic carrier acid mucopolysaccharides: 5 mg of hyaluronic acid, 2.5 mg each of chondroitin-4- and -6-sulfate, 2 mg of dermatan sulfate, 4 mg of heparan sulfates, and 2 mg of heparin. A total of 85–90% of the carrier glycosaminoglycans were recovered from pooled growth medium and cell digests on the basis of uronic acid assays. The glycosaminoglycans were fractionated (Schiller *et al.*, 1961), and the distributions of radioactivity among the fractions are shown in Table VI. The 0.4-M fractions contained less than 10% of the sulfate-S^{35}. One-half of the acetate-labeled glycosaminoglycans in cells were found in the 0.4-M salt fraction, but only 11% of those which occurred in the medium, indicating that little nonsulfated glycosaminoglycan formed was secreted into the medium. The polysaccharide in the 0.4-M fractions was shown to be hyaluronic acid by digestion with streptococcal hyaluronidase.

Over 60% of the labeled glycosaminoglycans obtained from the medium and sulfate-labeled cells and 27% of the labeled fraction from acetate-labeled cells were present in the 1.24-M salt fractions. A major portion of the labeled glycosaminoglycans which were associated with the cell fraction were not degraded with testicular hyaluronidase, whereas over 80% of the glycosaminoglycans in the medium were digested. This result suggested that heparan sulfate was indeed a major sulfated glycosaminoglycan in neuroblastoma cells.

To determine the percentage of heparan sulfates in the hyaluronidase-resistant labeled fraction, a portion of each fraction was subjected to nitrous acid degradation and the radioactive products were analyzed by gel filtration on Sephadex G50 according to Cifonelli (1968). The intracellular hyaluronidase-resistant materials were almost exclusively heparan sulfates, containing 30–50% N-sulfate groups. Less than 30% of the sulfate-labeled hyaluronidase-resistant material of the medium was degraded. It was concluded that this fraction was composed largely of glycoprotein, although the possibility that the extracellular product was dermatan sulfate could not be ruled out since testicular hyaluronidase does not completely degrade this compound. In summary, it appears that almost all of the heparan sulfate is cell associated and that little is secreted into the medium.

TABLE VI

Fractionation of Labeled Glycosaminoglycans Produced by NB41A Neuroblastoma Cells

Fraction	Sulfate-S^{35}				Acetate-C^{14}			
	Medium		Cells		Medium		Cells	
	cpm	%	cpm	%	cpm	%	cpm	%
Original	353,100	100	63,600	100	44,100	100	7,120	100
0.40 M	38,600	8	2,700	4	4,800	11	3,500	49
1.24 M	233,000	66	42,100	66	27,500	62	1,900	27
2.1 M	4,200	1	300	—	400	1	50	1
Total cpm recovered	265,800	75	45,100	70	32,700	74	5,450	77

IV. COLLAGEN SYNTHESIS

Since glycosaminoglycans and collagen are often synthesized by the same cells, preliminary studies of collagen synthesis by rat glial and neuroblastoma cells were carried out. Dehm and Prockop (1971) have shown that connective tissue cells can convert as much as one-third of incorporated proline-C^{14} into hydroxyproline-C^{14}. As anticipated, neither glial nor neuroblastoma cells produced significant amounts of collagen; the percentage of radioactive amino acids attributable to hydroxyproline-C^{14} was less than 0.5% in cells of both types. In contrast, Church *et al.* (1973) found that schwannoma cells synthesize sunstantial amounts of collagen.

V. CONCLUSIONS

The use of clonal cultures of cells of the central nervous system has permitted an investigation of the potentialities of such cells for synthesis of glycosphingolipids and glycosaminoglycans. The results obtained indicate that the spectrum of compounds produced is characteristic of individual cell types. Clonal strains of neuroblastoma synthesize a wide variety of glyco-sphingolipids including particularly the hexosamine-containing gangliosides characteristic of the central nervous system. Glial cell cultures synthesize principally hematoside, which is also the primary sialic acid–containing glycosphingolipid of human fibroblasts (Dawson *et al.*, 1972*b*, *c*). Schwan-noma cells produce hematoside, but preliminary experiments also indicate synthesis of myelin-specific galactosylceramide (together with small amounts of sulfatide). Glial cells, like fibroblasts, produce a spectrum of glycos-aminoglycans including hyaluronic acid, chondroitin sulfates, and heparan sulfates. Their rate of synthesis is much lower than that observed in chon-drocytes, and they appear to produce relatively more heparan sulfates than do skin fibroblasts. Preliminary results indicate that schwannoma cells also produce a spectrum of glycosaminoglycans, perhaps at a somewhat greater rate than do glial cells. In contrast, neuroblastoma cells produce only small amounts of glycosaminoglycans, a major portion of which is heparan sulfate. The latter compound appears to be produced by many cell types and may have a function in cell physiology different from that of other glycosaminoglycans. These results suggest that glycosaminoglycans of the brain are derived principally from glial elements. It remains to be determined whether these tissue culture studies accurately reflect normal brain metabolism, since recent studies with rat brain showed that a synaptosome fraction contained the highest concentration of sulfotransferase activity (Vos *et al.*, 1969; Saxena *et al.*, 1971) and substantial amounts of glycosaminoglycans (Vos *et al.*, 1969).

VI. REFERENCES

Abood, L. G., and Abul-Haj, S. K. 1956. Histochemistry and characterization of hyaluronic acid in axons of peripheral nerves. *J. Neurochem.* 1:119–125.

Andrews, J. M., Cancilla, P. A., Grippo, J., and Menkes, J. H. 1971. Globoid cell leukodystrophy (Krabbe's disease): morphological and biochemical studies. *Neurology* 21:337–353.

Arteta, J. L. 1956. Effect of hyaluronidase on the cat brain. *Proc. Soc. Exptl. Biol. Med.* 91:440–442.

Augusti-Tocco, G., and Sato, G. 1969. Establishment of functional clonal lines of neurons from mouse neuroblastoma. *Proc. Natl. Acad. Sci.* 64:311–315.

Austin, J. H., and Lehfeldt, D. 1965. Studies in globoid (Krabbe) leukodystrophy. III. Significance of experimentally-produced globoid-like elements in rat white matter and spleen. *J. Neuropathol. Exptl. Neurol.* 24:265–289.

Bachhawat, B. K., Balasubramanian, K. A., Balasubramanian, A. S., Singh, M., George, E., and Chandrasekaran, E. V. 1972. Chemistry and metabolism of glycosaminoglycans of the nervous system, pp. 51–71. *In* V. Zambotti, G. Tettamanti, and M. Arrigoni (eds.). Glycolipids, Glycoproteins, and Mucopolysaccharides of the Nervous System, Plenum Press, New York.

Baker, J. R., Cifonelli, J. A., Mathews, M. B., and Rodén, L. 1969. Mannose-containing glycopeptides from keratosulfate (KS). *Fed. Proc.* 28:605.

Baker, J. R., Rodén, L., and Stoolmiller, A. C. 1972. Biosynthesis of chondroitin sulfate proteoglycan. Xylosyl transfer to Smith-degraded cartilage proteoglycan and other exogenous acceptors. *J. Biol. Chem.* 247:3838–3847.

Balasubramanian, A. S., and Bachhawat, B. K. 1964. Enzymic transfer of sulphate from 3'-phosphoadenosine 5'-phosphosulphate to mucopolysaccharides in rat brain. *J. Neurochem.* 11:877–885.

Benda, P., Lightbody, J., Sato, G., Levine, L., and Sweet, W. 1968. Differentiated rat glial cell strain in tissue culture. *Science* 161:370–371.

Bhavanandan, V. P., and Meyer, K. 1968. Studies on keratosulfates: (methylation, desulfation, and acid hydrolysis studies on old human rib cartilage keratosulfate). *J. Biol. Chem.* 243:1052–1059.

Boström, H., and Odeblad, E. 1953. Autoradiographic observations on the uptake of S^{35}-labelled sodium sulphate in the nervous system of the adult rat. *Acta Psychiat. Neurol. Scand.* 28:5–8.

Brady, R. O., Johnson, W. G., and Uhlendorf, B. W. 1971. Identification of heterozygous carriers of lipid storage diseases. *Am. J. Med.* 51:423–431.

Brante, G. 1957. Hexosamine compounds in the nervous system. A preliminary report, pp. 112–120. *In* D. Richter (ed.). Metabolism of the Central Nervous System. Pergamon Press, London.

Brimacombe, J. S., and Webber, J. M. 1964. Mucopolysaccharides. Chemical Structure, Distribution and Isolation. B.B.A. Library, Vol. 6. Elsevier, Amsterdam. 181 pp.

Chandrasekaran, E. V., and Bachhawat, B. K. 1969. Isolation and characterization of glycosaminoglycans in peripheral nerve and spinal cord of monkey. *J. Neurochem.* 16:1529–1532.

Christensen-Lou, H. O., and Clausen, J. 1968. Polar lipids of oligodendrogliomas. *J. Neurochem.* 15:263–264.

Christensen-Lou, H. O., Clausen, J., and Biering, F. 1965. Phospholipids and glycolipids of tumors in the central nervous system. *J. Neurochem.* 12:619–627.

Church, R. L., Tanzer, M. L., and Pfeiffer, S. E. 1973. Collagen and procollagen production by a clonal line of Schwann cells, *Proc. Natl. Acad. Sci.* **70**:1943–1946.

Cifonelli, J. A. 1968. Reaction of heparitin sulfate with nitrous acid. *Carbohyd. Res.* **8**:233–242.

Cifonelli, J. A., and Dorfman, A. 1962. The uronic acid of heparin. *Biochem. Biophys. Res. Commun.* **7**:41–45.

Clausen, J., and Hansen, A. 1963. Acid mucopolysaccharides of human brain: Identification by means of infra-red analysis. *J. Neurochem.* **10**:165–168.

Cumar, F. A., Fishman, P. H., and Brady, R. O. 1972. Analogous reactions for the biosynthesis of monosialo- and disialo-gangliosides in brain. *J. Biol. Chem.* **246**:5075–5084.

Cunningham, W. L., and Goldberg, J. M. 1968. The determination of glycosaminoglycans present in various mammalian brains. *Biochem. J.* **110**:35P–36P.

D'Abramo, F., and Lipmann, F. 1957. The formation of adenosine-3'-phosphate-5'-phosphosulfate in extracts of chick embryo cartilage and its conversion into chondroitin sulfate. *Biochim. Biophys. Acta* **25**:211–213.

Dawson, G., Kemp, S. F., Stoolmiller, A. C., and Dorfman, A. 1971. Biosynthesis of glycosphingolipids by mouse neuroblastoma (NB41A), rat glia (RGC-6) and human glia (CHB-4) in cell culture. *Biochem. Biophys. Res. Commun.* **44**:687–694.

Dawson, G., Kemp, S. F., and Stoolmiller, A. C. 1972a. Biosynthesis of glycosphingolipids in cloned cell strains of neurological origin. *Trans. Am. Soc. Neurochem.* **3**:68.

Dawson, G., Matalon, R., and Dorfman, A. 1972b. Glycosphingolipids of cultured human skin fibroblasts. I. Characterization and metabolism in normal fibroblasts. *J. Biol. Chem.* **247**:5944–5950.

Dawson, G., Matalon, R., and Dorfman, A. 1972c. Glycosphingolipids of cultured human skin fibroblasts. II. Characterization and metabolism in fibroblasts from patients with inborn errors of glycosphingolipid and mucopolysaccharide metabolism. *J. Biol. Chem.* **247**:5951–5958.

Dehm, P., and Prockop, D. J. 1971. Synthesis and extrusion of collagen by freshly isolated cells from chick embryo tendon. *Biochim. Biophys. Acta* **240**:358–369.

Dekirmenjian, H., and Brunngraber, E. G. 1969. Distribution of protein-bound N-acetylneuraminic acid in subcellular particulate fractions prepared from rat whole brain. *Biochim. Biophys. Acta* **177**:1–10.

Den, H., Schultz, A. M., Basu, M., and Roseman, S. 1971. Glycosyltransferase activities in normal and polyoma-transformed BHK cells. *J. Biol. Chem.* **246**:2721–2723.

Derry, D. M., and Wolfe, L. 1967. Gangliosides in isolated neurons and glia. *Science* **158**:1450–1452.

DiCesare, J. L., and Dain, J. A. 1972. The enzymic synthesis of ganglioside. IV. UDP-N-acetylgalactosamine: (N-acetylneuraminyl)-galactosylglucosyl ceramide N-acetylgalactosaminyltransferase in rat brain. *Biochim. Biophys. Acta* **231**:385–393.

Dorfman, A., and Ho, P.-L. 1970. Synthesis of acid mucopolysaccharides by glial tumor cells in tissue culture. *Proc. Natl. Acad. Sci.* **66**:495–499.

Dorfman, A., and Matalon, R. 1972. The mucopolysaccharidoses, pp. 1218–1272. *In* J. B. Stanbury, J. B. Wyngaarden, and D. S. Fredrickson (eds.). The Metabolic Basis for Inherited Disease. McGraw-Hill, New York.

Eisenman, R. A., Balasubramanian, A. S., and Marx, W. 1967. 3'-Phosphoadenylylsulfate: desulfoheparin sulfotransferase associated with a postmicrosomal particulate mastocytoma fraction. *Arch. Biochem. Biophys.* **119**:387–397.

Elam, J. S., Goldberg, J. M., Radin, N. S., and Agranoff, B. W. 1970. Rapid axonal transport of sulfated mucopolysaccharide proteins. *Science* 170:458–460.

Embree, L. J., Hess, H. H., and Shein, H. M. 1972. Biochemical structural components of cloned *N*-nitrosomethylurea-induced astrocytoma cells grown subcutaneously. *Neurology* 194:201.

Fishman, P. H., McFarland, V. W., Mora, P. T., and Brady, R. O. 1972. Ganglioside biosynthesis in mouse cells: Glycosyltransferase activities in normal and virally transformed lines. *Biochem. Biophys. Res. Commun.* 48:48–57.

Forman, D. S., and Ledeen, R. 1972. Axonal transport of gangliosides in goldfish optic nerve. *Science* 177:630–633.

Fransson, L.-Å. 1970. Structure and metabolism of the proteoglycan of dermatan sulfate, pp. 823–842. *In* E. A. Balazs (ed.). NATO Advanced Study Institute on the Chemistry and Molecular Biology of the Intercellular Matrix, Vol. 2. Academic Press, London.

Fransson, L.-Å. and Rodén, L. 1967a. Structure of dermatan sulfate. I. Degradation by testicular hyaluronidase. *J. Biol. Chem.* 242:4161–4169.

Fransson, L.-Å., and Rodén, L. 1967b. Structure of dermatan sulfate. II. Characterization of products obtained by hyaluronidase digestion of dermatan sulfate. *J. Biol. Chem.* 242:4170–4175.

George, E., Singh, M., and Bachhawat, B. K. 1970. The nature of sulphation of uronic acid containing glycosaminoglycans catalysed by brain sulphotransferase. *J. Neurochem.* 17:189–200.

Godman, G. C., and Porter, K. R. 1960. Chondrogenesis, studied with the electron microscope. *J. Biophys. Biochem. Cytol.* 8:719–760.

Goldberg, J. M., and Cunningham, W. L. 1970. Incorporation of [^{35}S] sulphate into the glycosaminoglycans of rat brain. *Biochem. J.* 120:15P.

Gopal, K., Grossi, E., Paoletti, P., and Usardi, M. 1964. Lipid Composition of human intracranial tumors: A biochemical study. *Acta Neurochim. (Wien)* 11:333–341.

Grossfeld, H. 1957. Positive mucin clot test in supernates of cultures of avian embryonic brain. *Proc. Soc. Exptl. Biol. Med.* 96:844–846.

Guha, A., Northover, B. J., and Bacchawat, B. K. 1960. Incorporation of radioactive sulphate into chondroitin sulphate in the developing brain of rats. *J. Sci. Ind. Res.* 19C:287–289.

Hamberger, A., and Svennerholm, L. 1971. Composition of gangliosides and phospholipids of neuronal and glial cell enriched fractions. *J. Neurochem.* 18:1821–1829.

Hamerman, D. 1970. Protein–hyaluronate linkage. *New Engl. J. Med.* 282:165.

Hamerman, D., Rojkind, M., and Sandson, J. 1966. Analyses of the protein moiety of hyaluronate. *Fed. Proc.* 25:790.

Helting, T., and Lindahl, U. 1971. Occurrence and biosynthesis of β-glucuronidic linkages in heparin. *J. Biol. Chem.* 246:5442–5447.

Helting, T., and Rodén, L. 1968. Biosynthesis of chondroitin sulfate. I. Galactosyl transfer in the formation of the carbohydrate–protein linkage region. *J. Biol. Chem.* 244:2790–2798.

Helting, T., and Rodén, L. 1969. Biosynthesis of chondroitin sulfate. II. Glucuronosyl transfer in the formation of the carbohydrate–protein linkage region. *J. Biol. Chem.* 244:2799–2805.

Hess, A. 1953. The ground substance of the central nervous system revealed by histochemical staining. *J. Comp. Neurol.* 98:69–92.

Horner, A. A. 1971. Macromolecular heparin from rat skin. Isolation, characterization, and depolymerization with ascorbate. *J. Biol. Chem.* 246:231–239.

Horner, A. A. 1972. Enzymic depolymerization of macromolecular heparin as a factor in control of lipoprotein lipase activity. *Proc. Natl. Acad. Sci.* **69**:3469–3473.

Horwitz, A. L., and Dorfman, A. 1968. Subcellular sites for synthesis of chondromucoprotein of cartilage. *J. Cell Biol.* **38**:358–368.

Hydén, H., and Pigon, A. 1960. A cytophysiological study of the functional relationship between oligodendroglial cells and nerve cells of Deiters' nucleus. *J. Neurochem.* **6**: 57–72.

Jacobson, B., and Davidson, E. A. 1962. Biosynthesis of uronic acids by skin enzymes. II. Uridine diphosphate-D-glucuronic acid-5-epimerase. *J. Biol. Chem.* **237**:638–642.

Jones, J. P., Ramsey, R. B., Aexel, R. T., and Nicholas, H. J. 1972. Lipid biosynthesis in neuron-enriched and glial-enriched fractions of rat brain: Ganglioside biosynthesis. *Life Sci.* **11**:309–315.

Katzman, R. L. 1971. On arabinose as a constituent of hyaluronic acid from bovine brain. *J. Neurochem.* **18**:1187–1190.

Kaufman, B., Basu, S., and Roseman, S. 1967. Studies on the biosynthesis of gangliosides, pp. 187–213. *In* S. M. Aronson and B. W. Volk (eds.). Inborn Disorders of Sphingolipid Metabolism. Pergamon Press, Oxford.

Knecht, J., Cifonelli, J. A., and Dorfman, A. 1967. Structural studies on heparitin sulfate of normal and Hurler tissues. *J. Biol. Chem.* **242**:4652–4661.

Kornfeld, S., Kornfeld, R., Neufeld, E. F., and O'Brien, P. J. 1964. The feedback control of sugar nucleotide biosynthesis in liver. *Proc. Natl. Acad. Sci.* **52**:371–379.

Kraemer, P. M. 1971*a*. Heparan sulfates of cultured cells. I. Membrane associated and cell-sap species in Chinese hamster cells. *Biochemistry* **10**:1437–1445

Kraemer, P. M. 1971*b*. Heparan sulfates of cultured cells II. Acid-soluble and precipitable species of different cell lines. *Biochemistry* **10**:1445–1451.

Kraemer, P. M., and Tobey, R. A. 1972. Cell-cycle dependent desquamation of heparan sulfate from the cell surface. *J. Cell Biol.* **55**:713–717.

Lapetina, E. G., Soto, E. F., and DeRobertis, E. 1967. Gangliosides and acetylcholinesterase in isolated membranes of the rat brain cortex. *Biochim. Biophys. Acta* **135**: 33–41.

Ledeen, R. 1966. The chemistry of gangliosides. *J. Am. Oil. Chem. Soc.* **43**:57–66.

Lindahl, U. 1966. Further characterization of the heparin–protein linkage region. *Biochim. Biophys. Acta* **130**:368–382.

Lindahl, U. 1970. Structure of heparin, heparan sulfate and their related proteoglycans, pp. 943–960. *In* E. A. Balazs (ed.). NATO Advanced Study Institute on the Chemistry and Molecular Biology of the Intracellular Matrix, Vol. 2. Academic Press, London.

Lindahl, U., and Axelsson, O. 1971. Identification of iduronic acid as the major sulfated uronic acid of heparin. *J. Biol. Chem.* **246**:74–82.

Lindahl, U., and Bäckström, G. 1972. Biosynthesis of L-iduronic acid in heparin: Epimerization of D-glucuronic acid on the polymer level. *Biochem. Biophys. Res. Commun.* **46**:985–991.

Linker, A., Hoffman, P., Sampson, P., and Meyer, K. 1958. Heparatin sulfate. *Biochem. Biophys. Acta* **29**:443–444.

Maccioni, H. J., Arce, A., and Caputto, R. 1971. The biosynthesis of gangliosides. Labelling of rat brain gangliosides *in vivo*. *Biochem. J.* **125**:1131–1137.

Margolis, R. U. 1967. Acid mucopolysaccharides and proteins of bovine whole brain, white matter and myelin. *Biochim. Biophys. Acta* **141**:91–102.

Margolis, R. U. 1969. Mucopolysaccharides, pp. 245–260. *In* A. Lajtha (ed.). Handbook of Neurochemistry, Vol. I. Plenum Press, New York.

Margolis, R., and Atherton, D. M. 1972. The heparan sulfate of rat brain. *Biochim. Biophys. Acta* **273**:368–373.

Marshall, R. D. 1972. Glycoproteins. *Ann. Rev. Biochem.* **41**:673–702.

Mathews, M. B. 1967. Macromolecular evolution of connective tissue. *Biol. Rev.* **42**:499–551.

Meyer, K., Grumbach, M. M., Linker, A., and Hoffman, P. 1958. Excretion of sulfated mucopolysaccharide in gargolylism (Hurler's syndrome). *Proc. Soc. Exptl. Biol. Med.* **97**:275–279.

Mora, P. T., Brady, R. O., Bradley, R. M., and McFarland, V. W. 1969. Gangliosides in DNA virus-transformed and spontaneously transformed tumorigenic mouse cell lines. *Proc. Natl. Acad. Sci.* **63**:1290–1296.

Neufeld, E. F., and Hall, C. W. 1965. Inhibition of UDP-D-glucose dehydrogenase by UDP-D-xylose: A possible regulatory mechanism. *Biochem. Biophys. Res. Commun.* **19**:456–461.

Nevo, Z., and Dorfman, A. 1972. Stimulation of chondromucoprotein synthesis in chondrocytes by extracellular chondromucoprotein. *Proc. Natl. Acad. Sci.* **69**:2069–2072.

Nikaido, H., and Hassid, W. Z. 1971. Biosynthesis of saccharides from glycopyranosyl esters of nucleoside pyrophosphates ("sugar nucleotides"). *Advan. Carbohyd. Chem. Biochem.* **26**:351–483.

Norton, W. T., and Poduslo, S. E. 1971. Neuronal perikarya and astroglia in rat brain. Chemical composition during myelination. *J. Lipid Res.* **12**:84–90.

O'Brien, J. S., and Sampson, R. L. 1965. Lipid composition of the normal human brain: Gray matter, white matter, and myelin. *J. Lipid Res.* **6**:537–544.

Onodera, K., Hirona, S., Horiuchi, F., and Kashimura, N. 1966. A comparative study of some animal brains with regard to content of acidic mucopolysaccharide. *Carbohyd. Res.* **3**:234–238.

Parodi, A. J., Behrens, N. H., Leloir, L. F., and Carminatti, H. 1972. The role of polyprenol-bound saccharides as intermediates in glycoprotein synthesis in the liver. *Proc. Natl. Acad. Sci.* **69**:3268–3272.

Pfeiffer, S. E., and Dawson, G. 1972. Glycosphingolipid composition of a neoplastic clone of Schwann cells. *(Unpublished data)*.

Pfeiffer, S. E., and Wechsler, W. 1972. Biochemically differentiated neoplastic clone of Schwann cells. *Proc. Natl. Acad. Sci.* **69**:2885–2889.

Pigman, W. 1957. Introduction: Structure and stereochemistry of the monosaccharides, pp. 1–76. *In* W. Pigman (ed.). The Carbohydrates—Chemistry, Biochemistry, Physiology. Academic Press, New York.

Poduslo, S. E., and Norton, W. T. 1972. Isolation and some chemical properties of oligodendroglia from calf brain. *J. Neurochem.* **19**:727–736.

Radin, N. S. 1970. Brain cerebroside metabolism and possible implication for clinical problems, pp. 137–163. *In* J. Bernsohn and H. J. Grossman (eds.). Lipid Storage Diseases. Academic Press, New York.

Rapport, M. M., and Graf, L. 1969. Immunochemical reactions of lipids. *Progr. Allergy* **13**:273–331.

Ringertz, N. R. 1956. On the sulphate metabolism of the mouse brain. *Exptl. Cell Res.* **10**:230–233.

Robinson, J. D., Jr., and Green, J. P. 1962. Sulfomucopolysaccharides in brain. *Yale J. Biol. Med.* **35**:248–256.

Rodén, L. 1968. Linkage of acid mucopolysaccharides to protein, pp. 185–202. *In* Fourth International Conference on Cystic Fibrosis of the Pancreas (Mucoviscidosis), Berne/Grindelwald 1966, Part II. Karger, Basel.

Rodén, L. 1970. Biosynthesis of acidic glycosaminoglycans (mucopolysaccharides), pp. 345–442. *In* W. H. Fishman (ed.). Metabolic Conjugation and Metabolic Hydrolysis, Vol. II. Academic Press, New York.

Rodén L., Baker, J. R., Schwartz, N., Stoolmiller, A. C., Yamagata, S., and Yamagata, T. 1972. Some aspects of the structure and biosynthesis of connective tissue proteoglycans, pp. 345–385. *In* R. Piras and H. G. Pontis (eds.). Biochemistry of the Glycosidic Linkage: An Integrated View. Academic Press, New York.

Roseman, S. 1970. The synthesis of complex carbohydrates by multiglycosyltransferase systems and their potential function in intercellular adhesion. *Chem. Phys. Lipids* **5**:270–297.

Saxena, S., George, E., Kokrady, S., and Bachhawat, B. K. 1971. Sulfate metabolism in developing rat brain. Study with subcellular fractions. *Ind. J. Biochem. Biophys.* **8**: 1–8.

Scher, I., and Hamerman, D. 1972. Isolation of human synovial-fluid hyaluronate by density-gradient ultracentrifugation and evaluation of its protein content. *Biochem. J.* **126**:1073–1080.

Schiller, S., and Dorfman, A. 1959. The isolation of heparin from mast cells of the normal rat. *Biochim. Biophys. Acta* **31**:278–280.

Schiller, S., Slover, G. A., and Dorfman, A. 1961. A method for the separation of acid mucopolysaccharides: Its application to the isolation of heparin from the skin of rats. *J. Biol. Chem.* **236**:983–987.

Shapiro, D., and Flowers, H. M. 1961. Synthetic studies on sphingolipids. VI. The total synthesis of cerasine and phrenosine. *J. Am. Chem. Soc.* **83**:3327–3336.

Shein, H. M., Britva, A., Hess, H. H., and Selkoe, D. J. 1970. Isolation of hamster brain astroglia by *in vitro* cultivation and subcutaneous growth, and content of cerebroside, ganglioside, RNA and DNA. *Brain Res.* **19**:497–501.

Silbert, J. E. 1967. Biosynthesis of heparin. III. Formation of a sulfated glycosaminoglycan with a microsomal preparation from mast cell tumors. *J. Biol. Chem.* **242**:5146–5152.

Silbert, J. E., and DeLuca, S. 1969. Biosynthesis of chondroitin sulfate. III. Formation of a sulfated glycosaminoglycan with microsomal preparation from chick embryo cartilage. *J. Biol. Chem.* **244**:876–881.

Singh, M., and Bachhawat, B. K. 1965. The distribution and variation with age of different uronic acid–containing mucopolysaccharides in brain. *J. Neurochem.* **12**:519–525.

Singh, M., and Bachhawat, B. K. 1969. Isolation and characterization of glycosaminoglycans in human brain of different age groups. *J. Neurochem.* **15**:249–258.

Singh, M., Chandrasekaran, E. V., Cherian, R., and Bachhawat, B. K. 1969. Isolation and characterization of glycosaminoglycans in brain of different species. *J. Neurochem.* **16**:1157–1162.

Slagel, D. E., Dittmer, J. C., and Wilson, C. B. 1967. Lipid composition of human glial tumour and adjacent brain. *J. Neurochem.* **14**:789–798.

Snyder, R. A., Brady, R. O., and Kornblith, P. L. 1970. Ganglioside patterns of cultured human glioma cells. *Neurology* **20**:412 (abst.).

Sourander, P., Hansson, H.-A., Olsson, Y., and Svennerholm, L. 1966. Experimental studies on the pathogenesis of leucodystrophies. II. The effect of sphingolipids on various cell types in cultures from the nervous system. *Acta Neuropathol.* **6**:231–242.

Stary, Z., Wardi, A., and Turner, D. 1964. Galacturonic acid in hydrolysates of defatted human brain. *Biochim. Biophys. Acta* **83**:242–244.

Stoffel, W. 1971. Sphingolipids. *Ann. Rev. Biochem.* **40**:57–82.

Stoolmiller, A. C. 1972. Biosynthesis of mucopolysaccharides by neuroblastoma cells in tissue culture. *Fed. Proc.* **31**:910Abs.

Stoolmiller, A. C., and Bittner, S. J. 1972. Localization of sialyltransferase activity in the plasma membrane of cultured mouse neuroblastoma cells. *J. Cell Biol.* **55**:251a.

Stoolmiller, A. C., 3d Dorfman, A. 1969. Metabolism of glycosaminoglycans, pp. 241–275. *In* M. Florkin and E. Stotz (eds.). Carbohydrate Metabolism, Vol. 17. Elsevier, Amsterdam.

Stoolmiller, A. C., Dorfman, A., and Sato, G. 1972. Rat origin of CHB cells. *Science* **178**: 1308.

Suzuki, Y., and Suzuki, K. 1970. Krabbe's globoid cell leukodystrophy: Deficiency of galactocerebrosidase in serum, leukocytes and fibroblasts. *Science* **171**:73–75.

Suzuki, K., Poduslo, J. F., and Poduslo, S. E. 1968. Further evidence for a specific ganglioside fraction closely associated with myelin. *Biochim. Biophys. Acta* **152**:576–586.

Svennerholm, L. 1964. The gangliosides. *J. Lipid Res.* **5**:145–155.

Sweeley, C. C., and Dawson, G. 1969. Lipids of the erythrocyte, pp. 172–228. *In* G. A. Jamieson and T. W. Greenwalt (eds.). *Red Cell Membrane,* J. B. Lippincott, Philadelphia.

Szabo, M., and Roboz-Einstein, E. 1962. Acidic polysaccharides in the central nervous system. *Arch. Biochem. Biophys.* **98**:406–412.

Tamai, Y., Matsukawa, S., and Satake, M. 1970. Gangliosides in neuron. *J. Biochem. (Tokyo)* **69**:235–238.

Telser, A., Robinson, H. C., and Dorfman, A. 1966. The biosynthesis of chondroitin sulfate. *Arch. Biochem. Biophys.* **116**:458–465.

Vos, J., Kuriyama, K., and Roberts, E. 1969. Distribution of acid mucopolysaccharides in subcellular fractions of mouse brain. *Brain Res.* **12**:172–179.

Wardi, A. H., Allen, W. S., Turner, D. L., and Stary, Z. 1969. Hyaluronate–peptide linkage group. *Biochim. Biophys. Acta* **192**:151–154.

Wiegandt, H. 1967. The subcellular localization of gangliosides in the brain. *J. Neurochem.* **14**:671–674.

Wiegandt, H. 1970. Gangliosides of extraneuronal tissue. *Chem. Phys. Lipids* **5**:198–204.

Winterburn, P. J., and Phelps, C. F. 1970. Relevance of feedback inhibition applied to the biosynthesis of hexosamines. *Nature* **228**:1311–1313.

Yogeeswaran, G., Sheinin, R., Wherrett, J. R., and Murray, R. K. 1972. Studies on the glycosphingolipids of normal and virally transformed 3T3 mouse fibroblasts. *J. Biol. Chem.* **247**:5146–5158.

Young, I. J., and Custod, J. T. 1972. Isolation of glycosaminoglycans and variation with age in the feline brain. *J. Neurochem.* **19**:923–926.

Index

Note: Cell lines are indexed by first letter(s) and then in ascending numerical order.